Imaging Infections

Sanjay K. Jain
Editor

Imaging Infections

From Bench to Bedside

Springer

Editor
Sanjay K. Jain
Department of Pediatrics
Johns Hopkins University School of Medicine
Baltimore, MD, USA

ISBN 978-3-319-54590-5 ISBN 978-3-319-54592-9 (eBook)
DOI 10.1007/978-3-319-54592-9

Library of Congress Control Number: 2017941765

Printed on acid-free paper

This Springer imprint is published by Springer Nature
The registered company is Springer International Publishing AG
The registered company address is: Gewerbestrasse 11, 6330 Cham, Switzerland

This book is dedicated to all my amazing patients whose relentless battle with life-threatening infections has challenged me and nurtured my interest to develop new imaging technologies that could improve the care of future patients with infections.

I also want to thank my family, who have instilled the values I hold and who have strongly supported me in all my endeavors.

Contents

Contributors

Nathan K. Archer Department of Dermatology, Johns Hopkins University School of Medicine, Baltimore, MD, USA

Ulas Bagci Center for Research in Computer Vision, University of Central Florida, Orlando, FL, USA

Lauren E. Bambarger Department of Pediatrics, Johns Hopkins University School of Medicine, Baltimore, MD, USA

Center for Infection and Inflammation Imaging Research, Johns Hopkins University School of Medicine, Baltimore, MD, USA

Delphine L. Chen Mallinckrodt Institute of Radiology, Washington University School of Medicine, Saint Louis, MO, USA

Fereidoon Daryaee Institute for Chemical Biology and Drug Discovery, Department of Chemistry, Stony Brook University, Stony Brook, NY, USA

Department of Radiology, Stony Brook University School of Medicine, Stony Brook, NY, USA

Thomas Ebenhan Department of Nuclear Medicine, Steve Biko Academic Hospital, University of Pretoria, Pretoria, South Africa

Catherine A. Foss Russel H. Morgan Department of Radiology and Radiological Sciences, Johns Hopkins University School of Medicine, Baltimore, MD, USA

Kevin P. Francis Preclinical Imaging, Life Sciences, PerkinElmer, Inc., Hopkinton, MA, USA

Department of Orthopedic Surgery, David Geffen School of Medicine at UCLA, Los Angeles, CA, USA

Kayla R. Gogarty Institute for Chemical Biology and Drug Discovery, Department of Chemistry, Stony Brook University, Stony Brook, NY, USA

Department of Radiology, Stony Brook University School of Medicine, Stony Brook, NY, USA

Dima A. Hammoud Center for Infectious Disease Imaging, Radiology and Imaging Sciences, Clinical Center, U.S. National Institutes of Health, Bethesda, MD, USA

Nada M.S. Hammouda Icahn School of Medicine at Mount Sinai, New York, NY, USA

Sanjay K. Jain Department of Pediatrics, Johns Hopkins University School of Medicine, Baltimore, MD, USA

Center for Infection and Inflammation Imaging Research, Johns Hopkins University School of Medicine, Baltimore, MD, USA

Department of International Health, Johns Hopkins Bloomberg School of Public Health, Baltimore, MD, USA

Alvin S. Kalinda Department of Pediatrics, Johns Hopkins University School of Medicine, Baltimore, MD, USA

Center for Infection and Inflammation Imaging Research, Johns Hopkins University School of Medicine, Baltimore, MD, USA

Jun Li Vanderbilt Center for Molecular Probes and Molecular Imaging Research, Vanderbilt University, Nashville, TN, USA

H. Charles Manning Department of Radiology, Vanderbilt Center for Molecular Probes and Molecular Imaging Research, Vanderbilt University, Nashville, TN, USA

Lloyd S. Miller Department of Dermatology, Department of Medicine, Division of Infectious Diseases and Department of Orthopedic Surgery, Johns Hopkins University School of Medicine, Baltimore, MD, USA

Daniel J. Mollura Center for Infectious Disease Imaging, U.S. National Institutes of Health, Bethesda, MD, USA

Department of Radiology and Imaging Sciences, Clinical Center, U.S. National Institutes of Health, Bethesda, MD, USA

Niren Murthy Department of Bioengineering, University of California at Berkeley, Berkley, CA, USA

Alvaro A. Ordonez Department of Pediatrics, Johns Hopkins University School of Medicine, Baltimore, MD, USA

Center for Infection and Inflammation Imaging Research, Johns Hopkins University School of Medicine, Baltimore, MD, USA

Christopher J. Palestro Department of Radiology, Hofstra Northwell School of Medicine, Hempstead, NY, USA

Georgios Z. Papadakis Center for Infectious Disease Imaging, U.S. National Institutes of Health, Bethesda, MD, USA

Department of Radiology and Imaging Sciences, Clinical Center, U.S. National Institutes of Health, Bethesda, MD, USA

Mike Sathekge Department of Nuclear Medicine, Steve Biko Academic Hospital, University of Pretoria, Pretoria, South Africa

Philip M. Scherer Mallinckcrodt Institute of Radiology, Washington University School of Medicine, Saint Louis, MO, USA

Chentian Shen U.S. National Institutes of Health, Bethesda, MD, USA

Peter J. Tonge Institute for Chemical Biology and Drug Discovery, Department of Chemistry, Stony Brook University, Stony Brook, NY, USA

Department of Radiology, Stony Brook University School of Medicine, Stony Brook, NY, USA

Greetje Vande Velde Biomedical MRI Unit/MoSAIC, KU Leuven – University of Leuven, Leuven, Belgium

Carl Wagener Radiochemistry Group, Department of Applied Chemistry, South African Nuclear Energy Corporation SOC Limited, Pelindaba, South Africa

Edward A. Weinstein Department of Medicine, Johns Hopkins University School of Medicine, Baltimore, MD, USA

Center for Infection and Inflammation Imaging Research, Johns Hopkins University School of Medicine, Baltimore, MD, USA

Stefan Wiehr Department of Preclinical Imaging and Radiopharmacy, Werner Siemens Imaging Center, University Hospital Tuebingen, Tübingen, Germany

David M. Wilson Department of Radiology, University of California, San Francisco, San Francisco, CA, USA

Ziyue Xu Center for Infectious Disease Imaging, U.S. National Institutes of Health, Bethesda, MD, USA

Department of Radiology and Imaging Sciences, Clinical Center, U.S. National Institutes of Health, Bethesda, MD, USA

Jan Rijn Zeevaart Radiochemistry Group, Department of Applied Chemistry, South African Nuclear Energy Corporation SOC Limited, Pelindaba, South Africa

Zhuo Zhang Institute for Chemical Biology and Drug Discovery, Department of Chemistry, Stony Brook University, Stony Brook, NY, USA

Department of Radiology, Stony Brook University School of Medicine, Stony Brook, NY, USA

Chapter 1
Introduction

Sanjay K. Jain

1.1 Global Burden of Infectious Diseases

Infectious diseases have been a major scourge to humankind for centuries and are likely to continue to do so for centuries to come in both the USA and globally. For example, in 2011, about 722,000 Americans developed hospital-acquired infections (HAIs) with *Enterobacteriaceae* (26.8%), *Clostridium difficile* (12.1%), *Staphylococcus aureus* (10.7%), and *Pseudomonas aeruginosa* (7.1%) accounting for the majority of infections [1], resulting in 75,000 deaths [2]. HAIs cost the US healthcare system tens of billions of dollars in direct costs annually, and additional loses in lost wages extended hospital stays and premature deaths annually [3, 4]. While major efforts are being made to curb such infection, increasing rates of drug-resistant pathogens [5–9], increasing use of invasive techniques such as implants, and immunosuppressive and cancer therapies [10] remain a major challenge in controlling these infections. Multidrug-resistant (MDR) bacteria can also be notorious sources of life-threatening infections with high rates of death [5–9]. Similarly, viral infections such as influenza cause millions of new cases and several 1000 deaths annually in the USA [11]. The burden of hospital-acquired and other infections is substantially higher globally. In addition, global diseases such as tuberculosis (TB) continue to be major killers worldwide. In 2015, *Mycobacterium tuberculosis*, the causative agent of TB, was responsible for 10.4 new cases of TB and 1.8 million deaths [12]. It is also estimated that one third of the world's population is latently infected with *M. tuberculosis*, and many develop reactivation disease (relapse), years after the initial infection. It is expected that care and prevention of

S.K. Jain, MD (✉)
Department of Pediatrics, Johns Hopkins University School of Medicine, Baltimore, MD, USA

Center for Infection and Inflammation Imaging Research, Johns Hopkins University School of Medicine, Baltimore, MD, USA

Department of International Health, Johns Hopkins Bloomberg School of Public Health, Baltimore, MD, USA
e-mail: sjain5@jhmi.edu

S.K. Jain (ed.), *Imaging Infections*, DOI 10.1007/978-3-319-54592-9_1

tuberculosis (TB) patients in low and middle-income countries in 2016 alone will cost $8.3 billion. With alarming rise of MDR, extensively (XDR) and even totally drug-resistant (TDR) TB [13, 14], and poor treatment and monitoring options, we may be losing the battle, and *M. tuberculosis*, a single infectious agent, remains as one of the top ten causes of death worldwide [12]. Global travel and rapid spread of infections—swine flu, SARS-CoV, Ebola, and Zika virus—is also a major concern and led to several recent global pandemics [15, 16]. Finally, several infectious pathogens, e.g., *Yersinia pestis* (causes plague) from the *Enterobacteriaceae* family, are also recognized as biothreat agents [17].

1.2 Molecular Imaging

Molecular imaging focuses on understanding fundamental molecular pathways in live organisms and organ systems in a noninvasive manner. It is based on utilizing imaging biomarkers called "tracers" or "probes" which target specific molecular pathways by chemical interactions with the biological systems. The spatial localization of the biomarkers is determined by accurately measuring the source of the radionuclide attached to the biomarker, e.g., for nuclear medicine techniques such as single-photon emission computed tomography (SPECT) and positron emission tomography (PET), or by other methods (e.g., magnetic resonance spectroscopy (MRS)), providing two- or three-dimensional image representative of the molecular changes occurring within the area of interest. This allows exciting possibilities for medical application, including early detection and monitoring of diseases as well as study of basic biology and pathogenesis. Several molecular imaging techniques, e.g., PET, are also quantitative. Molecular imaging techniques are often used in conjunction with anatomic imaging, e.g., computed tomography (CT) and magnetic resonance imaging (MRI), for anatomic reference. The basic characteristics of common molecular imaging modalities are outlined in Table 1.1.

MRI is becoming widely available globally and has several advantages: (1) well established and widely available clinically, (2) does not utilize radiation, (3) capable of providing not only structural but also functional and metabolic information (e.g., MRS), (4) high tissue contrast and resolution, and (5) ability to provide both endogenous and exogenous contrast. However, current MRS techniques lack sensitivity, which are several magnitudes lower than that of nuclear medicine techniques (PET). One other limitation of MRI (compared to CT) is the relatively slower acquisition times. New MRI techniques are an area of active research and hold great promise.

While CT and nuclear medicine techniques are often perceived to deliver high levels of radiation, recent technological developments have significantly lowered radiation exposure and also allowed rapid acquisitions, which can avoid the need for sedation in children [18]. Figure 1.1 shows the risks of common imaging techniques compared with infections, nuclear medicine screening tests, and natural sources of radiation [19]. It should be noted that the risk of mortality for patients with drug-resistant infections can be similar to that due to cancers and substantially

Table 1.1 Characteristics of molecular imaging modalities

Modality	Agents	Sensitivity	Comments
Optical	Fluorescence, bio-luminance	Pico- to femtomolar	Excellent sensitivity but limited depth penetration and therefore applicable to imaging of small animals or superficial sites only; mostly two-dimensional
Nuclear SPECT PET	^{99m}Tc, $^{123/5}$I, ^{111}In ^{11}C, ^{18}F, ^{124}I	Nano- to picomolar	Excellent sensitivity and depth penetration with three-dimensional imaging, but radiation exposure; production facilities (e.g., cyclotron) for short half-life isotopes need to be close; relatively costly
MR spectroscopy	Endogenous	Micro- to millimolar	Excellent depth penetration with three-dimensional imaging without radiation exposure; low sensitivity and equipment is costly
Ultrasound	Functionalized microbubbles	Micro- to millimolar	Lower-cost imaging without radiation exposure; low sensitivity and generally operator dependent

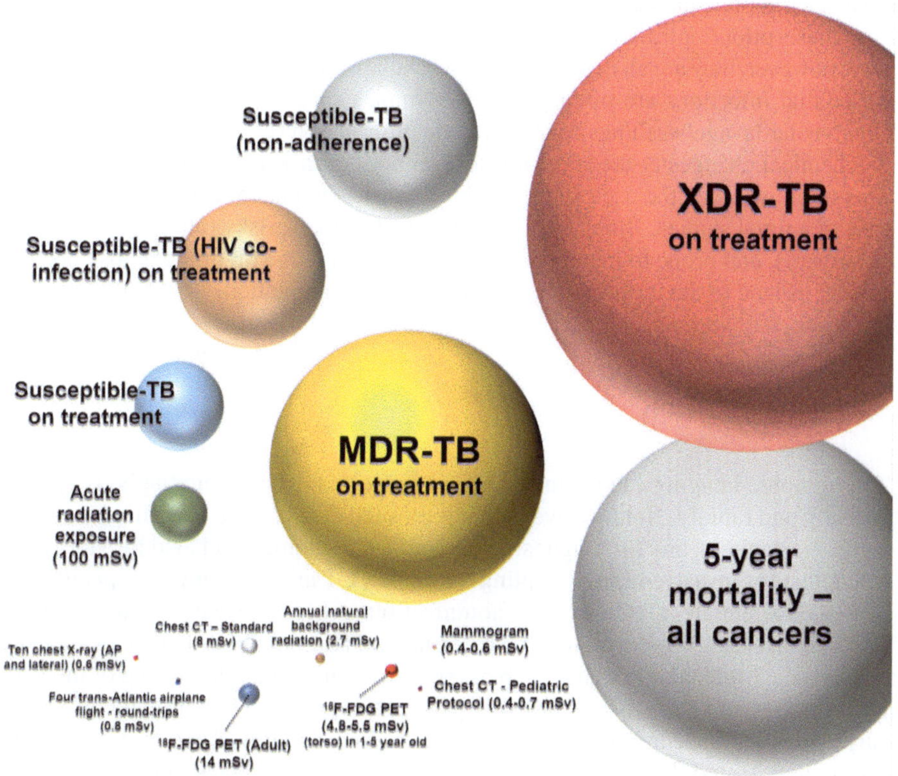

Figure 1.1 Risk of imaging. The risk of mortality due to infections (tuberculosis as an example) is compared to the risk of radiation-induced cancer due to commonly used imaging techniques. The risk of radiation-induced cancer and mortality have been theoretically estimated based on acute radiation exposure (100 mSv), and actual risks are likely to be much lower for smaller amounts of radiation. Adapted from Jain et al. [19]

higher than the theoretical risk due to radiation-induced cancers. Therefore, while no studies should be performed without an excellent rationale and clinical indication, we need to be pragmatic about the (minimal) risks of imaging, especially when dealing with infections due to drug-resistant organisms. Imaging tracers that are rapidly eliminated from the body could further limit radiation exposure.

1.3 The Problem

Traditional diagnostic tools, namely, microscopy, microbiology, and molecular techniques, are dependent upon sampling suspected sites of infection and then performing assays or tests. This approach is invasive, often terminal for animal experiments, and dangerous for deep-seated infections in humans, labor intensive, and time consuming (can take days), as well as subject to the uncertainties of incorrect sampling and contamination. Major advances have already been made in the use of molecular tools such as nucleic acid amplification (NAA), deep sequencing, matrix-assisted laser desorption/ionization, etc., for use in infectious disease research or patient care; however, they are all dependent on the availability of a relevant tissue sample(s). Given that infections are often localized, samples such as blood, urine, and bronchoalveolar lavage/washings cannot provide information on the crucial biological or biochemical changes at the sites of infection nor contribute to a specific diagnosis. This often warrants the use of invasive biopsies during patient care or necropsies in case of animal studies. Biopsies in patients can be costly, risky (anesthesia, dangers of surgery), and prone to incorrect sampling (limited to the tip of the biopsy needle) as well as lead to the introduction of artifacts or contamination.

1.4 The Solution

Tomographic imaging can evaluate disease processes deep within the body, noninvasively and rapidly. Noninvasive techniques, such as CT, MRI, and ultrasound, can provide a rapid means for diagnosing anatomical pathology and also provide a site of interest for invasive tissue sampling. However, CT and MRI are non-specific and cannot differentiate infections from noninfectious processes such as cancer or autoimmune diseases. Moreover, they reveal structural abnormalities that are often a late occurrence. Molecular imaging enables the visualization and monitoring of molecular processes and early events in living organisms noninvasively. It is therefore not surprising that nuclear molecular imaging tools such as SPECT and PET have powerfully augmented the investigation of various disease processes, both for research and patient care [20, 21]. Moreover, the ability to conduct noninvasive, longitudinal assessments in the same individual is a fundamental advantage over current methods utilized for infections. Other major advantages of imaging are its ability to provide a holistic, three-dimensional assessment of the whole organ or body, less likely to be limited by sampling errors and therefore correlating well with the overall disease process. Some examples of the potential uses of molecular imaging for infectious diseases are outlined in Table 1.2.

Noninvasive imaging can be used to study disease pathogenesis in an unprecedented fashion as discussed here [22, 23]. For example, standard methodologies for studying TB cannot reliably monitor and identify the spatial location of lesions and

Table 1.2 Role of imaging in infectious diseases

Advantages of tomographic imaging over traditional techniques used for infections		
Evaluate disease processes deep within the body, noninvasively and relatively rapidly Longitudinal assessments in the same individual—fundamental advantage over traditional tools Provide holistic, three-dimensional assessment of the whole organ or body representative of the overall disease (versus tip of a biopsy needle) and therefore less prone to sampling error		
Imaging in infectious diseases		
Role	Setting	Overall goal(s)
Pathogenesis	Preclinical	Unique insights into disease pathogenesis, e.g., assessing hideouts of infections, defining the diversity of the microbial populations (microbiome), etc. Studying multi-compartment antimicrobial pharmacokinetics Expedite bench-to-bedside translation of new therapeutics, e.g., surrogate end points to assess antimicrobial or vaccine efficacy or predict stable cure
	Clinical trials	Unique insights into disease pathogenesis—noninvasive visualization of processes deep inside the body Phase 0 studies to determine compartment-specific antimicrobial penetration/binding (sites of infection, necrotic/fibrotic lesions, privileged sites—CNS) to inform appropriate dosing of novel drugs and determine accumulation at nontarget sites to assess potential toxicities; current US Food and Drug Administration (FDA) guidelines require tissue drug distribution studies at the infected sites
	Patient settings	Enabling precision medicine by providing unique insights into disease pathogenesis, antimicrobial pharmacokinetics, etc.
Diagnosis	Clinical trials and patient settings	Rapidly and specifically distinguish an infectious process from other diseases (malignancy, sterile inflammatory processes, etc.) Determine the site (e.g., extension/metastasis to other organs or privileged sites) and extent of disease Provide information on the class of the infectious pathogen, which could help in targeted empiric antimicrobial treatments

(continued)

Table 1.2 (continued)

Role	Setting	Overall goal(s)
Monitoring and prognostication	Preclinical	Noninvasive longitudinal assessments especially in studies utilizing larger, more expensive animal species; serial assessments in the same animal could significantly reduce sample size, inter-animal variability (outbreed animals), and therefore cost of the studies
	Clinical trials	Early end points for treatment trials to assess activity of treatments and to predict stable cure Assessing host-directed treatments for infections Enable adaptive designs
	Patient settings	Rapidly detect treatment failures due to drug-resistant organisms or other reasons Rapidly monitor treatment responses in patients with drug-resistant organisms and individualize treatments Early end points for duration of treatment and predict stable cure enabling precision medicine
	Public health	Rapid determination of the infectious risk of a patient to the population based on response to treatment, extent, and location of disease Rapid diagnosis and monitoring of biothreat agents

Adapted from Jain et al. [19]

reactivation within the same animal because monitoring disease requires sacrificing animals. One study utilized ^{18}F-fluorodeoxyglucose (^{18}F-FDG) PET/CT to study the temporal evolution of reactivation (relapse) pulmonary TB [23]. The same cohort of infected mice that develops TB lesions akin to humans [24–26] were serially imaged through pretreatment, TB treatment, and subsequent development of relapse. A novel diffeomorphic image registration method was successfully used to monitor the spatial evolution of individual pulmonary lesions. They found that while the majority of lesions during relapse developed in the same regions as those noted during pretreatment, several lesions also arose de novo within regions with no prior lesions. Contrary to the commonly held belief, this study suggested that dormant bacteria may also reside outside TB lesions and cause relapse in regions where no apparent lesions were present initially, which could prove valuable in the development of novel therapeutics. Another interesting application of pathogen-specific imaging is the detection of viral dynamics and localization in the context of human immunodeficiency virus (HIV). Santangelo et al. developed a technique to image total-body simian immunodeficiency virus (SIV) replication using antibody-targeted PET. They utilized a ^{64}Cu-labeled SIV Gp120-specific antibody, and we were able to detect virus-specific PET signals in treated and untreated monkeys [27]. This real time, virus-specific imaging method could have important applications for studying HIV pathogenesis, development of novel therapeutics, and even potential for clinical use.

1.5 Biocontainment

Several pathogens are designated as biosafety level 3/4 (BSL-3/4) and require appropriate handling and containment. Furthermore, work with biothreat pathogens requires regulatory approvals, as well as highly trained personnel [28]. There are two major ways of achieving containment: (A) installing imaging equipment inside the BSL-3/4 barrier (e.g., NIAID, University of Pittsburg). While this is logistically advantageous, maintaining equipment within these barriers can be expensive. (B) Therefore, some groups have utilized portable biocontainment devices that can seal infected animals within, which can then be transported to the imaging suite (housed in standard environments) (Figure 1.2) [29–31], or polycarbonate plastic tubes extending from the biocontainment space to the imaging equipment [32]. Weinstein and Liu et al. have also described a tail vein catheter system for on-table drug delivery to infected animals, while sealed inside the biocontainment device [33, 34].

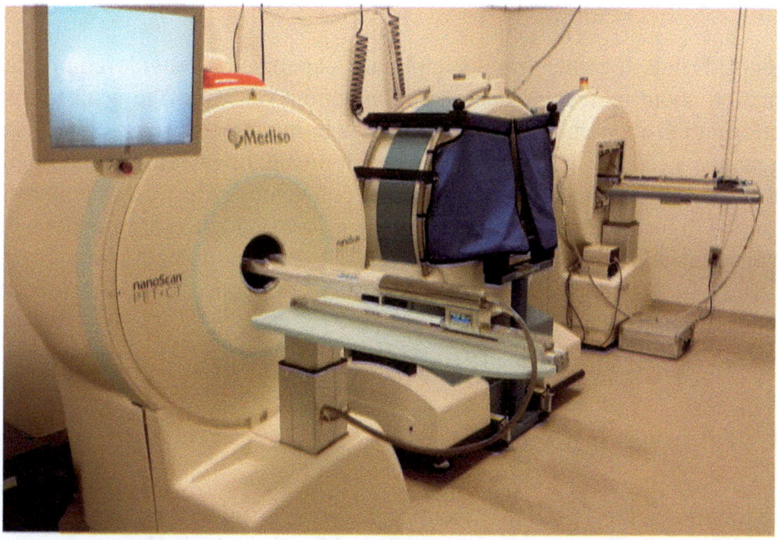

Figure 1.2 Biocontainment devices. The imaging suite at the Center for Infection and Inflammation Imaging Research at the Johns Hopkins University School of Medicine is shown here. The imaging equipment is located in a standard environment inside the animal vivarium and adjacent to a biosafety level 3 (BSL-3) facility. Animals infected with *Mycobacterium tuberculosis* (requiring BSL-3 handling) are isolated inside airtight, self-contained biocontainment devices. Standard small animal anesthesia machines are used to deliver a mixture of isoflurane and oxygen during transport and imaging, and two 0.22 μm filters are used in series at both the inlet and the outlet of the biocontainment device to contain the infectious agents. The external surface of the biocontainment device is decontaminated and transported to the imaging suite for imaging. During prolonged anesthesia, an infrared thermometer and a heat lamp are used to measure and maintain ambient air temperature inside the biocontainment device

Containment of animals rather than the imaging equipment allows for easier maintenance of the equipment, which can also be shared with other investigators that do not work within the BSL-3/4 barrier.

1.6 Human Translation of PET Tracers

Due to the use of sub-pharmacological doses used in most nuclear medicine studies, the risk to human subjects is limited due to the administration of the parent compound. Therefore, the requirements for preclinical safety testing are significantly simpler. The FDA currently accepts the use of extended (14-day) single-dose toxicity data in one mammalian species to support single-dose studies in humans [35], and this has streamlined this process for more rapid translation of new imaging agents to the clinic.

1.7 Imaging Infections: From Bench to Bedside

This book brings together multidisciplinary expertise to provide comprehensive information about molecular imaging of infectious diseases. We want to disseminate information about molecular imaging (to our infectious disease colleagues) and highlight the need for innovation and development of imaging technologies for infectious disease (to our molecular imaging colleagues). The overall goal is to spur interest and innovation to develop new imaging technologies for infectious disease and their translation to the clinic. Chapters 2–4 provide in-depth overviews, while Chapters 5–12 are more focused on discussing the concepts and techniques for infectious disease imaging.

1.7.1 Imaging in the Clinic

Unlike traditional tools used in infectious diseases, imaging can provide key spatial information about disease processes and enable whole-body detection and therapeutic monitoring of infections. This is especially relevant for patients with deep-seated infections or infections at unknown sites, for whom traditional clinical samples (e.g., blood, urine) would be insensitive, high risk, or impractical (e.g., bleeding risk, brain biopsy) or where rapid assessment of therapeutic effect is needed. In fact, oncology patients with fever and neutropenia or patients with fever of unknown origin (FUO) routinely undergo whole body imaging to look for foci of infection. Similarly patients with implants and orthopedic infections also utilize imaging extensively to guide management. Chapter 2 provides an authoritative overview of current imaging techniques used for infectious diseases, as well as the limitation of current tools, namely, that they are non-specific and dependent on host responses to infections.

1.7.2 Molecular Imaging Techniques

Optical imaging methods have been used extensively to study disease pathogenesis. Chapter 3 provides a detailed review of how in vivo optical imaging has permitted the noninvasive and longitudinal monitoring of host-pathogen interactions, including the dynamics of infection burden and dissemination, host immune responses, and the effects of treatments, all measured in the same live animals over time. These approaches have provided valuable information about microbial pathogenesis and treatment, while also significantly reducing animal numbers and cost. Although optical imaging was once considered to be applicable only to preclinical animal research, new methodologies such as photoacoustic imaging are advancing this technique into clinical practice.

While highly sensitive, optical imaging is limited by the depth of the signal, i.e., signals from deep inside the body cannot be visualized well, which however is not a limitation of nuclear medicine techniques. Chapter 4 provides a highly in-depth review of radiochemical methods to produce radiopharmaceuticals for SPECT and PET and also discusses the synthesis of several agents that have been used for infection imaging in the preclinical as well as clinical settings.

1.7.3 Imaging Host Responses

Chapter 5 discusses some of the emerging imaging techniques that measure host responses. These tracers can not only be used to study new biology but also to monitor disease. For example, imaging modalities targeting host inflammation, while non-specific, have been used to longitudinally monitor the natural history of some infections and/or responses to antimicrobial treatments in animal models as well as humans [18, 22, 23, 30, 36, 37]. Chen et al. reported that ^{18}F-2-fluoro-deoxy-D-glucose (^{18}FFDG) PET/CT imaging was superior to conventional (sputum) microbiology for monitoring response to treatments in adults with MDR-TB [38]. More recently, low-radiation exposure pulmonary CT imaging was used to monitor treatments for a highly drug-resistant form of TB (XDR-TB) in a 2-year-old child and guide an individualized drug regimen (Figure 1.3) [18]. Imaging agents with higher specificity for TB-associated inflammation have been shown to be even better at monitoring response to treatments in animal models [36].

1.7.4 Pathogen-Specific Tracers

An ideal imaging agent for diagnosing infections needs to be both sensitive and specific. However, current molecular imaging tools for infectious diseases are non-specific and dependent upon host responses that could be significantly altered in diseased states (e.g., cancer, AIDS). Therefore, there is a great need for the

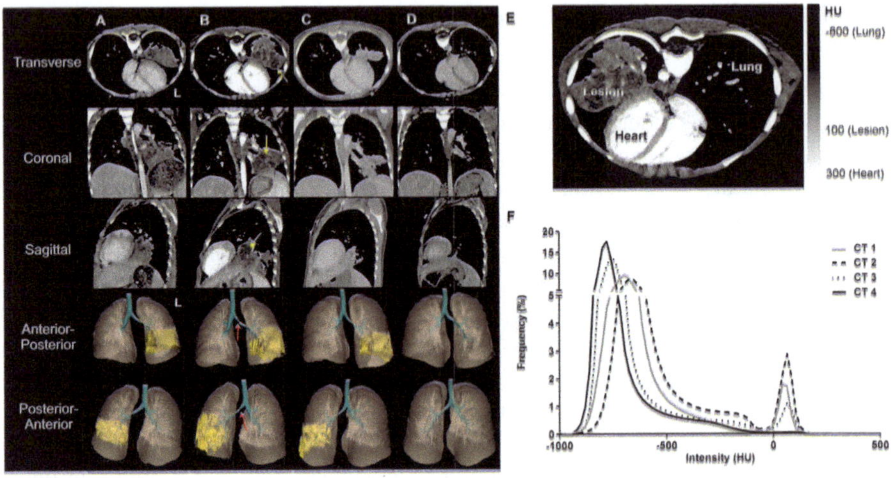

Figure 1.3 Serial CT to guide an individualized treatment in a 2-year-old with extensively drug-resistant (XDR) tuberculosis. (**a–d**) CT with intravenous contrast was performed using a protocol customized for children. The transverse, coronal, sagittal, and three-dimensional views of the lung parenchyma and the pulmonary infiltrates in the left lung are shown. Each panel corresponds to CT performed at initiation of first-line TB treatment (**a**, day 0), initiation of individualized XDR tuberculosis (TB) treatment (**b**, day 90), and 6 weeks (**c**, day 131) and 6 months (**d**, day 270) after initiation of XDR-TB treatment, respectively. Several necrotic (hypodense) central areas can be visualized in (**b**) (*yellow arrows*). Also, note the partial obstruction of the left main bronchus in (**b**) (*red arrows*). Marked improvement with resolution of necrotic areas is noted after 6 weeks (**c**) and near-complete resolution of the infiltrate after 6 months (**d**) of XDR-TB treatment, respectively. (**e**) Transverse CT image (post-contrast, day 90), showing the Hounsfield Unit (HU) densities in the chest cavity (lung, pulmonary lesion, and heart). (**f**) Histogram showing the HU densities of the segmented CT lung images. The pulmonary lesions correspond to −15 to 210 HU (smaller peaks on the right, which decrease with treatment). Lesion volumes were calculated at each time point by integrating the area under the corresponding curve. The lesion volumes were verified manually by drawing regions of interest. Each trace corresponds to CT performed at day 0 (CT1), day 90 (CT2), day 131 (CT3), and day 270 (CT4). *L* = left side. Adapted from Salazar-Austin et al. [18]

development of pathogen-specific imaging tracers. Chapters 6 and 7 focus on emerging targets and tracers for developing pathogen-specific imaging agents for bacterial and fungal infections, respectively. Chapter 7 also briefly discusses the use of imaging for select parasitic infections. There is also discussion on approaches for rationale selection of targets for pathogen-specific imaging tracers in Chapter 6. For example, there have been several recent studies showing the feasibility of pathogen-specific nuclear tracers in animal models [39–46]. MRI techniques have also been used to specifically image bacteria in mice [47]. It should be noted that clinically apparent (acute) infections often have high pathogen burden, e.g., 8.3 $\log_{10}$ CFU/ml of bacteria [48], and can be several centimeters in diameter with volumes of tens to hundreds of milliliters [49, 50]. Therefore, current pathogen-specific imaging agents in development could in principle provide early detection of infections in patients. In addition to diagnosis, pathogen-specific imaging can also be a great tool for predicting treatment responses [41, 42]. For example, ^{18}F-fluorodeoxysorbitol

(^{18}F-FDS) PET was able to rapidly (within 24 h) monitor the efficacy of antimicrobial treatment and identify therapeutic failures associated with drug-resistant, extended-spectrum β-lactamase (ESBL)-producing *E. coli* infections [42].

1.7.5 Neuroimaging

The field of neuroimaging is relatively advanced, and descriptions of cross-sectional imaging of the central nervous system (CNS) have been available for more than two decades. This has resulted in a large array of descriptive criteria capable, in most circumstances, of narrowing the differential diagnosis, detecting life-threatening complications, and establishing baseline for assessment of treatment response and is described briefly in Chapter 8. The availability of pathogen-specific imaging agents/ligands can have a great effect on the management of patients with CNS infection. Besides early diagnosis, avoidance of diagnostic brain biopsies can have significant effect on the mortality and morbidity of patients.

1.7.6 Antimicrobial Development

Vancomycin, a widely used antimicrobial to treat drug-resistant gram-positive bacteria, highlights some of the limitations of current tools for antimicrobial dosing. Methicillin-resistant *Staphylococcus aureus* (MRSA) pneumonia and methicillin-susceptible *S. aureus* (MSSA) pneumonia treated with vancomycin have been associated with mortality of 50% and 47%, respectively, versus only 5% for MSSA pneumonia treated with β-lactam antibiotics [51]. Vancomycin is a relatively large molecule and penetrates poorly into the alveolar lining fluid (ALF). As a result, levels attained in ALF are only one-sixth of the plasma concentration [52]. Conversely, high levels of vancomycin can cause nephrotoxicity. Based on these data, and recent studies demonstrating better efficacy with higher-dose vancomycin, new recommendations have been made for treating pulmonary infections [53]. Chapters 9 and 10 discuss the concepts behind developing PET imaging for multi-compartment pharmacokinetic and pharmacodynamics assessments of antimicrobials, with an eye toward clinical translation and as tools to optimize antimicrobial dosing strategies by achieving appropriate concentrations at the target, infected tissues.

1.7.7 Image Analyses

Current practice in the diagnosis and treatment of infections relies on radiologic image evaluation combined with clinical information. These tasks are challenging because radiologic manifestations of infections are associated with a large spectrum of non-specific patterns. The qualitative judgments of radiologists can be improved by quantitative image analysis techniques. These concepts as well as automated and computer-aided image analyses tools for infectious diseases are discussed in Chapter 11.

1.7.8 *Imaging in the Developing World*

During the past decade, developing countries, especially the BRICS nations (Brazil, Russia, India, China, South Africa), have witnessed significant increases in the installation and use of advanced imaging [54, 55]. Moreover, the costs of advanced imaging are substantially lower in some of these countries [32]. Mobile scanners and ^{68}Ga-PET agents that can be generated without the need of a cyclotron hold great promise, especially in these settings [56]. China has already overtaken the USA in purchasing power parity, with India also expected to do so by 2050 [57]. Since infections are rampant in the developing world, and these countries have huge populations living in big cities, advanced imaging has great potential. Chapter 12 discusses some of the challenges and opportunities of imaging of infections in the developing world.

1.8 Summary

Infectious diseases are a major cause of morbidity and mortality worldwide and in the USA. Overall costs and morbidity are expected to continue to rise due to increasing rates of drug-resistant pathogens, use of invasive techniques such as implants, as well as immunosuppressive and cancer therapies. Tomographic molecular imaging techniques enable rapid visualization and monitoring of molecular processes noninvasively and promise unparalleled opportunities for field of infectious diseases. These technologies are an emerging field of research, overcome several fundamental limitations of current tools, and could have a broad impact on both basic research and patient care. Beyond diagnosis and monitoring disease, these technologies could also provide a uniform cross-species platform for animal studies, allow unique insights into understanding disease pathogenesis, and expedite bench-to-bedside translation of new therapeutics. Finally, since molecular imaging is readily available for humans, validated tracers could also become valuable tools for clinical applications and for enabling personalized medicine for infectious diseases.

References

1. Magill, S.S., et al., *Multistate point-prevalence survey of health care-associated infections*. N Engl J Med, 2014. **370**(13): p. 1198-208.
2. CDC. *HAI Data and Statistics*. [cited 2016 December 29, 2016]; Available from: https://www.cdc.gov/hai/surveillance/.
3. IDSA. *Facts about Antibiotic Resistance*. 2011 November 13, 2016]; Available from: https://www.idsociety.org/AR_Facts/.
4. McCaughey, B. *Unnecessary Deaths: The Human and Financial Costs of Hospital Infections*. 2nd Edition November 13, 2016]; Available from: http://emerald.tufts.edu/med/apua/consumers/faqs_2_4154863510.pdf.

5. Keen, E.F., III, et al., *Changes in the incidences of multidrug-resistant and extensively drug-resistant organisms isolated in a military medical center.* Infect.Control Hosp.Epidemiol., 2010. **31**(7): p. 728-732.
6. Murray, C.K., et al., *Infections complicating the care of combat casualties during operations Iraqi Freedom and Enduring Freedom.* J.Trauma, 2011. **71**(1 Suppl): p. S62-S73.
7. McKenna, M., *Antibiotic resistance: the last resort.* Nature, 2013. **499**(7459): p. 394-6.
8. Nordmann, P., L. Dortet, and L. Poirel, *Carbapenem resistance in Enterobacteriaceae: here is the storm!* Trends Mol Med, 2012. **18**(5): p. 263-72.
9. Melzer, M. and I. Petersen, *Mortality following bacteraemic infection caused by extended spectrum beta-lactamase (ESBL) producing E. coli compared to non-ESBL producing E. coli.* J Infect, 2007. **55**(3): p. 254-9.
10. Kohn, L.T., J.M. Corrigan, and M.S. Donaldson, *To Err Is Human: Building a Safer Health System.* 2000, NATIONAL ACADEMY PRESS, Washington, D.C.
11. CDC. *Seasonal Influenza-Associated Hospitalizations in the United States.* [cited 2016 December 27, 2016]; Available from: https://www.cdc.gov/flu/about/qa/hospital.htm.
12. WHO. *Global tuberculosis report 2016.* [cited 2016 November 12]; Available from: http://www.who.int/tb/publications/global_report/gtbr2016_executive_summary.pdf?ua=1.
13. *Emergence of Mycobacterium tuberculosis with extensive resistance to second-line drugs--worldwide, 2000-2004.* MMWR Morb Mortal Wkly Rep, 2006. **55**(11): p. 301-5.
14. Velayati, A.A., et al., *Emergence of new forms of totally drug-resistant tuberculosis bacilli: super extensively drug-resistant tuberculosis or totally drug-resistant strains in iran.* Chest, 2009. **136**(2): p. 420-5.
15. Rota, P.A., et al., *Characterization of a novel coronavirus associated with severe acute respiratory syndrome.* Science, 2003. **300**(5624): p. 1394-9.
16. WHO. *Zika virus.* 2016 December 29, 2016]; Available from: http://www.who.int/mediacentre/factsheets/zika/en/.
17. Donnenberg, M.S., *Enterobacteriaceae*, in *Mandell, Douglas, and Bennett's principles and practice of infectious diseases.*, J.E.B. Gerald L. Mandell, and Raphael Dolin, Editor. 2010, Elsevier Inc: Philadelphia, PA. p. 2815-2833.
18. Salazar-Austin, N., et al., *Extensively drug-resistant tuberculosis in a young child after travel to India.* Lancet Infect Dis, 2015. **15**(12): p. 1485-91.
19. Jain, S.K., *The Promise of Molecular Imaging in the Study and Treatment of Infectious Diseases.* Mol Imaging Biol, 2017.
20. Higgins, L.J. and M.G. Pomper, *The evolution of imaging in cancer: current state and future challenges.* Semin Oncol, 2011. **38**(1): p. 3-15.
21. James, M.L. and S.S. Gambhir, *A molecular imaging primer: modalities, imaging agents, and applications.* Physiol Rev, 2012. **92**(2): p. 897-965.
22. Lin, P.L., et al., *Sterilization of granulomas is common in active and latent tuberculosis despite within-host variability in bacterial killing.* Nat Med, 2014. **20**(1): p. 75-9.
23. Murawski, A.M., et al., *Imaging the evolution of reactivation pulmonary tuberculosis in mice using 18F-FDG PET.* J Nucl Med, 2014. **55**(10): p. 1726-9.
24. Harper, J., et al., *Mouse model of necrotic tuberculosis granulomas develops hypoxic lesions.* J Infect Dis, 2012. **205**(4): p. 595-602.
25. Pan, H., et al., *Ipr1 gene mediates innate immunity to tuberculosis.* Nature, 2005. **434**(7034): p. 767-72.
26. Ordonez, A.A., et al., *Mouse model of pulmonary cavitary tuberculosis and expression of matrix metalloproteinase-9.* Disease Models and Mechanisms, 2016. **9**(7): p. 779-788.
27. Santangelo, P.J., et al., *Whole-body immunoPET reveals active SIV dynamics in viremic and antiretroviral therapy-treated macaques.* Nat Methods, 2015. **12**(5): p. 427-32.
28. Bocan, T.M., R.G. Panchal, and S. Bavari, *Applications of in vivo imaging in the evaluation of the pathophysiology of viral and bacterial infections and in development of countermeasures to BSL3/4 pathogens.* Mol Imaging Biol, 2015. **17**(1): p. 4-17.
29. Davis, S.L., et al., *Bacterial thymidine kinase as a non-invasive imaging reporter for Mycobacterium tuberculosis in live animals.* PLoS One, 2009. **4**(7): p. e6297.

30. Davis, S.L., et al., *Noninvasive pulmonary [18F]-2-fluoro-deoxy-D-glucose positron emission tomography correlates with bactericidal activity of tuberculosis drug treatment.* Antimicrob Agents Chemother, 2009. **53**(11): p. 4879-84.
31. Tucker, E.W., et al., *Microglia activation in a pediatric rabbit model of tuberculous meningitis.* Dis Model Mech, 2016. **9**(12): p. 1497-1506.
32. Lackemeyer, M.G., et al., *ABSL-4 aerobiology biosafety and technology at the NIH/NIAID integrated research facility at Fort Detrick.* Viruses, 2014. **6**(1): p. 137-50.
33. Weinstein, E.A., et al., *Noninvasive determination of 2-[18F]-fluoroisonicotinic acid hydrazide pharmacokinetics by positron emission tomography in Mycobacterium tuberculosis-infected mice.* Antimicrob Agents Chemother, 2012. **56**(12): p. 6284-90.
34. DeMarco, V.P., et al., *Determination of [11C]rifampin pharmacokinetics within Mycobacterium tuberculosis-infected mice by using dynamic positron emission tomography bioimaging.* Antimicrob Agents Chemother, 2015. **59**(9): p. 5768-74.
35. FDA. *Guidance for Industry, Investigators, and Reviewers: Exploratory IND Studies.* 2006 [cited November 10, 2012.; Available from: http://www.fda.gov/downloads/Drugs/GuidanceComplianceRegulatoryInformation/Guidances/ucm078933.pdf.
36. Ordonez, A.A., et al., *Radioiodinated DPA-713 imaging correlates with bactericidal activity of tuberculosis treatments in mice.* Antimicrob Agents Chemother, 2015. **59**(1): p. 642-9.
37. Sathekge, M., et al., *Use of 18F-FDG PET to predict response to first-line tuberculostatics in HIV-associated tuberculosis.* J Nucl Med, 2011. **52**(6): p. 880-5.
38. Chen, R.Y., et al., *PET/CT imaging correlates with treatment outcome in patients with multidrug-resistant tuberculosis.* Sci Transl Med, 2014. **6**(265): p. 265ra166.
39. Bettegowda, C., et al., *Imaging bacterial infections with radiolabeled 1-(2'-deoxy-2'-fluoro-beta-D-arabinofuranosyl)-5-iodouracil.* Proc Natl Acad Sci U S A, 2005. **102**(4): p. 1145-50.
40. Gowrishankar, G., et al., *Investigation of 6-[18F]-fluoromaltose as a novel PET tracer for imaging bacterial infection.* PLoS One, 2014. **9**(9): p. e107951.
41. Ning, X., et al., *PET imaging of bacterial infections with fluorine-18-labeled maltohexaose.* Angew Chem Int Ed Engl, 2014. **53**(51): p. 14096-101.
42. Weinstein, E.A., et al., *Imaging Enterobacteriaceae infection in vivo with 18F-fluorodeoxysorbitol positron emission tomography.* Sci Transl Med, 2014. **6**(259): p. 259ra146.
43. Wiehr, S., et al., *New pathogen-specific immunoPET/MR tracer for molecular imaging of a systemic bacterial infection.* Oncotarget, 2016. **7**(10): p. 10990-1001.
44. Rolle, A.M., et al., *ImmunoPET/MR imaging allows specific detection of Aspergillus fumigatus lung infection in vivo.* Proc Natl Acad Sci U S A, 2016. **113**(8): p. E1026-33.
45. Wang, Y., et al., *Detection of Aspergillus fumigatus pulmonary fungal infections in mice with (99m)Tc-labeled MORF oligomers targeting ribosomal RNA.* Nucl Med Biol, 2013. **40**(1): p. 89-96.
46. Petrik, M., et al., *68Ga-siderophores for PET imaging of invasive pulmonary aspergillosis: proof of principle.* J Nucl Med, 2010. **51**(4): p. 639-45.
47. Liu, G., et al., *Noninvasive imaging of infection after treatment with tumor-homing bacteria using Chemical Exchange Saturation Transfer (CEST) MRI.* Magn Reson Med, 2013. **70**(6): p. 1690-8.
48. Konig, C., H.P. Simmen, and J. Blaser, *Bacterial concentrations in pus and infected peritoneal fluid--implications for bactericidal activity of antibiotics.* J Antimicrob Chemother, 1998. **42**(2): p. 227-32.
49. Jang, K., et al., *Treatment of prostatic abscess: case collection and comparison of treatment methods.* Korean J Urol, 2012. **53**(12): p. 860-4.
50. Yamamoto, M., et al., *Treatment of bacterial brain abscess by repeated aspiration--follow up by serial computed tomography.* Neurol Med Chir (Tokyo), 2000. **40**(2): p. 98-104; discussion 104-5.
51. Gonzalez, C., et al., *Bacteremic pneumonia due to Staphylococcus aureus: A comparison of disease caused by methicillin-resistant and methicillin-susceptible organisms.* Clin Infect Dis, 1999. **29**(5): p. 1171-7.

52. Scheetz, M.H., et al., *Potential impact of vancomycin pulmonary distribution on treatment outcomes in patients with methicillin-resistant Staphylococcus aureus pneumonia.* Pharmacotherapy, 2006. **26**(4): p. 539-50.
53. Stein, G.E. and E.M. Wells, *The importance of tissue penetration in achieving successful antimicrobial treatment of nosocomial pneumonia and complicated skin and soft-tissue infections caused by methicillin-resistant Staphylococcus aureus: vancomycin and linezolid.* Curr Med Res Opin, 2010. **26**(3): p. 571-88.
54. Jankharia, G.R., *Commentary - radiology in India: the next decade.* The Indian journal of radiology & imaging, 2008. **18**(3): p. 189-91.
55. Jha, S.. *(2015) Radiology in India: Trends in medical imaging technology.* 2015 December 28, 2016]; Available from: http://www.auntminnie.com/index.aspx?sec=ser&sub=def&pag=dis&ItemID=110035.
56. Ebenhan, T., et al., *Preclinical evaluation of 68Ga-labeled 1,4,7-triazacyclononane-1,4,7-triacetic acid-ubiquicidin as a radioligand for PET infection imaging.* J Nucl Med, 2014. **55**(2): p. 308-14.
57. *The World in 2050.* 2015 December 29, 2016]; Available from: http://www.pwc.com/gx/en/issues/the-economy/assets/world-in-2050-february-2015.pdf.

Chapter 2
Clinical Imaging

Delphine L. Chen, Philip M. Scherer, and Christopher J. Palestro

2.1 Introduction

Despite significant advances in the understanding of its pathogenesis, infection remains a major cause of patient morbidity and mortality. Although symptoms and signs such as fever, pain, general malaise, and abnormal laboratory test results may suggest the presence of infection, the diagnosis can be elusive, and imaging tests often are used for confirmation and localization. Imaging tests can be divided into two groups: those that identify infections based on changes in anatomy or morphology and those that identify infections based on changes in function at the organ, cellular, and molecular levels. Anatomical imaging tests include radiographs, computed tomography, magnetic resonance imaging, and ultrasonography. These tests reveal structural alterations in tissues and organs caused by a combination of the infection itself and the inflammatory response of the host. Functional, or molecular, imaging tests most often use small quantities, or tracer amounts, of radioactive material. These agents, which reflect the physiological changes that are part of the inflammatory process, are taken up directly by cells, tissues, and organs or are attached to native substances that subsequently migrate to the region of interest. Indium-111, for example, is trapped intracellularly in leukocytes and is used to monitor leukocyte accumulation at foci of infection. Other molecular imaging agents used for localizing infection include gallium-67 and gallium-68, as well as ^{18}F-2-fluoro-deoxy-D-glucose (^{18}F-FDG).

D.L. Chen • P.M. Scherer
Mallinckcrodt Institute of Radiology, Washington University School of Medicine, Saint Louis, MO, USA

C.J. Palestro (✉)
Department of Radiology, Hofstra Northwell School of Medicine, Hempstead, NY, USA
e-mail: Palestro@northwell.edu

S.K. Jain (ed.), *Imaging Infections*, DOI 10.1007/978-3-319-54592-9_2

2.2 Anatomical Imaging Tests

2.2.1 *Computed Tomography*

Computed tomography (CT) uses attenuation of X-rays to display various densities. As the density of the structure through which the X-rays pass increases, the brightness of the structure increases on the CT image. The acute inflammatory response incited by an infection alters the normal density of the host tissue and hence its characteristic appearance on CT images. The normal air-filled lung parenchyma, for example, is usually black. In bacterial pneumonia, however, a water density or soft tissue density exudate replaces the air in the alveoli, and the affected areas of the lung become denser on the CT image (Figure 2.1) [1].

2.2.2 *Magnetic Resonance Imaging*

Magnetic resonance imaging (MRI) uses changes induced by magnetization, instead of ionizing radiation, to generate images. The region of the body to be imaged is placed in a homogeneous magnetic field, which causes the protons of the tissues to uniformly align with the magnetic field. Radio-frequency waves are pulsed through the tissues, changing the direction of this alignment. Coils in the scanner detect the

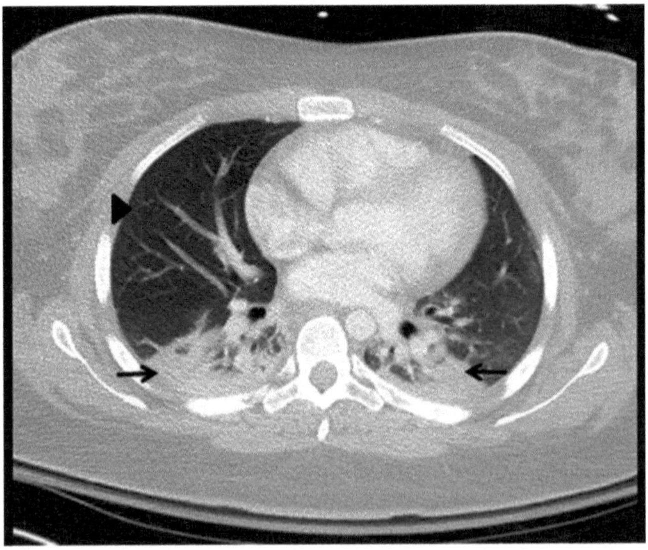

Figure 2.1 Pneumonia. The *gray* appearance of the bilateral lower lung consolidation (*arrows*) on the axial CT image is caused by replacement of the normally air-filled lung (*arrowhead*), which appears *black*, by water or soft tissue density exudates containing both fluid and cells

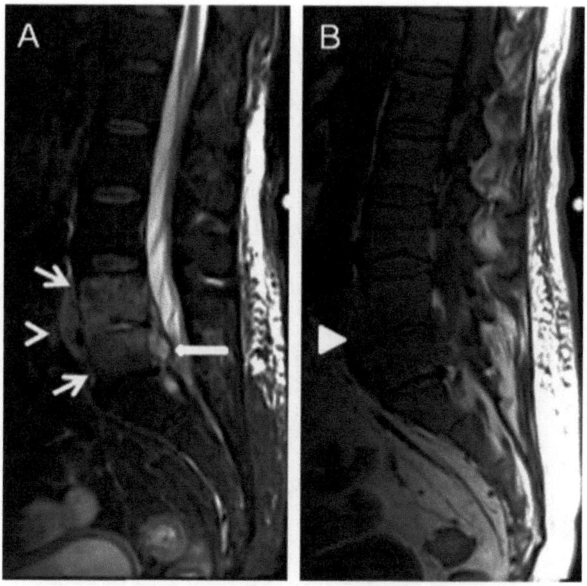

Figure 2.2 Spondylodiscitis. On the pretreatment sagittal STIR MRI image of the lumbar spine (**a**), there is L4-L5 disc space narrowing and edema with L4 and L5 vertebral body edema (*arrows*). There are fluid collections in the paravertebral region (*arrowhead*) and anterior spinal canal (*solid arrow*). On the sagittal noncontrast T1 MRI image of the lumbar spine (**b**), there is corresponding decreased signal in the L4 and L5 vertebral bodies and L4–L5 disc space (*solid arrowhead*). Biopsy confirmed acute osteomyelitis with paravertebral abscess and ventral epidural abscess

energy emitted by the protons as they return to their low-energy state of normal alignment [1]. MRI provides excellent anatomic detail, is useful for evaluating both bone and soft tissue, and is the anatomical imaging test of choice for diagnosing osteomyelitis. The earliest findings of osteomyelitis, for example, which can appear by 2 days after the onset of infection, are changes in signal intensity caused by inflammatory marrow edema (Figure 2.2). Intravenous gadolinium-containing contrast agents are also useful for evaluating soft tissue abscesses and for distinguishing synovial thickening from synovial fluid [1].

2.2.3 *Ultrasonography*

Like MRI, ultrasonography does not use ionizing radiation. Tissues attenuate and reflect sound waves differently. By taking advantage of these differences, images can be generated. An abscess, for example, presents as a focal area of decreased echoes, i.e., a hypoechoic area. Although ultrasonography is useful for evaluation of

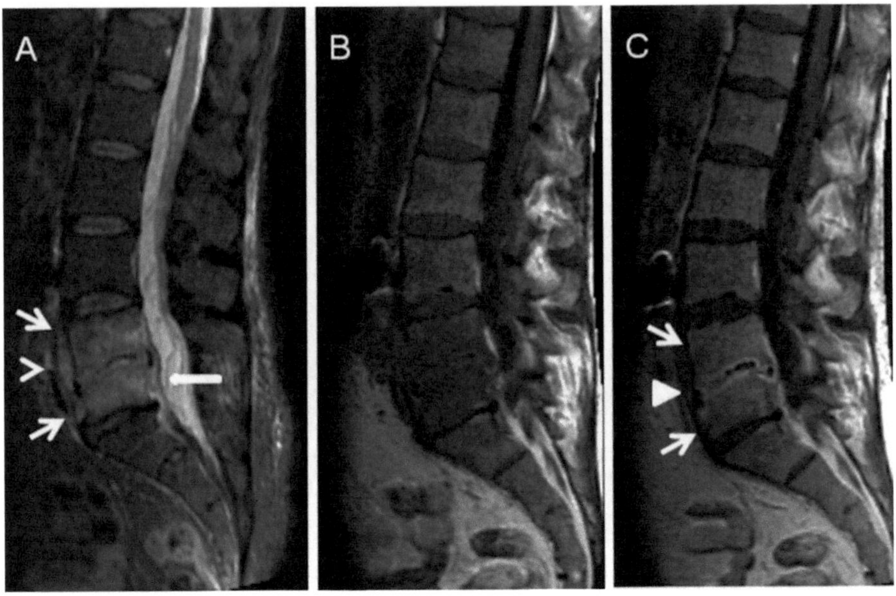

Figure 2.3 Spondylodiscitis (posttreatment). On the posttreatment sagittal STIR (**a**), precontrast T1 (**b**), and postcontrast T1 (**c**) MRI images of the lumbar spine, there is interval decrease in size of the paravertebral (*arrowhead*) and ventral epidural (*solid arrow*) abscesses, consistent with treatment response. There is continued abnormal signal and postcontrast enhancement in the L4 and L5 vertebral bodies and L4–L5 disc space (*arrows*) with slight progression of end plate irregularity (*solid arrowhead*), which may reflect expected evolution of infection

a suspected septic joint, it is less useful for diagnosing osteomyelitis, because it cannot image beyond the cortex of the bone [1].

There are limitations to anatomical imaging tests. While sensitive for bacterial and fungal infections, they are much less sensitive for detecting viral infections, which often cause very subtle or no structural changes. Moreover, they lack specificity and cannot reliably differentiate noninfectious processes (e.g., sterile inflammation, oncologic processes) from infection, nor can they reliably differentiate one infectious etiology from another. The role of morphologic imaging for assessing response to treatment and detecting recurrent infection also is limited because structural abnormalities can persist with little or no change for some time after the infection has resolved. In patients with spondylodiscitis, for example, while a decrease in soft tissue involvement on MRI correlates to some degree with response to treatment, the bony findings of destruction, sclerosis, and marrow edema can persist, and in some cases progress, even after the infection has resolved. Thus, the persistence of bone and disc abnormalities on MRI does not necessarily represent treatment failure (Figure 2.3) [2, 3].

2.3 Molecular Imaging Tests

2.3.1 Nonspecific Agents

2.3.1.1 Single-Photon-Emitting (SPECT) Radiopharmaceuticals

Gallium-67 Citrate

The ability of gallium-67 citrate (^{67}Ga) to concentrate in infection and inflammation was first appreciated nearly 50 years ago. Several factors govern uptake of this radiopharmaceutical in infection. About 90% of circulating gallium is in the plasma, bound almost entirely to transferrin. Increased blood flow and vascular membrane permeability result in increased delivery and accumulation of transferrin-bound ^{67}Ga to foci of infection. ^{67}Ga also binds to lactoferrin, which is present in high concentrations in infection and which has a high affinity for this radiopharmaceutical. Direct bacterial uptake of ^{67}Ga has also been observed in vitro. Siderophores, small chelates produced by bacteria, have a high affinity for ^{67}Ga. The siderophore-^{67}Ga complex is transported into the bacterium and eventually phagocytized by macrophages. Although some ^{67}Ga may be directly transported by leukocytes, this radiopharmaceutical accumulates in infection even in the absence of circulating white cells [4]. While ^{67}Ga has been replaced by other radiopharmaceuticals for most indications, it remains useful in select circumstances. This radiopharmaceutical is a sensitive indicator of pulmonary inflammation and accumulates in opportunistic infections, interstitial pneumonitis, drug reactions, pneumoconioses, and sarcoidosis. Intensity of uptake correlates loosely with disease activity and response to treatment (Figure 2.4).

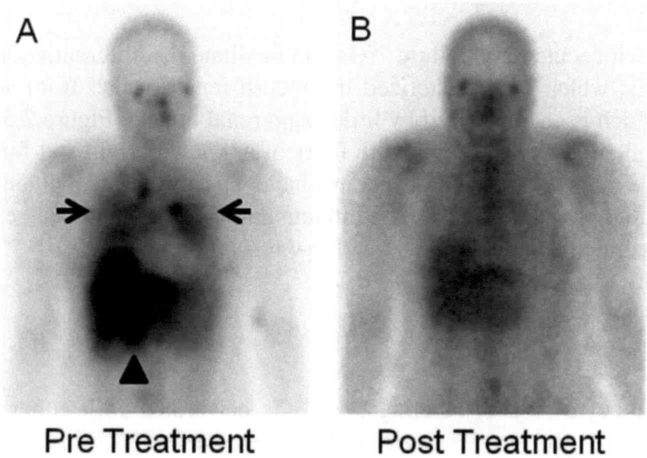

Figure 2.4 Sarcoidosis. On the pretreatment gallium-67 image (**a**), there is patchy radiopharmaceutical uptake in both lungs (*arrows*) and in the celiac/periportal region (*arrowhead*). On the posttreatment image (**b**) the abnormalities have resolved

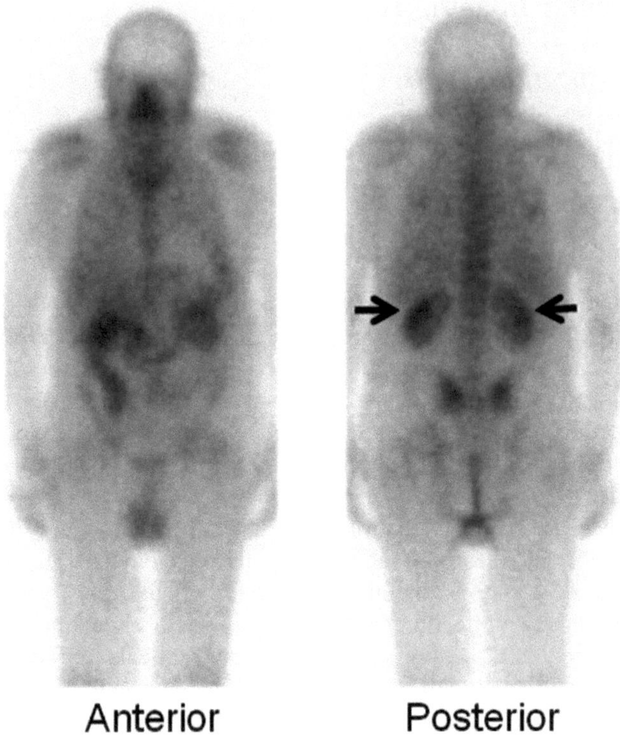

Figure 2.5 Interstitial nephritis. There is intense renal uptake of gallium-67 in both kidneys (*arrows*). Acute tubular necrosis, in contrast, is characterized by faint or no renal uptake of this radiopharmaceutical

In patients with acute renal failure, ^{67}Ga can facilitate the differentiation of interstitial nephritis, which is characterized by intense renal uptake, from acute tubular necrosis, which is characterized by little or no renal uptake (Figure 2.5). ^{67}Ga is an acceptable alternative in patients with fever of unknown origin and for diagnosing spondylodiscitis when ^{18}F-FDG is not available. Disadvantages include nonspecific uptake in tumors, trauma, and aseptic inflammation, the long interval between injection and imaging (usually 48–72 h), and low-resolution images [4].

Labeled Leukocytes

In vitro leukocyte (WBC) labeling usually is performed with either indium-111 oxyquinolone (^{111}In) or technetium-99m-exametazime (^{99m}Tc). WBC uptake depends on intact chemotaxis (which is preserved with standard in vitro labeling procedures), the number and types of cells labeled, and the cellular response to the specific infection. A total circulating leukocyte count of at least 2000/uL is needed

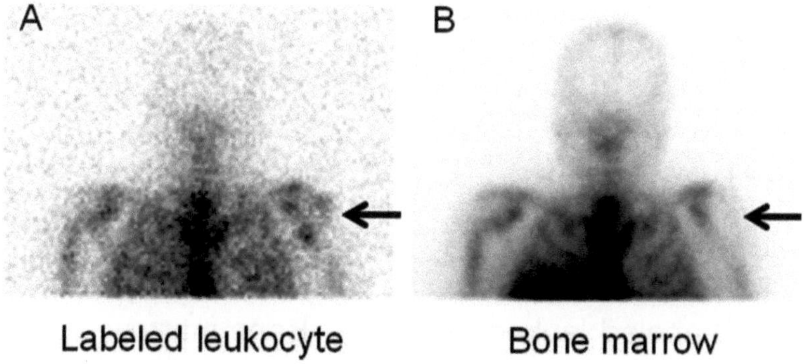

Figure 2.6 Osteomyelitis left shoulder. On the indium-111-labeled autologous leukocyte image (**a**), there is subtly increased activity in the left shoulder (*arrow*), which could easily be overlooked. On the technetium-99m sulfur colloid bone marrow image (**b**), however, there is no corresponding activity in this region (*arrow*). The combined study is positive for osteomyelitis

to obtain satisfactory images. In most clinical scenarios, the majority of WBCs labeled are neutrophils, and the test is most sensitive for identifying neutrophil-mediated inflammatory processes, such as bacterial infections. WBC imaging is much less sensitive for infections in which the predominant cellular response is not neutrophilic, such as tuberculosis [5]. WBC imaging remains the most commonly performed molecular imaging test for most infections in the immunocompetent population. It can be used either as the primary imaging test or an adjunct to other imaging or laboratory tests to diagnose infections nearly anywhere in the body, including both primary and complicating osteomyelitis, infective endocarditis, vascular graft infections, and abscesses. When performed for suspected osteomyelitis, WBC imaging is frequently performed in conjunction with ^{99m}Tc sulfur colloid bone marrow imaging. This is because leukocytes accumulate in the normal bone marrow as well as in infection. The normal distribution of hematopoietically active bone marrow is variable, and it is not always possible to differentiate infection from marrow on WBC images. Performing bone marrow imaging facilitates the differentiation. WBCs and sulfur colloid both accumulate in marrow; WBCs accumulate in infection, and sulfur colloid does not. The combined study is positive for infection when activity is present on the WBC image without corresponding activity on the marrow image (Figures 6 and 7). This test, which has been most extensively investigated in prosthetic joint infection, is useful in any condition that potentially affects marrow distribution and has an overall accuracy of approximately 90% [6]. In contrast to other areas of the skeleton, WBC imaging is not useful for diagnosing spondylodiscitis. For reasons that are not well understood, 50% or more of all cases present as areas of decreased or absent activity on WBC images (Figure 2.8). This pattern, which is associated with numerous conditions, is not specific for spinal infection [7].

There are significant disadvantages to in vitro labeled leukocyte imaging. The labeling procedure is labor intensive, involves contact with blood products, and may

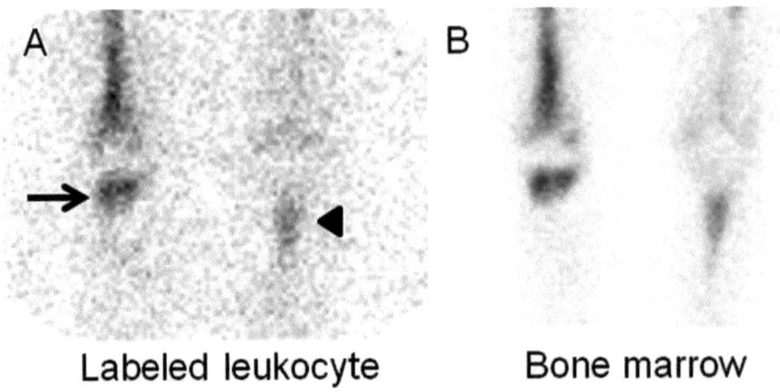

Figure 2.7 Focal hypercellular bone marrow. On the indium-111-labeled autologous leukocyte image (**a**), there are focal areas of increased activity in the right tibial metaphysis (*arrow*) and left tibial shaft (*arrowhead*). These foci could be interpreted as being indicative of osteomyelitis. The distribution of activity on the technetium-99m sulfur colloid bone marrow image (**b**), however, is virtually identical to that on the labeled leukocyte study, indicating that the labeled leukocyte uptake reflects marrow activity, not infection

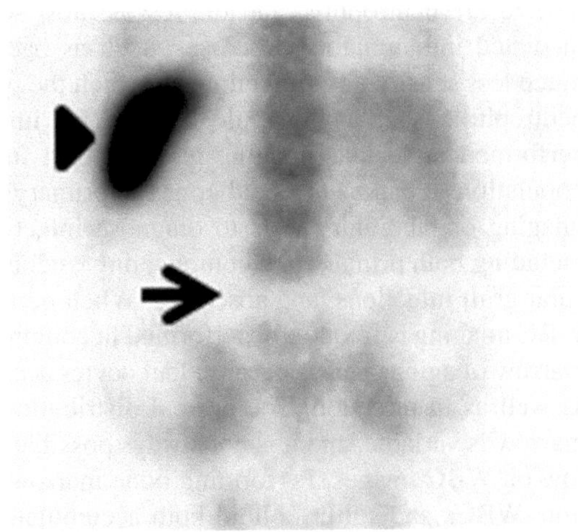

Figure 2.8 Spinal osteomyelitis. Note the absent activity in the lower lumbar spine (*arrow*) on the indium-111-labeled autologous leukocyte image, which is not specific for spinal osteomyelitis. The area of intense activity in the left upper quadrant (*arrowhead*) is the normal spleen

be difficult to perform in leukopenic patients and children. In an effort to overcome the disadvantages of the in vitro procedure, in vivo leukocyte labeling methods have been investigated. Besilesomab (Scintimum®), a 150 kDa murine monoclonal antibody of the IgG1 kappa isotype, binds to nonspecific cross-reacting antigen-95 (NCA-95), an epitope expressed on cell membranes of granulocytes and granulocyte precursors. About 10% of injected activity is neutrophil bound within 45 min. Twenty percent remains in the circulation, presumably localizing in inflammatory foci through nonspecific mechanisms. This agent has demonstrated reasonable accuracy for diagnosing musculoskeletal infections and appendicitis. A significant disadvantage of ^{99m}Tc-besilesomab is the incidence of human antimurine antibody

(HAMA) response, which ranges from less than 5% in patients receiving a single dose of 125 μg of antibody to more than 30% in patients receiving repeated injections. Consequently, patients should be prescreened for HAMA, should receive no more than 50 μg of antibody, and should not undergo repeat injections [8].

Antibody fragments, which do not induce a HAMA response, are a potential alternative to whole antibodies. ^{99m}Tc-sulesomab (Leukoscan®) is a 50 kDa fragment antigen-binding (Fab) portion of an IgG1 class murine monoclonal antibody that binds to normal cross-reactive antigen-90 (NCA-90) present on leukocytes. Approximately 3–6% of the injected activity is associated with circulating neutrophils; at 24 h after injection, about 35% of the remaining activity is in the bone marrow. Initial investigations suggested that sulesomab bound to both circulating neutrophils that migrate to foci of infection and to neutrophils already present at the site of infection. Subsequent data, however, suggested that the accumulation in infection is nonspecific. ^{99m}Tc-sulesomab is sensitive for diagnosing musculoskeletal infection; specificity, however, is variable. The test is reasonably accurate for diagnosing soft tissue infections and fever of unknown origin [8].

Radiolabeled cytokines, which are low molecular weight proteins that interact with specific cell-surface receptors on specific cell populations, also have been investigated as in vivo leukocyte labeling agents, but no large-scale investigations have been conducted [9, 10].

2.3.1.2 Positron-Emitting Radiopharmaceuticals

Positron emission tomography (PET) offers several advantages over single-photon-emitting radiopharmaceuticals. PET provides high-resolution three-dimensional images of the whole body that, especially when performed as PET/CT, facilitates precise localization of abnormalities. Other advantages of PET include the short interval between radiopharmaceutical injection and imaging with rapid, same-day results in most cases. The relatively short half-life of most PET radiopharmaceuticals permits administration of greater amounts of activity, which improves image quality. Semiquantitative analysis, which is more feasible with PET than with SPECT, potentially could be useful for differentiating infectious from noninfectious conditions and for monitoring response to treatment [11].

^{18}F-FDG

An analog of 2-deoxyglucose with a half-life of 109 min, ^{18}F-FDG is the most widely used PET radiopharmaceutical. It enters cells by active transport via glucose transporters and, to a lesser extent, by passive diffusion. ^{18}F-FDG accumulates in virtually all leukocytes, and its uptake in these cells is dependent on their metabolic rate and the number of glucose transporters. There is increased expression of glucose transporters by activated inflammatory cells. There is an increased affinity of these transporters for ^{18}F-FDG in inflammation, probably due to the effects of

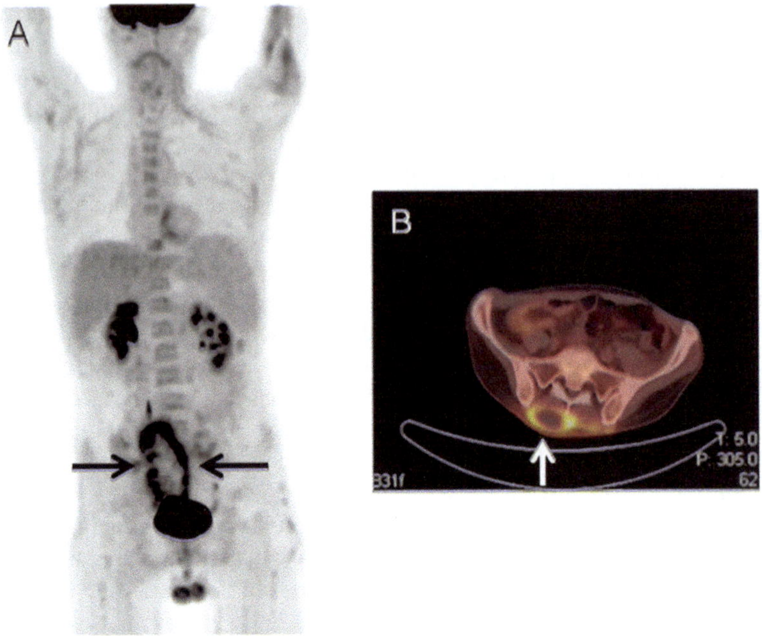

Figure 2.9 Soft tissue abscess in a patient with suspected relapsed lymphoma. On the maximum-intensity-projection PET image (**a**), there is a large oval-shaped area of peripherally increased ^{18}F-FDG accumulation in the lower abdomen/pelvis (*arrows*). This pattern is not typical of the nodal ^{18}F-FDG uptake associated with lymphoma. On the axial PET/CT image (**b**), the abnormal ^{18}F-FDG activity is confined to the soft tissues (*arrow*). An abscess subsequently was drained

circulating cytokines and growth factors [11]. While ^{18}F-FDG is an established radiopharmaceutical for oncologic, cardiac, and neurologic PET studies, increased glycolysis in inflammatory cells as well as in bacteria themselves also leads to increased ^{18}F-FDG uptake, making it a very sensitive test for detecting infectious and inflammatory processes. Despite the fact that ^{18}F-FDG cannot consistently distinguish between sterile and infectious inflammatory processes, a growing number of studies indicate that this radiopharmaceutical may be useful for both diagnosing infection and monitoring response to treatment. ^{18}F-FDG has proven clinically helpful in approximately two-thirds of patients with suspected focal infection or a localized inflammatory process [12] and can also contribute to the diagnosis of superimposed infection in postsurgical fluid collections, in cysts in solid organs such as the kidney or liver, and peripancreatic fluid collections, abdominal and pelvis abscesses, colitis, and diverticulitis [13]. Even when performed for oncologic indications, ^{18}F-FDG identifies unsuspected sites of inflammation and infection (Figure 2.9). Some of the more commonly identified abnormalities include wound infections, sinusitis, pneumonia, esophagitis, enteritis, acute appendicitis, infectious and inflammatory colitis, and mycobacterial infections [14].

Sensitivity in excess of 95% and specificity ranging from 75 to 99% has been reported for ^{18}F-FDG in acute and subacute bone and soft tissue infection

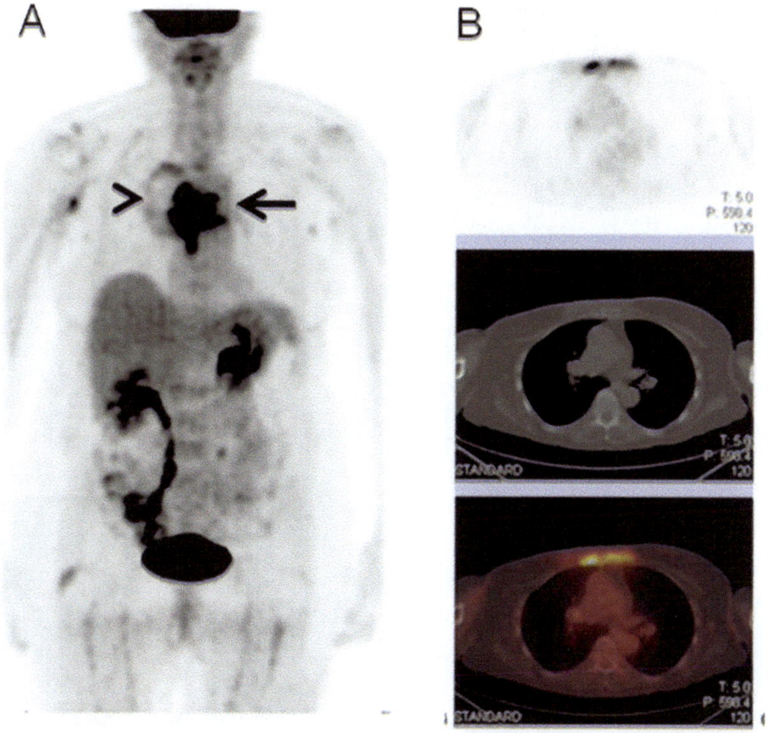

Figure 2.10 Sternal osteomyelitis with soft tissue involvement. On the maximum-intensity-projection PET image (**a**), there is a large focus of intensely increased ^{18}F-FDG uptake in the mid chest (*arrow*). There is a circumferential area of faintly increased activity just to the right of the midline (*arrowhead*). On the axial PET/CT images (**b**), the abnormal uptake involves both bone and soft tissue

(Figure 2.10). ^{18}F-FDG has also been useful for diagnosing chronic and low-grade musculoskeletal infection because this radiopharmaceutical accumulates in activated macrophages, the predominant cell type present in chronic infection [7, 15, 16]. ^{18}F-FDG also compares favorably with MRI for diagnosing spinal infections [17–23] and may be useful for monitoring response to treatment in patients with spondylodiscitis (Figure 2.11). Some investigators have found that changes in the standardized uptake value before and after treatment are useful for determining the efficacy of therapy and persistence of residual disease [22, 24, 25]. Riccio et al. [26] analyzed imaging findings and found that patients who responded poorly to treatment for hematogenous spondylodiscitis had persistent ^{18}F-FDG uptake in bone and soft tissue.

^{18}F-FDG will be less useful in some situations. It is likely that ^{18}F-FDG will be less reliable for differentiating infection from tumor and infection superimposed on tumor. Moreover, significant focal ^{18}F-FDG uptake can occur in degenerative spinal disease, and nonspecific, increased ^{18}F-FDG uptake can occur around uninfected

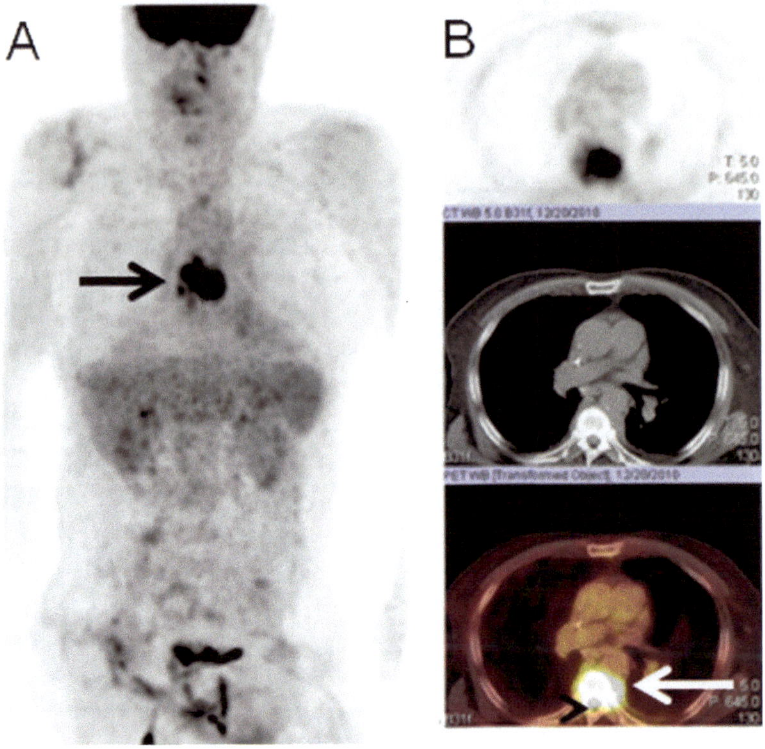

Figure 2.11 Spondylodiscitis. On the maximum-intensity-projection PET image (**a**), there is abnormal ^{18}F-FDG uptake in the mid thorax (*arrow*). On the axial PET/CT images (**b**), the infection involves bone (seventh and eighth thorax vertebrae) and extends into the adjacent soft tissues (*arrow*) and spinal canal (*arrowhead*)

spinal implants, both of which may adversely affect specificity [7]. Regardless of any limitations, the data accumulated to date demonstrate that ^{18}F-FDG accurately diagnoses spondylodiscitis and support its role as the molecular imaging test of choice for this entity.

In contrast to the results reported for spondylodiscitis, the results of ^{18}F-FDG for diagnosing diabetic pedal osteomyelitis have been variable. Some investigators have reported that the test is both sensitive and specific [27–30]. Other investigators have found that the test is not sensitive, and in one investigation, it was less sensitive than planar ^{99m}Tc-WBC imaging [31, 32]. Variations in sensitivity may have been related to varying degrees of vascular insufficiency among the study populations, yet these data are lacking [33].

^{18}F-FDG has also generated considerable interest for diagnosing prosthetic joint infection, but the results have been variable. In an early investigation, Zhuang et al. [34] reported that the test was 89.5% and 77.8% accurate for diagnosing hip and knee arthroplasty infection, respectively, and accurate diagnosis depended on location, not intensity, of ^{18}F-FDG uptake. While several other studies reported similar results [35–39], other investigators have reported less satisfactory results [40–45]. García-Barrecheguren et al. [43] reported that ^{18}F-FDG PET was neither sensitive (64%) nor specific (67%) for prosthetic hip infection. In another investigation, increased ^{18}F-FDG uptake in the synovial membrane was present in 27/28 painful knee arthroplasties, including 24/25 uninfected devices [46]. Studies comparing ^{18}F-FDG and bone or WBC imaging have yielded contradictory results [36, 37, 41, 45]. The failure of ^{18}F-FDG to consistently differentiate between aseptic loosening and infection of a prosthetic joint should not be surprising because both of these conditions can be accompanied by an inflammatory response in which leukocytes participate.

The role of ^{18}F-FDG in the diagnosis of infective endocarditis (IE) and cardiovascular implantable electronic device (CIED) infections has also been investigated. In a recent meta-analysis, which included 246 patients, pooled sensitivity and specificity of ^{18}F-FDG for diagnosing IE were 61 and 88%, respectively. Despite the low overall sensitivity, ^{18}F-FDG may be useful in the subset of patients with prosthetic cardiac valves [47, 48]. Published data also suggest that ^{18}F-FDG is more sensitive but less specific than WBC imaging for diagnosing IE in patients with prosthetic valves. It has been suggested that WBC imaging be reserved for those cases in which results of ^{18}F-FDG are inconclusive and within the first 2 months after cardiac surgery [49]. Results of ^{18}F-FDG for diagnosing CIED infections such as pacemakers and left ventricular assist devices also are encouraging [47, 48, 50–54]. False-negative results for IE and CIED have been attributed to small lesions below the limits of resolution of current PET/CT systems. Sensitivity may also be adversely affected by performing imaging after institution of antibiotic treatment, especially if the patient has been on treatment for more than 1 week. False-positive results may be associated with postoperative inflammation and the presence of severe prosthetic valve thrombosis [48]. ^{18}F-FDG is potentially useful for diagnosing left ventricular assist device (LVAD) infections, determining its extent, and monitoring response to therapy (Figure 2.12) [53, 54].

^{18}F-FDG appears to be useful for diagnosing prosthetic vascular graft infection, especially when performed as a PET/CT study (Figure 2.13) [55, 56], and for monitoring response to treatment in patients with prosthetic vascular graft infections [57]. However, prosthetic vascular grafts can induce a foreign-body inflammatory reaction, which can be associated with increased ^{18}F-FDG activity, even in the absence of infection. Knowledge of typical ^{18}F-FDG uptake patterns associated with infection and foreign body reaction can improve the specificity of the test. Vascular graft infection typically presents as a focal or heterogeneous pattern of ^{18}F-FDG uptake projecting over the vessel on CT, while linear, diffuse, homogeneous uptake along the graft favors foreign body reaction [58, 59].

Fever of unknown origin (FUO) is one of the more frustrating conditions for both clinicians and patients, with no definite diagnosis established in up to 50% of cases. The differential diagnosis for FUO is wide but can be divided into four major cate-

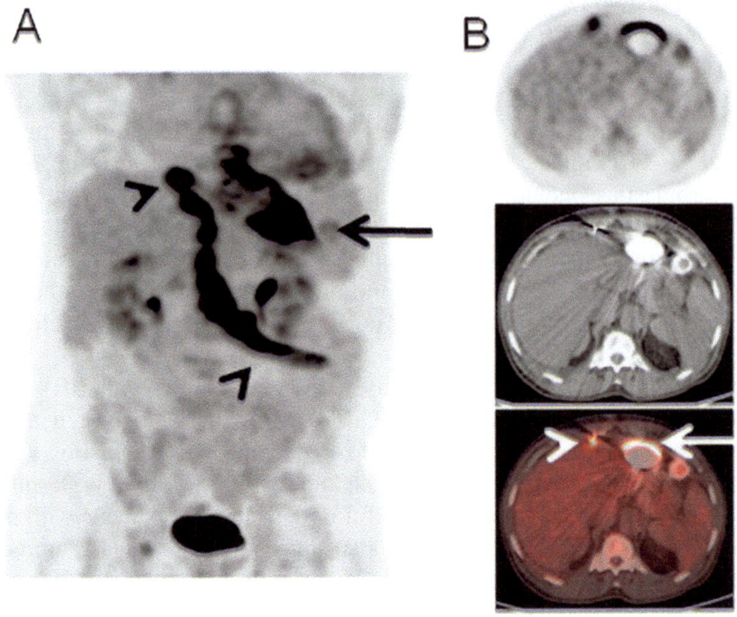

Figure 2.12 Infected left ventricular assist device. On the maximum-intensity-projection PET image (**a**), there is increased ^{18}F-FDG uptake along the device (*arrow*) and its driveline (*arrowheads*). Axial PET-CT images of the upper abdomen (**b**) demonstrate increased uptake along the device (*arrow*) and its driveline (*arrowhead*) in the anterior abdominal wall. Driveline cultures grew *Staphylococcus aureus*

gories: infection (20–40%), malignancy (20–30%), noninfectious inflammatory diseases (10–30%), and miscellaneous (10–20%). In developing countries, infections are the major cause of FUO; in developed countries, noninfectious inflammatory diseases are the most common cause [60]. The workup of the patient with FUO should begin with a comprehensive history and physical examination including a complete blood count, chest radiograph, urinalysis and culture, electrolyte panel, liver enzymes, erythrocyte sedimentation rate, and C-reactive protein level. Additional imaging procedures, serum antibodies, and tissue biopsies are included as second-line procedures. The selection of imaging procedures should be guided by results of previous tests, with the ultimate goal being to identify abnormal tissue to culture or biopsy for definitive diagnosis [60]. When there is no clear etiology of the FUO, ^{18}F-FDG may be especially useful to localize a possible lesion or area of interest (Figure 2.14) [61]. While highly sensitive, false-negative results have been reported in systemic lupus erythematosus, cytomegalovirus infection, toxoplasmosis, urinary infection, septicemia, pyelonephritis, and Crohn's disease [12, 62–67]. In a multicenter trial of 75 patients with FUO, ^{18}F-FDG PET, chest CT, abdominal CT, abdominal ultrasound, and chest X-ray were diagnostically helpful in 33%, 20%, 20%, 10%, and 8% of cases, respectively [63]. Other studies have reported

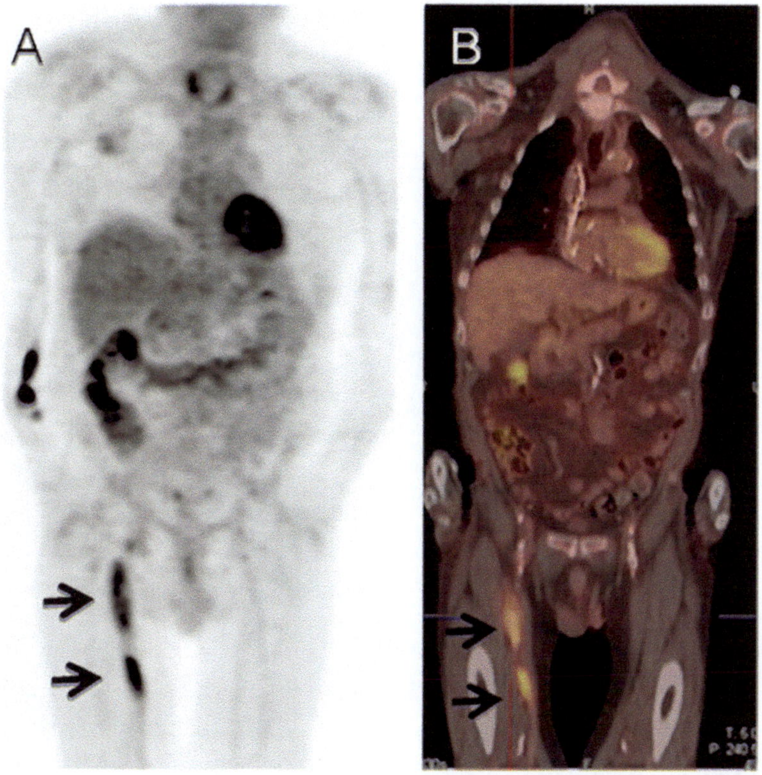

Figure 2.13 Infected femoral/popliteal vascular graft. There is a long segment of increased ^{18}F-FDG uptake (*arrows*) on the maximum-intensity-projection PET image (**a**) and the coronal PET/CT (**b**) image. Culture of the excised graft grew methicillin-sensitive *Staphylococcus aureus*

that ^{18}F-FDG contributed useful information in about 54–74% versus 39–62% for chest/abdominal CT [64, 67]. ^{18}F-FDG is also useful for FUO in children [68–70] (Figure 2.15). These data suggest that ^{18}F-FDG is superior to CT and that early imaging may be useful for clinical management [71, 72]. ^{18}F-FDG can also provide useful information in patients with occult bacteremia by identifying the site of origin of the bacteremia, remote foci of infection, and complications such as thromboembolic phenomena, though this may be complicated due to nonspecific uptake in sites of sterile inflammation [73, 74].

In summary, ^{18}F-FDG is a very useful imaging technique for infectious diseases and has been used extensively. This technique has high sensitivity and is superior to CT imaging, especially in the setting of FUO. However, the lack of specificity and difficulties in interpreting some of the studies due to differences in protocols, patient populations, selection criteria, and definitions of what constitutes an infection,

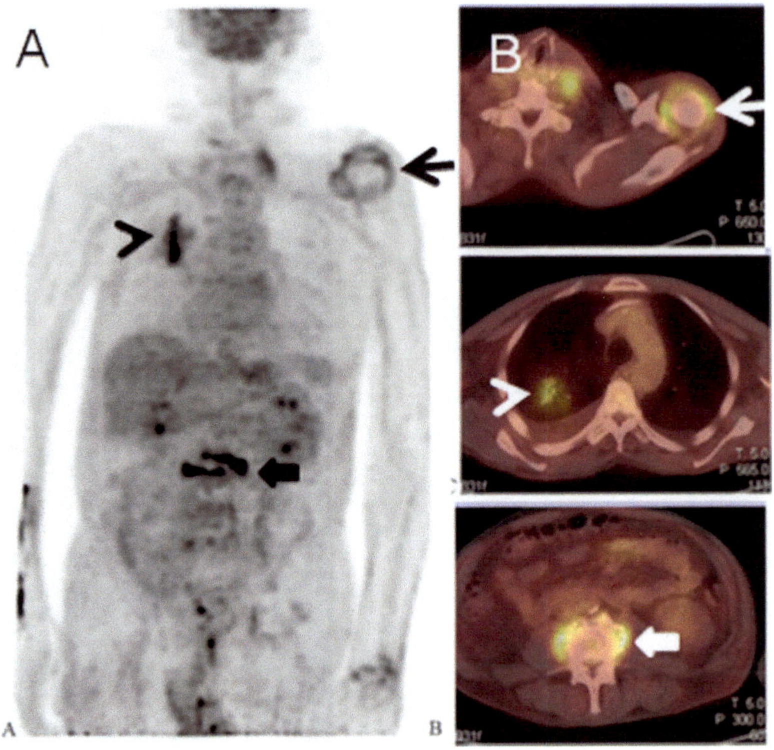

Figure 2.14 Multifocal infection in a patient with fever of unknown origin. 66-year-old man presented with altered mental status, intermittent fevers, and recent pneumococcal bacteremia. On the maximum-intensity-projection PET image (**a**) and axial PET/CT images (**b**), there are areas of increased ^{18}F-FDG uptake in the left shoulder (*arrow*), right upper lung (*arrowhead*), and mid lumbar spine (*solid arrow*), consistent with septic arthritis, pneumonia, and spondylodiscitis, respectively. Left shoulder and bronchial lavage cultures grew *Mycobacterium chelonae*

remain as obstacles. Thus, more specific imaging techniques for identifying infections are still needed.

Other PET Radiopharmaceuticals

Investigators have studied both in vitro and in vivo leukocyte labeling with various PET agents. Although published results using leukocytes labeled in vitro with ^{18}F-FDG (^{18}F-FDG-WBC) were encouraging, it is unlikely that ^{18}F-FDG-WBC imaging ever will enter clinical practice. The 109-min half-life of fluorine-18 (^{18}F) makes it impractical for labeling to be performed off-site, so the test would be limited to institutions capable of performing the labeling in-house. The short half-life of ^{18}F also precludes imaging much beyond 4–5 h after injection; thus delayed imaging is

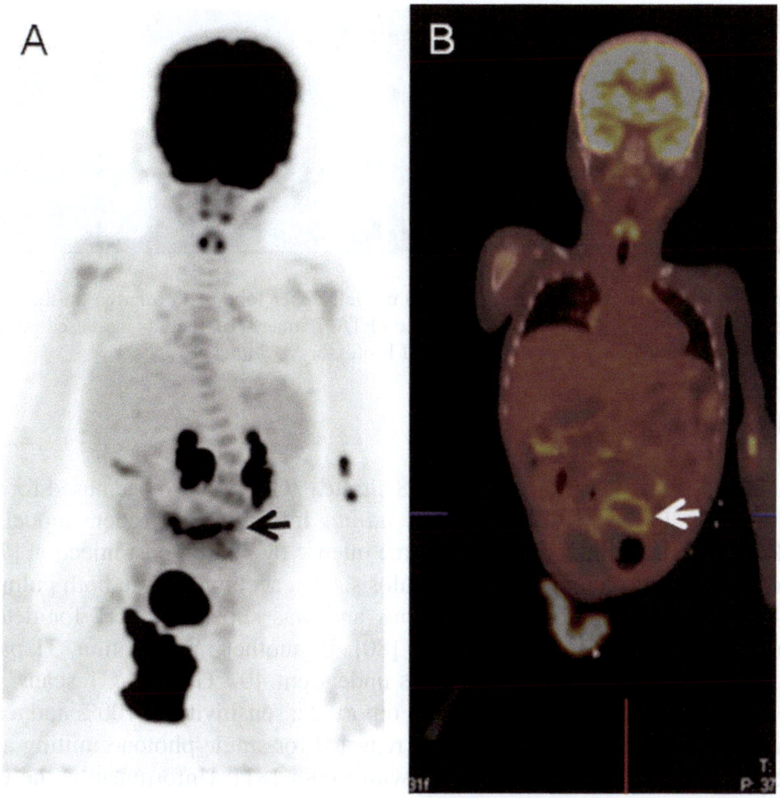

Figure 2.15 Infected ventriculoperitoneal shunt in a 5-year-old boy with Chiari 2 malformation and myelomeningocele presenting with hydrocephalus and fever of unknown origin. On the maximum-intensity-projection PET image (**a**), there is increased ^{18}F-FDG uptake in the mid abdomen (*arrow*). On the coronal PET/CT image (**b**), this activity is within a rim of soft tissue surrounding a fluid collection (*arrow*). Cerebrospinal fluid cultures from the shunt grew *Staphylococcus epidermidis*

not an option. Labeling efficiency is significantly lower and more variable than with ^{111}In-oxine and ^{18}F-FDG rapidly elutes from leukocytes [75–77].

The positron-emitting radionuclide copper-64 (^{64}Cu) has been used to label leukocytes both in vitro and in vivo. The physical half-life of ^{64}Cu is nearly 13 h, which is sufficiently long for both the in vitro labeling procedure and for obtaining delayed images. In vitro labeling efficiency is similar to what can be achieved with ^{111}In-WBC. Label stability is less than what is achieved with ^{111}In-WBC but similar to that of ^{99m}Tc-WBC [77]. No clinical or preclinical investigations have been conducted with this agent. A ^{64}Cu-labeled peptide, cFLFLFK-PEG that targets the formyl peptide receptor (FPR) on leukocytes, was studied in a murine model of *Klebsiella pneumoniae*. At 18 h post injection, pulmonary uptake of this agent was 5–6 times higher than that of controls [78]. No clinical investigations have been conducted with this agent.

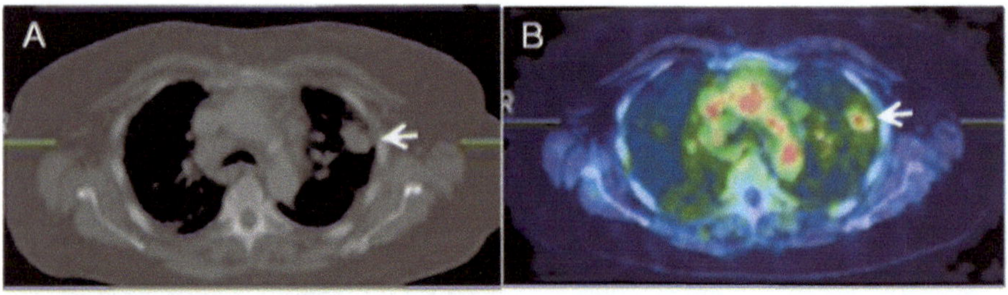

Figure 2.16 Tuberculosis. There is a 3.5 × 3 cm left upper lobe mass (*arrow*) on the axial CT image (**a**) of a patient with tuberculosis. On the PET/CT image (**b**), there is increased gallium-68 uptake in this lesion (*arrow*). (Case courtesy of Professor M. Sathekge)

Gallium-68 Citrate

Similar to gallium-67 citrate, gallium-68 citrate (^{68}Ga) has also been used for imaging infection. In an investigation of *S. aureus* infection in a rodent model, ^{68}Ga uptake was seen within 5 min and became intense by 30 min post injection [79]. In a pilot study of 13 patients with tuberculosis, ^{68}Ga accumulated in both pulmonary and extra-pulmonary tuberculous lesions and was superior to CT for detecting extra-pulmonary disease (Figure 2.16) [80]. In another investigation, 31 patients with suspected osteomyelitis or discitis underwent 40 ^{68}Ga PET/CT scans. There were 23 cases of infection. The authors reported a sensitivity of 100% and a specificity of 76%, similar to what has been reported for single-photon-emitting agents. False-positive results were associated with tumor [81]. Unfortunately, the uptake mechanisms of ^{68}Ga in inflammation and infection are the same nonspecific mechanisms responsible for uptake of ^{67}Ga. Although ^{68}Ga offers the advantages of superior image quality and same-day imaging, the other limitations associated with ^{67}Ga remain, making this a less than ideal radiopharmaceutical for imaging infection.

2.3.2 *Infection-Specific Agents*

2.3.2.1 SPECT Radiopharmaceuticals

Radiolabeled Antibiotics

Although useful, none of the clinically available radiopharmaceuticals is specific for infection, and the search continues for such an agent. Radiolabeled antibiotics have been investigated as "infection-specific" radiopharmaceuticals. Presumably, the labeled antibiotic is incorporated into and metabolized by bacteria, thereby accurately and specifically localizing infection. The most extensively investigated of these compounds is ^{99m}Tc-ciprofloxacin. Initial investigations reported high sensitivity and specificity; subsequent studies, however, cast serious doubts about its specificity, and much of the original enthusiasm for radiolabeled antibiotics as an infection-specific test has faded [82–84].

^{111}In-Biotin

Biotin, or vitamin B7, plays a key role in glucose metabolism including regulation of hepatic glucose uptake, gluconeogenesis, and lipogenesis, insulin receptor transcription, and pancreatic β-cell function. Biotin also is used as a growth factor by certain bacteria [85]. ^{111}In-Biotin, alone and in combination with streptavidin, has been used for imaging musculoskeletal infection. Advantages of this radiopharmaceutical include same-day imaging, minimal bone marrow uptake, and less patient radiation than with labeled leukocyte and ^{67}Ga studies. Antibiotic therapy does not appear to affect test sensitivity [86, 87]. Although the reported results have been encouraging, this radiopharmaceutical is available in only a very few centers outside the United States.

Radiolabeled Antimicrobial Peptides

Antimicrobial peptides (AMPs) are an important component of the natural defenses of most living organisms. Most AMPs are small, cationic, and amphipathic (hydrophilic and hydrophobic) and attack pathogens by multiple mechanisms. They exhibit broad-spectrum activity against Gram-positive and Gram-negative bacteria, yeasts, fungi, and enveloped viruses. They also are involved in apoptosis, wound healing, and immune modulation. Their expression may be constant or induced on contact with microbes; they also may be transported by circulating leukocytes to sites of infection [8, 88]. Ubiquicidin (UBI) is a murine antimicrobial peptide (AMP) found in the cytosolic fraction of macrophages [89]. Radiolabeled synthetic fragments of UBI have been investigated as infection-specific imaging agents. ^{99m}Tc-UBI-29-41 appears to be both sensitive and specific for a variety of infections and has shown promise for monitoring response to treatment [90]. A recent meta-analysis reported that pooled sensitivity, specificity, and accuracy were 94.5%, 92.7%, and 93.7% [91].

^{99m}Tc-labeled recombinant human beta-defensin-3, an AMP that exerts bactericidal effects on Gram-positive and Gram-negative bacteria, also has been investigated. By 3 h after injection, uptake in a *Staphylococcus aureus* infection model was significantly higher than uptake in sterile inflammation [92]. These approaches still need to be further tested in clinical trials.

2.3.2.2 PET Radiopharmaceuticals

While some investigators have explored the potential of ^{68}Ga-citrate for imaging infection, other investigators, in an attempt to develop an infection-specific imaging agent, have complexed ^{68}Ga with peptides [93–96]. In one study, UBI29-41 and UBI30-41, synthetic fragments of the AMP ubiquicidin, were labeled with ^{68}Ga. The in vitro binding of the radiolabeled fragments was significantly higher in *S. aureus* than in human leukocytes [93]. In a rabbit model, uptake of ^{68}Ga-NOTA-UBI29-41 was significantly higher in sites of *S. aureus* infection than in sites of sterile, turpentine-induced inflammation [94]. Vascular adhesion protein 1 (VAP-1) is a human endothelial protein whose cell surface expression is induced under inflammatory conditions. ^{68}Ga-DOTA-VAP-P1, which targets the VAP-1, was compared in infection (osteomyelitis) and inflammation (aseptic healing cortical bone defects) in rats. Animals with healing bones (inflammation) showed transient radiopharmaceutical uptake at 24 h post injection, which normalized over 7 days. In the infected bone, however, radiopharmaceutical uptake continued to increase over time. The authors concluded that these results indicate that ^{68}Ga-DOTA-VAP-P1 can, in the experimental setting, detect the effects of anti-inflammatory agents on bone healing and response to treatment [95].

The thymidine analogue fialuridine (FIAU) is a specific substrate of γ-herpesvirus and bacterial thymidine kinase [97]. Localized bacterial infections have been imaged successfully with ^{125}I-FIAU [98, 99]. In a pilot study ^{124}I-FIAU PET/CT was used for diagnosing musculoskeletal infection. All eight patients with proven musculoskeletal infections demonstrated radiopharmaceutical accumulation at the site of infection within 2 h after injection. There was no abnormal uptake in the one control [100]. Results of subsequent investigations, however, have been disappointing. An investigation of painful lower extremity joint replacements was terminated because poor image quality precluded image analysis [101]. A diabetic pedal osteomyelitis study was terminated because there was no correlation between radiopharmaceutical uptake and bone biopsy results.

Several other infection-specific agents are currently under development. ^{18}F-labeled maltose and maltohexaose [102, 103] and ^{18}F-fluordeoxysorbitol [104] are radiofluorinated sugars that have demonstrated specificity for bacterial pathogens. Recently, in a study of healthy volunteers, ^{18}F-FDS was found to be safe, well tolerated, and rapidly cleared, following a single, intravenous dose [105], suggesting significant potential for use in humans. A ^{64}Cu-NODAGA-labeled antibody was also evaluated in a *Yersinia* murine model [106], though antibodies may require much longer to clear from nontarget sites.

2.4 Summary

At the present time clinically available imaging modalities, both anatomical and functional, rely primarily on the host immune response to diagnose infection. These methods, though useful, are not specific for infection and cannot consistently distinguish infectious from sterile inflammatory processes or, in some cases, from tumor. Furthermore, the ability of these various modalities to monitor response to treatment is limited. There clearly is a need to develop imaging techniques that not only are specific for infection but also can identify the pathogen and can reliably monitor response to treatment. Investigations into new imaging agents that fulfill these criteria are ongoing. None of these agents has been incorporated into clinical practice, however. Therefore, further work is needed to identify and evaluate imaging approaches that will result in improved clinical outcomes in the diagnosis and management of infections.

References

1. Palestro, C.J., C. Love, and T.T. Miller, *Diagnostic imaging tests and microbial infections.* Cell Microbiol, 2007. **9**(10): p. 2323-33.
2. Kowalski, T.J., et al., *Follow-up MR imaging in patients with pyogenic spine infections: lack of correlation with clinical features.* AJNR Am J Neuroradiol, 2007. **28**(4): p. 693-9.
3. Euba, G., et al., *Long-term clinical and radiological magnetic resonance imaging outcome of abscess-associated spontaneous pyogenic vertebral osteomyelitis under conservative management.* Semin Arthritis Rheum, 2008. **38**(1): p. 28-40.
4. Palestro, C.J., *Scintigraphic diagnosis of inflammation and infection*, in *Fundamentals of Diagnostic Radiology*, H.C. Brant WE, Editor. 2012, Lippincott, Williams and Wilkins.: Philadelphia. p. 1339-52.
5. Palestro, C.J., C. Love, and K.K. Bhargava, *Labeled leukocyte imaging: current status and future directions.* Q J Nucl Med Mol Imaging, 2009. **53**(1): p. 105-23.
6. Palestro, C.J., et al., *Combined labeled leukocyte and technetium 99m sulfur colloid bone marrow imaging for diagnosing musculoskeletal infection.* Radiographics, 2006. **26**(3): p. 859-70.
7. Palestro, C.J., *Radionuclide Imaging of Musculoskeletal Infection: A Review.* J Nucl Med, 2016. **57**(9): p. 1406-12.
8. Palestro, C.J., A.W.J.M. Glaudemans, and R.A.J.O. Dierckx, *Multiagent imaging of inflammation and infection with radionuclides.* Clinical and Translational Imaging, 2013. **1**(6): p. 385-396.
9. Bleeker-Rovers, C.P., et al., *99mTc-labeled interleukin 8 for the scintigraphic detection of infection and inflammation: first clinical evaluation.* J Nucl Med, 2007. **48**(3): p. 337-43.
10. Gratz, S., et al., *(99m)Tc-interleukin-8 for imaging acute osteomyelitis.* J Nucl Med, 2001. **42**(8): p. 1257-64.
11. Love, C., et al., *FDG PET of infection and inflammation.* Radiographics, 2005. **25**(5): p. 1357-68.
12. Bleeker-Rovers, C.P., et al., *Clinical value of FDG PET in patients with fever of unknown origin and patients suspected of focal infection or inflammation.* Eur J Nucl Med Mol Imaging, 2004. **31**(1): p. 29-37.
13. Petruzzi, N., N. Shanthly, and M. Thakur, *Recent trends in soft-tissue infection imaging.* Semin Nucl Med, 2009. **39**(2): p. 115-23.
14. Wong, P.S., et al., *Clinically important detection of infection as an 'incidental' finding during cancer staging using FDG-PET/CT.* Intern Med J, 2012. **42**(2): p. 176-83.
15. Guhlmann, A., et al., *Chronic osteomyelitis: detection with FDG PET and correlation with histopathologic findings.* Radiology, 1998. **206**(3): p. 749-54.
16. de Winter, F., et al., *Fluorine-18 fluorodeoxyglucose-position emission tomography: a highly accurate imaging modality for the diagnosis of chronic musculoskeletal infections.* J Bone Joint Surg Am, 2001. **83-A**(5): p. 651-60.
17. Ohtori, S., et al., *18F-fluorodeoxyglucose-PET for patients with suspected spondylitis showing Modic change.* Spine (Phila Pa 1976), 2010. **35**(26): p. E1599-603.
18. Stumpe, K.D., et al., *FDG positron emission tomography for differentiation of degenerative and infectious endplate abnormalities in the lumbar spine detected on MR imaging.* AJR Am J Roentgenol, 2002. **179**(5): p. 1151-7.
19. Seifen, T., et al., *Prolonged back pain attributed to suspected spondylodiscitis. The value of (1)(8)F-FDG PET/CT imaging in the diagnostic work-up of patients.* Nuklearmedizin, 2012. **51**(5): p. 194-200.
20. Fuster, D., et al., *Prospective comparison of whole-body (18)F-FDG PET/CT and MRI of the spine in the diagnosis of haematogenous spondylodiscitis.* Eur J Nucl Med Mol Imaging, 2015. **42**(2): p. 264-71.
21. Skanjeti, A., et al., *PET in the clinical work-up of patients with spondylodiscitis: a new tool for the clinician?* Q J Nucl Med Mol Imaging, 2012. **56**(6): p. 569-76.

22. Ioannou, S., et al., *Fluorine-18 fluoro-2-deoxy-D-glucose positron emission tomography/computed tomography scan contributes to the diagnosis and management of brucellar spondylodiskitis.* BMC Infect Dis, 2013. **13**: p. 73.
23. Nakahara, M., et al., *18F-FDG-PET/CT better localizes active spinal infection than MRI for successful minimally invasive surgery.* Acta Radiol, 2015. **56**(7): p. 829-36.
24. Kim, S.J., et al., *Prediction of residual disease of spine infection using F-18 FDG PET/CT.* Spine (Phila Pa 1976), 2009. **34**(22): p. 2424-30.
25. Nanni, C., et al., *FDG PET/CT is useful for the interim evaluation of response to therapy in patients affected by haematogenous spondylodiscitis.* Eur J Nucl Med Mol Imaging, 2012. **39**(10): p. 1538-44.
26. Riccio, S.A., et al., *Fluorodeoxyglucose Positron Emission Tomography/Computed Tomography Interpretation Criteria for Assessment of Antibiotic Treatment Response in Pyogenic Spine Infection.* Can Assoc Radiol J, 2015. **66**(2): p. 145-52.
27. Nawaz, A., et al., *Diagnostic performance of FDG-PET, MRI, and plain film radiography (PFR) for the diagnosis of osteomyelitis in the diabetic foot.* Mol Imaging Biol, 2010. **12**(3): p. 335-42.
28. Kagna, O., et al., *FDG PET/CT imaging in the diagnosis of osteomyelitis in the diabetic foot.* Eur J Nucl Med Mol Imaging, 2012. **39**(10): p. 1545-50.
29. Yang, H., et al., *Mild-to-moderate hyperglycemia will not decrease the sensitivity of 18F-FDG PET imaging in the detection of pedal osteomyelitis in diabetic patients.* Nucl Med Commun, 2016. **37**(3): p. 259-62.
30. Shagos, G.S., et al., *18-F flourodeoxy glucose positron emission tomography-computed tomography imaging: A viable alternative to three phase bone scan in evaluating diabetic foot complications?* Indian J Nucl Med, 2015. **30**(2): p. 97-103.
31. Schwegler, B., et al., *Unsuspected osteomyelitis is frequent in persistent diabetic foot ulcer and better diagnosed by MRI than by 18F-FDG PET or 99mTc-MOAB.* J Intern Med, 2008. **263**(1): p. 99-106.
32. Familiari, D., et al., *Can sequential 18F-FDG PET/CT replace WBC imaging in the diabetic foot?* J Nucl Med, 2011. **52**(7): p. 1012-9.
33. Palestro, C.J., *18F-FDG and diabetic foot infections: the verdict is.* J Nucl Med, 2011. **52**(7): p. 1009-11.
34. Zhuang, H., et al., *The promising role of 18F-FDG PET in detecting infected lower limb prosthesis implants.* J Nucl Med, 2001. **42**(1): p. 44-8.
35. Chacko, T.K., et al., *The importance of the location of fluorodeoxyglucose uptake in periprosthetic infection in painful hip prostheses.* Nucl Med Commun, 2002. **23**(9): p. 851-5.
36. Reinartz, P., et al., *Radionuclide imaging of the painful hip arthroplasty: positron-emission tomography versus triple-phase bone scanning.* J Bone Joint Surg Br, 2005. **87**(4): p. 465-70.
37. Pill, S.G., et al., *Comparison of fluorodeoxyglucose positron emission tomography and (111) indium-white blood cell imaging in the diagnosis of periprosthetic infection of the hip.* J Arthroplasty, 2006. **21**(6 Suppl 2): p. 91-7.
38. Cremerius, U., et al., *[Analysis of (18)F-FDG uptake patterns in PET for diagnosis of septic and aseptic loosening after total hip arthroplasty].* Nuklearmedizin, 2003. **42**(6): p. 234-9.
39. Gravius, S., et al., *[Analysis of 18F-FDG uptake pattern in PET for diagnosis of aseptic loosening versus prosthesis infection after total knee arthroplasty. A prospective pilot study].* Nuklearmedizin, 2010. **49**(3): p. 115-23.
40. Stumpe, K.D., et al., *FDG PET for differentiation of infection and aseptic loosening in total hip replacements: comparison with conventional radiography and three-phase bone scintigraphy.* Radiology, 2004. **231**(2): p. 333-41.
41. Van Acker, F., et al., *FDG-PET, 99mtc-HMPAO white blood cell SPET and bone scintigraphy in the evaluation of painful total knee arthroplasties.* Eur J Nucl Med, 2001. **28**(10): p. 1496-504.
42. Vanquickenborne, B., et al., *The value of (18)FDG-PET for the detection of infected hip prosthesis.* Eur J Nucl Med Mol Imaging, 2003. **30**(5): p. 705-15.

43. Garcia-Barrecheguren, E., et al., *[FDG-PET: a new diagnostic approach in hip prosthetic replacement].* Rev Esp Med Nucl, 2007. **26**(4): p. 208-20.
44. Delank, K.S., et al., *The implications of 18F-FDG PET for the diagnosis of endoprosthetic loosening and infection in hip and knee arthroplasty: results from a prospective, blinded study.* BMC Musculoskelet Disord, 2006. **7**: p. 20.
45. Love, C., et al., *Diagnosing infection in the failed joint replacement: a comparison of coincidence detection 18F-FDG and 111In-labeled leukocyte/99mTc-sulfur colloid marrow imaging.* J Nucl Med, 2004. **45**(11): p. 1864-71.
46. Stumpe, K.D., et al., *The value of FDG-PET in patients with painful total knee arthroplasty.* Eur J Nucl Med Mol Imaging, 2006. **33**(10): p. 1218-25.
47. Yan, J., et al., *The role of 18F-FDG PET/CT in infectious endocarditis: a systematic review and meta-analysis.* Int J Clin Pharmacol Ther, 2016. **54**(5): p. 337-42.
48. Pizzi, M.N., et al., *Improving the Diagnosis of Infective Endocarditis in Prosthetic Valves and Intracardiac Devices With 18F-Fluordeoxyglucose Positron Emission Tomography/Computed Tomography Angiography: Initial Results at an Infective Endocarditis Referral Center.* Circulation, 2015. **132**(12): p. 1113-26.
49. Rouzet, F., et al., *Respective performance of 18F-FDG PET and radiolabeled leukocyte scintigraphy for the diagnosis of prosthetic valve endocarditis.* J Nucl Med, 2014. **55**(12): p. 1980-5.
50. Bensimhon, L., et al., *Whole body [(18) F]fluorodeoxyglucose positron emission tomography imaging for the diagnosis of pacemaker or implantable cardioverter defibrillator infection: a preliminary prospective study.* Clin Microbiol Infect, 2011. **17**(6): p. 836-44.
51. Sarrazin, J.F., et al., *Usefulness of fluorine-18 positron emission tomography/computed tomography for identification of cardiovascular implantable electronic device infections.* J Am Coll Cardiol, 2012. **59**(18): p. 1616-25.
52. Graziosi, M., et al., *Role of (1)(8)F-FDG PET/CT in the diagnosis of infective endocarditis in patients with an implanted cardiac device: a prospective study.* Eur J Nucl Med Mol Imaging, 2014. **41**(8): p. 1617-23.
53. Dell'Aquila, A.M., et al., *Contributory Role of Fluorine 18-Fluorodeoxyglucose Positron Emission Tomography/Computed Tomography in the Diagnosis and Clinical Management of Infections in Patients Supported With a Continuous-Flow Left Ventricular Assist Device.* Ann Thorac Surg, 2016. **101**(1): p. 87-94.; discussion 94.
54. Kim, J., et al., *FDG PET/CT imaging for LVAD associated infections.* JACC Cardiovasc Imaging, 2014. **7**(8): p. 839-42.
55. Keidar, Z., et al., *Prosthetic vascular graft infection: the role of 18F-FDG PET/CT.* J Nucl Med, 2007. **48**(8): p. 1230-6.
56. Sah, B.R., et al., *Diagnostic performance of 18F-FDG-PET/CT in vascular graft infections.* Eur J Vasc Endovasc Surg, 2015. **49**(4): p. 455-64.
57. Husmann, L., et al., *(1)(8)F-FDG PET/CT for Therapy Control in Vascular Graft Infections: A First Feasibility Study.* J Nucl Med, 2015. **56**(7): p. 1024-9.
58. Keidar, Z., et al., *18F-FDG uptake in noninfected prosthetic vascular grafts: incidence, patterns, and changes over time.* J Nucl Med, 2014. **55**(3): p. 392-5.
59. Saleem, B.R., et al., *18F-Fluorodeoxyglucose positron emission tomography/CT scanning in diagnosing vascular prosthetic graft infection.* Biomed Res Int, 2014. **2014**: p. 471971.
60. Hersch, E.C. and R.C. Oh, *Prolonged febrile illness and fever of unknown origin in adults.* Am Fam Physician, 2014. **90**(2): p. 91-6.
61. Sioka, C., A. Assimakopoulos, and A. Fotopoulos, *The diagnostic role of (18)F fluorodeoxyglucose positron emission tomography in patients with fever of unknown origin.* Eur J Clin Invest, 2015. **45**(6): p. 601-8.
62. Gafter-Gvili, A., et al., *[18F]FDG-PET/CT for the diagnosis of patients with fever of unknown origin.* QJM, 2015. **108**(4): p. 289-98.
63. Bleeker-Rovers, C.P., et al., *A prospective multicenter study on fever of unknown origin: the yield of a structured diagnostic protocol.* Medicine (Baltimore), 2007. **86**(1): p. 26-38.

64. Crouzet, J., et al., *Place of (18)F-FDG-PET with computed tomography in the diagnostic algorithm of patients with fever of unknown origin.* Eur J Clin Microbiol Infect Dis, 2012. **31**(8): p. 1727-33.
65. Kubota, K., et al., *FDG-PET for the diagnosis of fever of unknown origin: a Japanese multi-center study.* Ann Nucl Med, 2011. **25**(5): p. 355-64.
66. Buysschaert, I., et al., *Contribution of (18)fluoro-deoxyglucose positron emission tomography to the work-up of patients with fever of unknown origin.* Eur J Intern Med, 2004. **15**(3): p. 151-156.
67. Federici, L., et al., *Value of (18)F-FDG-PET/CT in patients with fever of unknown origin and unexplained prolonged inflammatory syndrome: a single centre analysis experience.* Int J Clin Pract, 2010. **64**(1): p. 55-60.
68. Jasper, N., et al., *Diagnostic value of [(18)F]-FDG PET/CT in children with fever of unknown origin or unexplained signs of inflammation.* Eur J Nucl Med Mol Imaging, 2010. **37**(1): p. 136-45.
69. Blokhuis, G.J., et al., *Diagnostic value of FDG-PET/(CT) in children with fever of unknown origin and unexplained fever during immune suppression.* Eur J Nucl Med Mol Imaging, 2014. **41**(10): p. 1916-23.
70. Sturm, E., et al., *Fluordeoxyglucose positron emission tomography contributes to management of pediatric liver transplantation candidates with fever of unknown origin.* Liver Transpl, 2006. **12**(11): p. 1698-704.
71. Becerra Nakayo, E.M., et al., *[Analysis of cost-effectiveness in the diagnosis of fever of unknown origin and the role of (18)F-FDG PET-CT: a proposal of diagnostic algorithm].* Rev Esp Med Nucl Imagen Mol, 2012. **31**(4): p. 178-86.
72. Pereira, A.M., et al., *Determinants of diagnostic performance of 18F-FDG PET/CT in patients with fever of unknown origin.* Nucl Med Commun, 2016. **37**(1): p. 57-65.
73. Vos, F.J., et al., *Cost-effectiveness of routine (18)F-FDG PET/CT in high-risk patients with gram-positive bacteremia.* J Nucl Med, 2011. **52**(11): p. 1673-8.
74. Vos, F.J., et al., *Metastatic infectious disease and clinical outcome in Staphylococcus aureus and Streptococcus species bacteremia.* Medicine (Baltimore), 2012. **91**(2): p. 86-94.
75. Dumarey, N., et al., *Imaging infection with 18F-FDG-labeled leukocyte PET/CT: initial experience in 21 patients.* J Nucl Med, 2006. **47**(4): p. 625-32.
76. Rini, J.N., et al., *PET with FDG-labeled leukocytes versus scintigraphy with 111In-oxine-labeled leukocytes for detection of infection.* Radiology, 2006. **238**(3): p. 978-87.
77. Bhargava, K.K., et al., *In vitro human leukocyte labeling with (64)Cu: an intraindividual comparison with (111)In-oxine and (18)F-FDG.* Nucl Med Biol, 2009. **36**(5): p. 545-9.
78. Locke, L.W., et al., *A novel neutrophil-specific PET imaging agent: cFLFLFK-PEG-64Cu.* J Nucl Med, 2009. **50**(5): p. 790-7.
79. Kumar, V., et al., *(68)Ga-Citrate-PET for diagnostic imaging of infection in rats and for intra-abdominal infection in a patient.* Curr Radiopharm, 2012. **5**(1): p. 71-5.
80. Vorster, M., et al., *68Ga-citrate PET/CT in Tuberculosis: A pilot study.*. Q J Nucl Med Mol Imaging, 2014.
81. Nanni, C., et al., *68Ga-citrate PET/CT for evaluating patients with infections of the bone: preliminary results.* J Nucl Med, 2010. **51**(12): p. 1932-6.
82. Britton, K.E., et al., *Imaging bacterial infection with (99m)Tc-ciprofloxacin (Infecton).* J Clin Pathol, 2002. **55**(11): p. 817-23.
83. De Winter, F., et al., *Biodistribution and dosimetry of 99mTc-ciprofloxacin, a promising agent for the diagnosis of bacterial infection.* Eur J Nucl Med, 2001. **28**(5): p. 570-4.
84. Sarda, L., et al., *Inability of 99mTc-ciprofloxacin scintigraphy to discriminate between septic and sterile osteoarticular diseases.* J Nucl Med, 2003. **44**(6): p. 920-6.
85. Kennedy, D.O., *B Vitamins and the Brain: Mechanisms, Dose and Efficacy--A Review.* Nutrients, 2016. **8**(2): p. 68.
86. Lazzeri, E., et al., *Clinical feasibility of two-step streptavidin/111In-biotin scintigraphy in patients with suspected vertebral osteomyelitis.* Eur J Nucl Med Mol Imaging, 2004. **31**(11): p. 1505-11.

87. Lazzeri, E., et al., *Clinical impact of SPECT/CT with In-111 biotin on the management of patients with suspected spine infection.* Clin Nucl Med, 2010. **35**(1): p. 12-7.
88. Wang, G., *Human antimicrobial peptides and proteins.* Pharmaceuticals (Basel), 2014. **7**(5): p. 545-94.
89. Hiemstra, P.S., et al., *Ubiquicidin, a novel murine microbicidal protein present in the cytosolic fraction of macrophages.* J Leukoc Biol, 1999. **66**(3): p. 423-8.
90. Lupetti, A., et al., *99mTc-antimicrobial peptides: promising candidates for infection imaging.* Q J Nucl Med, 2003. **47**(4): p. 238-45.
91. Ostovar, A., et al., *A pooled analysis of diagnostic value of (99m)Tc-ubiquicidin (UBI) scintigraphy in detection of an infectious process.* Clin Nucl Med, 2013. **38**(6): p. 413-6.
92. Liberatore, M., et al., *Microbial targeting of 99mTc-labeled recombinant human beta-defensin-3 in an animal model of infection: a feasibility pilot study.* J Nucl Med, 2009. **50**(5): p. 823-6.
93. Ebenhan, T., et al., *Peptide synthesis, characterization and (6)(8)Ga-radiolabeling of NOTA-conjugated ubiquicidin fragments for prospective infection imaging with PET/CT.* Nucl Med Biol, 2014. **41**(5): p. 390-400.
94. Ebenhan, T., et al., *Preclinical evaluation of 68Ga-labeled 1,4,7-triazacyclononane-1,4,7-triacetic acid-ubiquicidin as a radioligand for PET infection imaging.* J Nucl Med, 2014. **55**(2): p. 308-14.
95. Lankinen, P., et al., *(68)Ga-DOTAVAP-P1 PET imaging capable of demonstrating the phase of inflammation in healing bones and the progress of infection in osteomyelitic bones.* Eur J Nucl Med Mol Imaging, 2008. **35**(2): p. 352-64.
96. Vilche, M., et al., *68Ga-NOTA-UBI-29-41 as a PET Tracer for Detection of Bacterial Infection.* J Nucl Med, 2016. **57**(4): p. 622-7.
97. Boerman, O.C., P. Laverman, and W.J. Oyen, *FIAU: From reporter gene imaging to imaging of bacterial proliferation.* Am J Nucl Med Mol Imaging, 2012. **2**(3): p. 271-2.
98. Bettegowda, C., et al., *Imaging bacterial infections with radiolabeled 1-(2'-deoxy-2'-fluoro-beta-D-arabinofuranosyl)-5-iodouracil.* Proc Natl Acad Sci U S A, 2005. **102**(4): p. 1145-50.
99. Pullambhatla, M., et al., *[(125)I]FIAU imaging in a preclinical model of lung infection: quantification of bacterial load.* Am J Nucl Med Mol Imaging, 2012. **2**(3): p. 260-70.
100. Diaz, L.A., Jr., et al., *Imaging of musculoskeletal bacterial infections by [124I]FIAU-PET/CT.* PLoS One, 2007. **2**(10): p. e1007.
101. Zhang, X.M., et al., *[(124)I]FIAU: Human dosimetry and infection imaging in patients with suspected prosthetic joint infection.* Nucl Med Biol, 2016. **43**(5): p. 273-9.
102. Gowrishankar, G., et al., *Investigation of 6-[(1)(8)F]-fluoromaltose as a novel PET tracer for imaging bacterial infection.* PLoS One, 2014. **9**(9): p. e107951.
103. Ning, X., et al., *PET imaging of bacterial infections with fluorine-18-labeled maltohexaose.* Angew Chem Int Ed Engl, 2014. **53**(51): p. 14096-101.
104. Weinstein, E.A., et al., *Imaging Enterobacteriaceae infection in vivo with 18F-fluorodeoxysorbitol positron emission tomography.* Sci Transl Med, 2014. **6**(259): p. 259ra146.
105. Zhu, W., et al., *Biodistribution and Radiation Dosimetry of the Enterobacteriaceae-Specific Imaging Probe [F]Fluorodeoxysorbitol Determined by PET/CT in Healthy Human Volunteers.*. Mol Imaging Biol, 2016.
106. Wiehr, S., et al., *New pathogen-specific immunoPET/MR tracer for molecular imaging of a systemic bacterial infection.* Oncotarget, 2016. **7**(10): p. 10990-1001.

Chapter 3
Optical Imaging

Nathan K. Archer, Kevin P. Francis, and Lloyd S. Miller

3.1 Introduction

In vivo whole-animal optical imaging is a noninvasive and nontoxic approach that employs the detection and visualization of photons of light arising from an enzymatic or chemical reaction resulting in bioluminescent or chemiluminescent light or from the emission of photons following the excitation of a fluorescent molecule resulting in fluorescence [1, 2]. To facilitate the detection of light, in vivo whole-animal optical imaging typically involves the use of dark chambers in which anesthetized animals can be placed and the photons generated from either luminescence or fluorescence can be detected using highly sensitive photon detectors, such as cooled (and intensified) charge-coupled device (CCD) cameras (Figure 3.1a) [1, 2]. Using these techniques, it is possible to visualize and quantify the intensity and spatial and anatomical localization of the light passing through different tissue types in live animals, including the skin, subcutaneous tissues, muscles, bone, and internal organs. In addition, the same animals can be visualized at different time points,

N.K. Archer
Department of Dermatology, Johns Hopkins University School of Medicine,
Baltimore, MD, USA

K.P. Francis
Preclinical Imaging, Life Sciences, PerkinElmer, Inc., Hopkinton, MA, USA

Department of Orthopedic Surgery, David Geffen School of Medicine at UCLA,
Los Angeles, CA, USA

L.S. Miller (✉)
Department of Dermatology, Department of Medicine, Division of Infectious Diseases and Department of Orthopedic Surgery, Johns Hopkins University School of Medicine, Baltimore, MD, USA
e-mail: lloydmiller@jhmi.edu

S.K. Jain (ed.), *Imaging Infections*, DOI 10.1007/978-3-319-54592-9_3

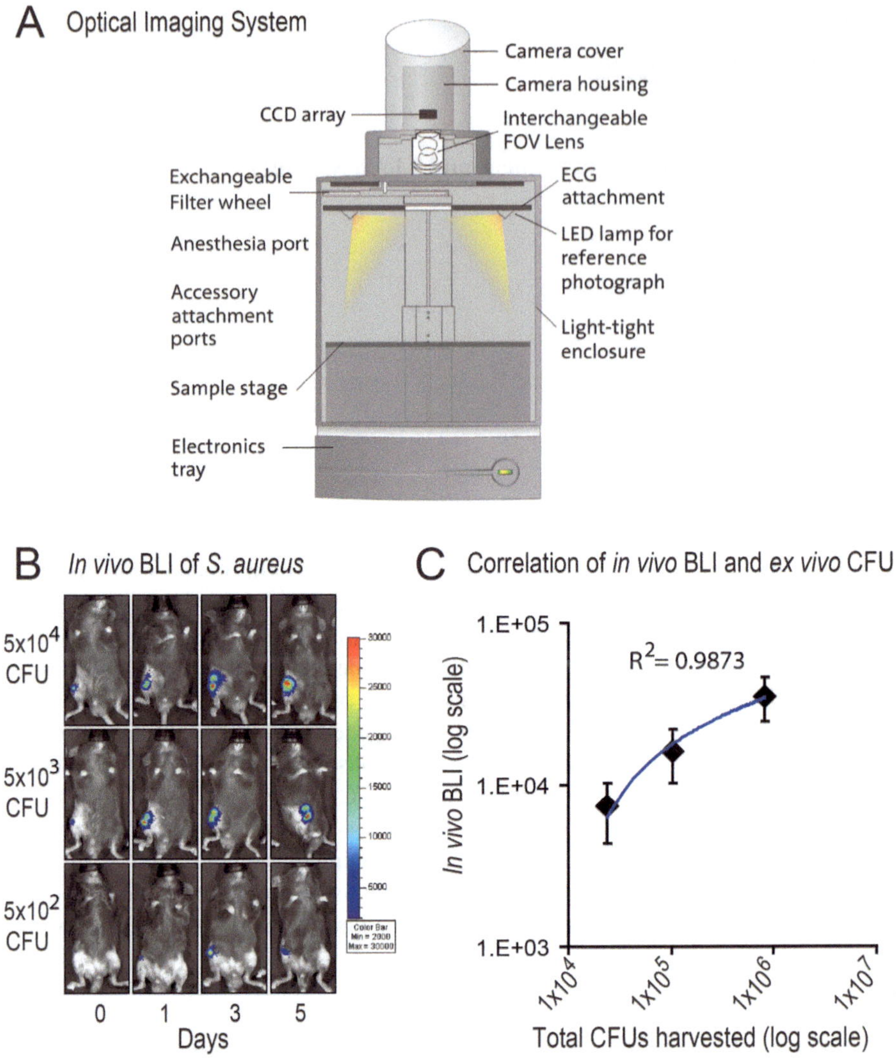

Figure 3.1 In vivo optical imaging system for infectious disease research. (**a**) Representative schematic of a typical in vivo optical imaging system, consisting of a light–tight (*dark*) chamber with an adjustable sample stage (e.g., for placement of anesthetized animals) and a cooled integrating CCD camera to facilitate acquiring the inherent low optical signal generated from the subject (e.g., in vivo bioluminescence/fluorescence) as well as the reference grayscale photograph (during LED illumination). (**b**) Representative image of a bioluminescent strain of *S. aureus* (detected from different infecting inocula) in the right knee joints of mice possessing a titanium Kirschner-wire implant extending from the femoral intramedullary canal as a mouse model of an orthopedic implant infection [3]. (**c**) High correlation observed of in vivo BLI signals and ex vivo CFU from the homogenized bone/joint tissue obtained from euthanized mice on day 5 after infection (R^2 = 0.9873) [3]

allowing dynamics of the light signals to be temporally visualized, providing longitudinal information about the light signals over time. An example of the longitudinal 5-day course of in vivo bioluminescence imaging (BLI) signals from an orthopedic implant infection in the right knee joints of mice is shown for different inocula of *Staphylococcus aureus* (Figure 3.1b) [3]. Of note, the in vivo BLI signals correlated well with ex vivo colony-forming units (CFU) of bacteria in this model (Figure 3.1c) [3].

With relevance to infectious disease studies, pathogenic microorganisms have different routes of infection and disease mechanisms and trigger a multitude of host–pathogen interactions and immune responses, all of which are important and active areas of research [1, 2]. In vivo optical imaging provides an approach to monitor these processes both noninvasively and longitudinally. For example, bioluminescently engineered microorganisms can be imaged in mice possessing fluorescent reporters for specific mammalian cell types or protein expression, providing the ability to visualize both the infectious agent and host immune responses simultaneously in vivo. We have recently used such an approach to noninvasively and longitudinally quantify the bacterial burden of a *S. aureus* skin infection while simultaneously monitoring the expression of IL-1β and neutrophil recruitment (Figure 3.2a) [4]. This was accomplished by combining in vivo optical imaging with bioluminescent bacteria (Figure 3.2b) [5], a transgenic mouse that expresses dsRed fluorescence based on IL-1β-promoter activity (pIL1-DsRed mice) (Figure 3.2c) [6] as well as a knockin mouse strain that possesses green fluorescent neutrophils (LysEGFP mice) (Figure 3.2d) [7]. It should be mentioned that in vivo optical imaging techniques help promote the ethical use of animals in which practices facilitate the three R's: replacement, reduction, and refinement [1]. Although animals are not replaced with in vivo optical imaging, the numbers of animals can be substantially reduced since euthanasia is not required to obtain information about the infectious burden or host immune responses. In addition, in vivo optical imaging promotes the refinement of methods to minimize animal pain or distress as it can provide noninvasive data of various different endpoints such as infectious burden, localization of the infection, and host immune responses that would otherwise need to be obtained by invasive sampling techniques to obtain specimens of blood, tissues, organs, or bodily fluids. Furthermore, the information gained from in vivo optical imaging can be used to determine the most relevant time points to perform any additional sampling or experiments on the animals, thereby minimizing any stress or discomfort by performing repeated procedures.

More recently, advances in this technology have demonstrated the potential for optical imaging to be translated into clinical practice [8]. This has been made possible in part by advances in fluorescent probe chemistries and photoacoustic imaging techniques that can detect signals several centimeters into tissue, permitting detection of optical signals at some depth within animal and human subjects [9–12]. This technology could be used in combination with optical pathogen-specific probes to diagnose an infection or monitor the response to treatment. Furthermore, photodynamic therapy combines the use of pathogen-specific photosensitizers that generate cytotoxic reactive oxygen species when activated, which could be used as a non-antibiotic-based approach to induce killing of pathogens in infected tissues [13, 14].

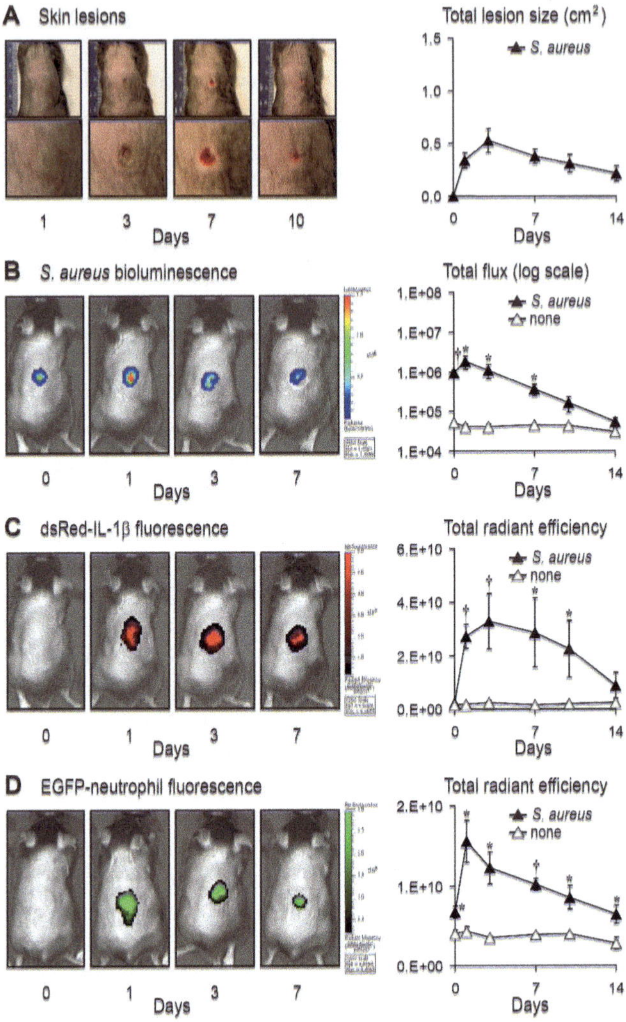

Figure 3.2 Combining in vivo BLI and in vivo FLI to monitor bacterial burden, IL-1β expression, and neutrophil recruitment during a *S. aureus* skin infection. A bioluminescent *S. aureus* strain was inoculated intradermally into pIL-1-DsRed reporter mice (a transgenic mouse strain that produces DsRed driven by the IL-1β promoter) or LysEGFP mice (a mouse knockin strain of EGFP in the lysozyme promoter) [4]. (**a**) Representative skin lesions of the *S. aureus*-infected mice (*left*) and mean lesion size (cm^2) ± s.e.m. (*right*). (**b**) Representative in vivo BLI of *S. aureus* (*left*) and mean total flux (photons/s) ± s.e.m. (*right*). (**c**) Representative in vivo FLI of IL-1β-DsRed fluorescence (*left*) and mean total radiant efficiency (photons/s)/(μW/cm^2) ± s.e.m. (*right*). (**d**) Representative in vivo FLI of EGFP-neutrophil fluorescence (*left*) and mean total radiant efficiency (photons/s)/(μW/cm^2) ± s.e.m. (*right*). $*p < 0.05$, $^{\dagger}p < 0.01$, *S. aureus*-infected mice versus none (sham injection alone) (Student's *t*-test)

3.2 Bioluminescent Imaging

Bioluminescence is naturally found in many different types of organisms and involves the production of light from luciferase enzymes and a specific luciferin substrate in the presence of energy (e.g., $FMNH_2$ and ATP) and oxygen [1, 2, 15, 16]. To date, the most applicable bioluminescent system for infectious disease research has been the *lux* operon from the bacterial insect pathogen, *Photorhabdus luminescens*. This *lux CDABE* operon is comprised of a heterodimeric α and β subunit bacterial luciferase enzyme, encoded by the *luxA* and *luxB* genes, respectively, and does not require an exogenous substrate as the *luxC*, *luxD*, and *luxE* genes encode the aldehyde substrate required for light production [1, 2, 15, 16]. The luciferase catalyzes the oxidation of long-chain aldehydes and flavin mononucleotide ($FMNH_2$), resulting in production of light at a peak wavelength of 490 nm [1, 2, 15, 16]. Modified versions of this *lux* operon have been stably integrated into many different bacterial species to be used for in vivo bioluminescence imaging (BLI) (Table 3.1).

Table 3.1 Bioluminescent bacteria

Groups	Microorganism	Reporter	References
Gram positive	*Bacillus anthracis*	*lux*	[48–50, 103, 104]
	Bifidobacterium breve	*lux*	[105, 106]
	Listeria monocytogenes	*lux*	[33, 43, 107, 108]
	Staphylococcus aureus	*lux*	[4, 5, 29, 34, 36, 37, 40, 41, 109, 110]
	Staphylococcus epidermidis	*lux*	[32, 111]
	Streptococcus pneumoniae	*lux*	[19, 27, 112]
	Streptococcus pyogenes	*lux*	[30, 113]
Gram negative	*Acinetobacter baumannii*	*lux*	[114, 115]
	Brucella melitensis	*lux*	[44, 45, 116]
	Burkholderia pseudomallei	*lux*	[117, 118]
	Citrobacter rodentium	*lux*	[46, 47, 119–121]
	Edwardsiella ictaluri	*lux*	[122, 123]
	Escherichia coli	*lux, fluc*	[124–126]
	Chlamydia muridarum	*fluc*	[127]
	Haemophilus influenzae	*lux*	[128, 129]
	Leptospira interrogans	*fluc*	[130]
	Neisseria meningitidis	*lux*	[131]
	Proteus mirabilis	*lux*	[132–134]
	Pseudomonas aeruginosa	*lux*	[135–137]
	Pseudomonas fluorescens	*lux*	[138, 139]
	Salmonella enterica typhimurium	*lux*	[26, 106, 107]
	Salmonella enteritidis	*lux*	[140]
Mycobacteria	*Mycobacterium bovis* BCG	*lux*	[18, 141]
	Mycobacterium smegmatis	*lux, fluc*	[142]
	Mycobacterium tuberculosis	*lux, fluc*	[142, 143]
Other	*Borrelia burgdorferi*	*fluc*	[144]

As an alternative approach, luciferase enzymes from other organisms have been utilized, including those from firefly (e.g., *Photinus pyralis*), click beetle (*Pyrophorus plagiophtalamus*), the sea pansy (*Renilla reniformis*), and the marine copepod (*Gaussia princeps*) [1, 2, 15, 16]. Microorganisms and eukaryotic cells can be engineered to express these luciferases for BLI. However, the substrates for these enzymes need to be exogenously administered for the luciferase enzymes to act as reporters for BLI. The luminescence reactions for the firefly and click beetle involve a monomeric luciferase enzyme, *luc*, which requires the oxidation of an exogenous luciferin substrate, benzothiazoyl-thiazole luciferin [1, 2, 15, 16]. The emission peak of firefly luciferase (encoded by *fluc*) is approximately 560 nm at 20 °C but shifts to around 610 nm at 37 °C, whereas the peak emission for click beetle luciferase is either 540 (click beetle green luciferase, encoded by *CBGluc*) or 615 (click beetle red luciferase, encoded by *CBRluc*), with neither wavelength varying significantly with temperature [1, 2, 15–17]. For the most part, exogenously administered luciferin (most commonly via subcutaneous, intraperitoneal, or intravenous routes) is well distributed throughout the animal, and substrate availability is typically not a limiting factor for small animal in vivo BLI. The sea pansy and copepod luciferases, encoded by *rluc* and *gluc*, respectively, emit blue light (~480 nm) upon exposure of exogenous coelenterazine. One important factor that has limited the widespread use of *rluc* and *gluc* for in vivo BLI is that coelenterazine has an inherent background luminescence and is actively transported out of mammalian cells by the action of a multidrug residence *P*-glycoprotein (MDR1) [1, 2]. Thus, unlike luciferin, bioavailability of coelenterazine can be a concern that is particularly relevant for detecting luciferase-produced bioluminescent signals from microorganisms inside of cells [1, 2].

Bioluminescent signals from different luciferases can be separated in vivo by a number of different methodologies, allowing two or more reporters to be monitored sequentially in the same animal. For signals located at shallow depths, specific wavelength filters can be used to spectrally unmix the peak emissions and profiles of two or more different bioluminescent readouts [2, 18]. For example, the signals generated by *lux* (490 nm) could be distinguished from signals generated by *fluc* (610 nm), as demonstrated by Kadurugamuwa et al. using a streptococcal meningitis model that simultaneously allows both bacterial burden (*lux*) and astrocyte damage (*fluc*) to be visualized [19]. Alternatively, sequential substrate delivery could be used to gain defined peak signals from each luciferase in vivo, even at depth (e.g., imaging *fluc* and *rluc*/*gluc* using sequential injection of luciferin and coelenterazine, respectively) [2]. However, differences in the delivery and pharmacokinetics of each substrate and the subsequent duration of each bioluminescent signal need to be taken into account. For example, after intraperitoneal or subcutaneous administration of luciferin, bioluminescence produced by *fluc* peaks at around 10 min and can remain constant for 20 plus min, whereas intravenous administration of coelenterazine peaks at 1 min, and the bioluminescent signal rapidly diminishes in 10 min [2]. Finally, although lower wavelength signals in the blue–green spectrum are brighter, their ability to penetrate through tissue is decreased due to attenuation of the shorter wavelengths of light, predominantly through absorption by hemoglobin [2]. Thus, the longer-wavelength bioluminescence generated by firefly and click beetle luciferase has greater tissue penetration than *lux*, *rluc*, and *gluc*, and these differences in sensitively also need to be taken into account when performing dual or multi-reporter BLI.

In conjunction with the use of bioluminescent reporters in vivo (typically in mice), instrumentation to detect bioluminescence involves the use of CCD cameras and dark chambers [1, 2, 15, 16] (Figure 3.1a). Detection of BLI is generally rapid and straightforward with low background signals, which might only include signals from the mouse intestines that have chow containing chlorophyll and other pigments that produce low amounts of light or reactive oxygen species from macrophage and neutrophils (through inflammation) that can also add to this background through chemiluminescent emission. The spatial resolution of BLI depends very much on the depth of tissue that the signal is emanating from, but is usually within the range of 1–3 mm from the foci (point source) and can be acquired both two and three dimensionally (2D and 3D) [1, 2, 15, 16]. There are also software reconstruction techniques that are able to convert 2D into 3D images of BLI data. BLI is mostly used in preclinical small animal imaging as it cannot be used to detect light beyond a few centimeters of tissue (depending on the intensity and wavelength of the light). Thus, BLI in humans is not currently possible, except for surface and perhaps subcutaneous infections.

3.3 Fluorescence Imaging

Fluorescent compounds have an inherent property in which irradiation at a specific "excitation" wavelength of light results in excitation of an electron in the molecule to a higher energy state, followed by the return of the electron to a lower energy states that results in the "emission" of red-shifted fluorescent light [1]. There are numerous fluorescent compounds available for in vivo fluorescence imaging (FLI) [1]. Some of the notable discoveries of fluorescent proteins include the discovery of green fluorescent protein (GFP) from the *Aequorea victoria* jellyfish [20], DsRed protein from the coral *Discosoma* species [21], and TurboRFP modified from a protein from the sea anemone *Entacmaea quadricolor* [22] of which many other fluorescent proteins were generated with different excitation and emission wavelengths. Other nonprotein fluorescent molecules have also been used. Notably, a prior study linked the near-infrared (NIR) carbocyanine fluorophore to zinc(II)dipicolylamine (Zn-DPA), which binds to the negatively charged anionic surfaces of bacteria as an NIR imaging probe to detect *S. aureus* bacteria in an in vivo mouse thigh infection model [23, 24]. Moreover, it is now becoming a commonplace to conjugate chemical fluorochromes (e.g., cyanine dyes, especially those in the NIR range) to antibodies and peptides to target infective processes, both directly (microbe) or indirectly (upregulation of a host marker in response to infection). Finally, quantum dots, which are small fluorescent nanocrystals, have high brightness and photostability and narrow emission spectra [1, 25]. The fluorescent excitation and emission wavelengths can be modified by changing the size the particles, making quantum dots extremely versatile. Quantum dots can be linked to probes to target bacteria or by linking the quantum dots to luciferases or other fluorescent compounds to amplify the light signals [1, 25]. For any of these fluorescent compounds to perform successfully as an in vivo FLI agent, longer wavelengths are generally more efficient due to their enhanced tissue penetration with red-shifted and NIR fluorescent compounds (>650 nm) often having bright signals and excellent tissue penetration [1]. It should be noted that FLI often has inherent problems with sensitivity due to background autofluorescence and light has to penetrate into tissue for both excitation and emission, and this creates problems due to tissue absorption and scattering of the light [1].

3.4 Development of Bioluminescent and Fluorescent Microorganisms

The development of bioluminescent or fluorescent genetic constructs that can be integrated into microorganisms provides an approach to monitor the infectious burden and pathogenesis [1, 2, 15, 16]. Constructs that do not have toxic effects that might impact fitness or affect virulence are ideal. In general, it is better to stably integrate a reporter gene(s) into the chromosome of the microorganism, since plasmid-based constructs are often lost, especially for plasmids that require selection to be maintained [1, 2, 15, 16]. There have been several successful strategies that continue to pave the way for the generation of more and more bioluminescent and fluorescent reporter microorganisms.

One of the initial studies demonstrating the feasibility of using the *lux* operon from *P. luminescens* to monitor infection was conducted by Contag et al. in which a plasmid-based construct was used to create a bioluminescent strain of *Salmonella typhimurium* [26]. This group used this strain along with in vivo BLI to study the infectious course, to compare virulence among different bacterial strains, and to monitor the response to antibiotic therapy. Although these initial studies provided the proof of concept for generating and employing bioluminescent bacteria, the plasmid constructs proved unstable, and as a result, progeny lost this plasmid during replication of the bacteria in vivo [26]. One of the first techniques used to integrate the *lux* operon into the bacterial chromosome to generate a stable bioluminescent bacterial strain in which the bioluminescent signal is not lost is the use of transposons such as the Tn*4001* transposon that we used [27] and the mini-Tn*5* transposon used by Winson et al. [28]. However, these methods result in random insertion of the *lux* operon into the chromosome, so careful analysis for any impact on bacterial fitness and virulence needs to be determined.

Unlike Gram-negative bacteria, the *lux* operon from *P. luminescens* is not efficiently translated in Gram-positive bacteria. Francis et al. sought to overcome this technical difficulty by generating a modified *luxABCDE* operon in which stronger

Gram-positive ribosome binding sites were introduced upstream of each of the *lux* genes so that each Lux polypeptide was efficiently synthesized by Gram-positive bacteria [29]. This construct was successfully integrated into the chromosome of a wide range of Gram-positive bacteria, including *S. aureus* (e.g., Xen29) [29], *S. pneumoniae* (e.g., Xen10) [27], group A *Streptococcus* (Xen20) [30], *S. epidermidis* (Xen43) [31, 32], and *L. monocytogenes* (Xen19) [33] and into a stable bacterial plasmid of *S. aureus* (Xen36) as well as into numerous other Gram-positive bacteria (Table 3.1).

Another strategy used to create stable bioluminescent bacterial strains is to perform targeted integration into sites on the chromosome that are known to not impact virulence. Although these targeted strategies in theory might be better, the results are often unpredictable as the expression of the *lux* genes might not be optimal and/or the integration of the gene at the sites might also have unanticipated consequences on fitness and virulence. Nonetheless, there are several successful examples of such strategies. For example, Plaut et al. inserted a similarly modified *lux* operon at a targeted pseudogene site of a community-acquired methicillin-resistant *S. aureus* (MRSA) strain, which resulted in a 10- to 50-fold brighter strain compared to prior Tn*4001 luxABCDE* transposon insertion strains. Moreover, this *lux* operon insertion did not negatively impact the virulence of the bacteria [34].

The choice of using bioluminescent- versus fluorescent-labeled microorganisms is an important decision that is dependent upon a number of factors. If bioluminescence is preferred, in general, *lux* is typically used because an exogenous substrate is not required. However, the bioluminescence signals from the *lux* luciferase are dependent on products of bacterial metabolism (i.e., $FMNH_2$ and ATP) [1, 2, 15, 16]. Thus, under certain circumstances when the bacterial metabolism is decreased, such as in the case of bacteria in stationary phase in in vitro cultures or in in vivo biofilms, the bioluminescent signals might be substantially diminished even though CFU of bacteria might be present in large numbers [15]. As an example of this, the *S. epidermidis* strain Xen43 had bioluminescent signals that decreased to background levels when the bacteria formed in vivo biofilms in two different infection models [31, 32].

To report signals from certain eukaryotic microorganisms, including fungi and parasites, or to report signals from viral infections in eukaryotic cells, the *luc* reporter constructs with exogenous substrate administration are used, as *lux* constructs have not been optimized sufficiently to allow significant bioluminescence in eukaryotic cells, especially at depth [1, 2]. However, Close et al. recently was able to codon optimize *lux* for expression into a human embryonic kidney cell line (HEK293), which resulted in autonomous and persistent in vitro and in vivo light production, providing a potential alternative for using *luc* reporter constructs in eukaryotic cells [35]. It should be noted that the dependence of bioluminescent signals on metabolites for *lux* and coleopteran luciferases (*fluc*, *CBGluc*, *CBRluc*) is not as apparent for the *gluc* and *rluc* in those cases in which bacterial metabolism might be an issue. In these cases, an approach using *gluc* or *rluc* expression could provide a viable alternative [1, 2].

If a fluorescent reporter is desired, there are several important factors that need to be taken into account, including the appropriate excitation/emission wavelengths, maturation speed, duration of fluorescence, and photostability, which all contribute to brightness [1]. These are critical as in general the fluorescent signals are dimmer compared to bioluminescent signals from microorganisms in vivo. Fluorescent signals will also likely be less dependent upon metabolic activity and products of metabolism than bioluminescent constructs and could offer an advantage in certain circumstances, although in most cases oxygen is still vital to allow the correct folding and function of fluorescent proteins. One potential concern with fluorescence reporter microorganisms is that it might be difficult to distinguish fluorescence signals from live versus dead microorganisms and this needs to be accounted for in the interpretation of data obtained using in vivo FLI of fluorescent microorganisms.

Ultimately, if successful, bioluminescent and fluorescent microorganisms provide the opportunity of using BLI and FLI to noninvasively and longitudinally monitor the infectious burden, the anatomic localization of the infection, tracking dissemination of the infection, and microorganism gene expression during an in vivo infection [1, 2, 15, 16]. In addition, the combination of bioluminescent and fluorescent reporter microorganisms with genetically engineered reporter mouse lines possessing fluorescent or bioluminescent reporter host cells or reporters for host protein expression can provide extremely valuable information regarding the pathogen and host responses that occur during the course of an infection in vivo. A description of some of the key information obtained from using BLI and FLI is described below.

3.5 Bacterial Imaging

Since the initial report by Contag et al. in 1995 demonstrated that a bioluminescent *S. typhimurium* possessing the *lux* operon could be used for in vivo BLI and provide information about the infection and disease pathogenesis [26], there are many examples of how BLI and FLI have been used to study bacterial infections (Table 3.1). Below are a few specific examples.

Our group has been studying the pathogenesis of *S. aureus* infections using in vivo BLI in various models of infection. For example, using a *S. aureus* skin infection model, we discovered a key role for IL-1β, which was a more important determinant for MyD88-dependent neutrophil recruitment and host defense than TLR2 [5]. We further discovered that IL-1β-mediated neutrophil recruitment was mediated by induction of IL-17 and that the predominant source of IL-1β was from the recruited neutrophils [4, 36, 37]. In addition, we have used in vivo BLI to compare the efficacy of various different systemic and topical antibiotics against an MRSA skin infection [38]. Our studies have also used an orthopedic implant *S. aureus* infection model, and in vivo BLI was used to study the pathogenesis of these biofilm-associated infections, the response to antibiotic therapy, and the efficacy of an antibiotic-releasing implant coating [3, 39–42]. In these models, the in vivo BLI signals closely approximated the actual numbers of CFU at the different sites of *S. aureus* infection (Figure 3.1c) [5, 36, 38, 40–42]. In addition, we were able to monitor both the bacteria burden and the degree of neutrophil infiltration by performing experiments using LysEGFP mice and sequential in vivo BLI and FLI (Figure 3.3a, b). We could also follow individual responses among different mice, and three mice are shown as examples (Figure 3.3c). Mouse #1 and Mouse #2 had high bacterial in vivo BLI signals that peaked on ~21 days after infection with concomitant decreased EGFP-neutrophil fluorescent signals at about the same time. In contrast, Mouse #3 had increasing bacterial in vivo BLI signals for the 48-day duration of the experiment and had EGFP-neutrophil fluorescent signals that diminished rapidly to baseline by 14 days after infection.

Hardy et al. using a bioluminescent *Listeria monocytogenes* strain in mice found that after the oral or intravenous inoculation of mice with *L. monocytogenes* possessing the *lux* construct in the bacterial chromosome, the bacteria localized to a signal near the thoracic region [33, 43]. After dissection, they found that the source of the bioluminescent signal was in the gallbladder and they further showed that the bacteria replicated in the lumen of the gallbladder [33, 43]. This finding was unexpected because the environment in the gallbladder is inhospitable to many different bacteria and provided a potentially new anatomical location of where *L. monocytogenes* might cause infections and disease in humans.

Another example of information about the anatomical localization of infection was obtained using a bioluminescent *Brucella melitensis* strain, which causes a disease called brucellosis that can affect different tissues and organs. Rajashekara et al. found that during an acute infection via an intraperitoneal inoculation, the bacteria localized to expected areas, including the draining inguinal lymph nodes, spleen, and liver, as well as previously unrecognized areas, including the submandibular region and the testes [44, 45].

Wiles et al. used a bioluminescent strain of *Citrobacter rodentium*, a mouse intestinal pathogen, to study the pathogenesis of this infection after oral inoculation [46]. They found that *C. rodentium* first colonized the cecum for several days before colonizing and causing disease in the rest of the colon [46]. In addition, the cecum was the first anatomic location of bacteria clearance before the bacteria were cleared from the remainder of the colon. In subsequent work, they also showed that *C. rodentium* shed in infected stool of mice was hypervirulent and had a 1000-fold lower infectious dose when inoculated into naïve mice [47]. In addition, the hypervirulent *C. rodentium* was also able to directly infect the entire colon and did not require an initial incubation period in the cecum [47]. These findings might relate to the pathogenesis of gastrointestinal pathogenic bacteria in humans.

One final example of how in vivo BLI provided new insights into the pathogenesis involved the study of a bioluminescent strain of *Bacillus anthracis*, a Gram-positive sporulating bacterium that causes anthrax. Glomski et al. investigated the three major routes of infection, cutaneous, inhalational, and gastrointestinal [48–50]. As the spores of *B. anthracis* are metabolically inactive, the bacteria will only emit bioluminescent signals after germination. After cutaneous and inhalational inoculation, they found that germination occurred at the site of inoculation, whereas after

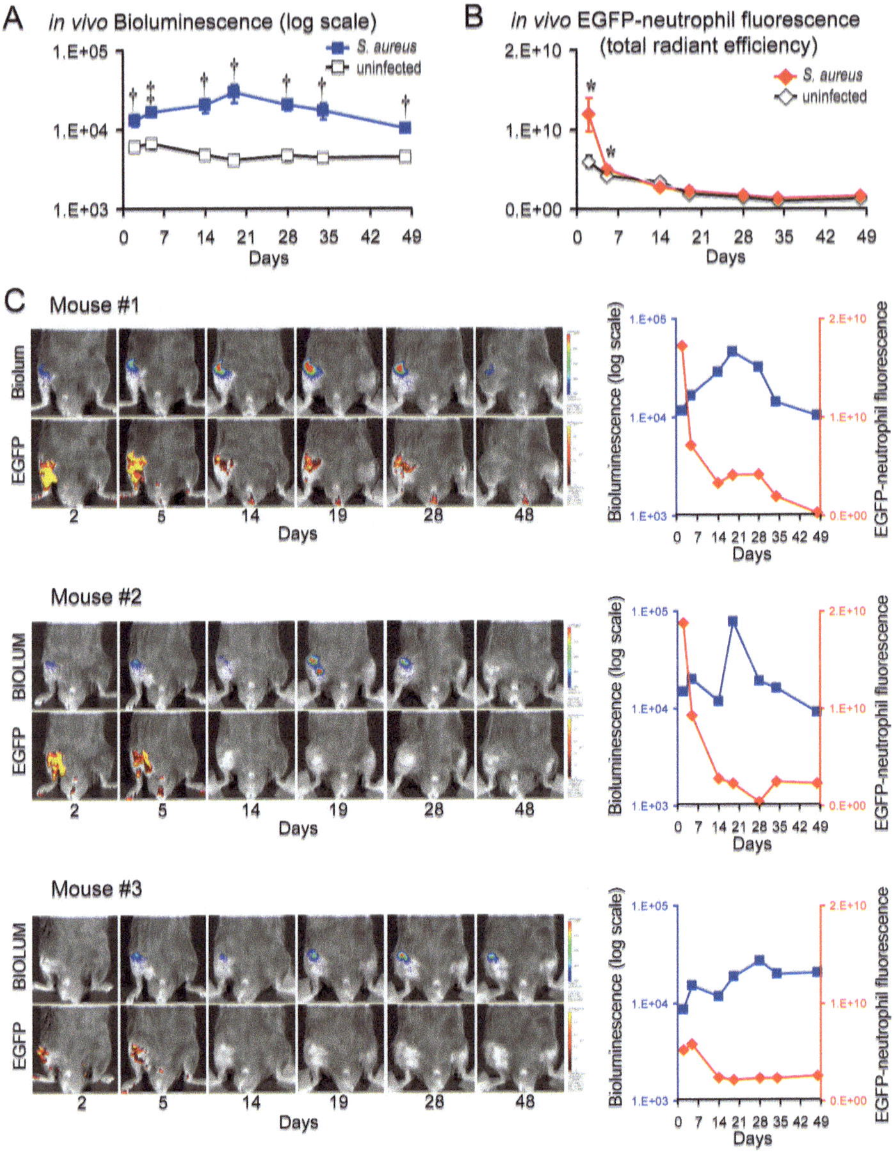

Figure 3.3 In vivo BLI and FLI to monitor the bacterial burden and neutrophil recruitment during an orthopedic implant infection. An orthopedic infection model was used in which a bioluminescent strain of *S. aureus* or no bacteria (uninfected) was inoculated in the right knee joints of mice in the presence of a titanium K-wire implant extending from the femoral intramedullary canal [40, 41]. (**a**) In vivo BLI of *S. aureus* (mean total flux [photons/s] ± s.e.m.). (**b**) In vivo FLI of EGFP-neutrophil fluorescence (mean total radiant efficiency [photons/s]/[μW/cm^2] ± s.e.m.). $*p < 0.05$, $\dagger p < 0.01$, $\ddagger p < 0.001$ *S. aureus*-infected mice versus uninfected mice (Student's *t*-test [two tailed]). (**c**) (*Left*) Representative images of in vivo BLI (*upper panels*) and in vivo FLI (*lower panels*) from the three individual *S. aureus*-infected mice. (*Right*) In vivo BLI of *S. aureus* (photons/s) (*blue*) and in vivo FLI ([photons/s]/[μW/cm^2]) (*red*)

gastrointestinal inoculation, germination occurred in the Peyer's patches in the walls of the intestines [48–50]. All three infectious routes resulted in systemic disease with bacterial dissemination to the draining lymph nodes, spleen, lungs, and blood [48–50]. Of note, there were different levels of bioluminescent signals detected depending on the depth of penetration of the light and tissue attenuation. They found that the limit of detection of the in vivo BLI signals in the superficial skin of the ear was in the 10^3 CFU range, whereas in the spleen, the limit of detection of in vivo BLI signals was in the 10^5 CFU range, and there was a lot of quenching of the signals from the lungs and heart [48–50]. Therefore, the studies using in vivo BLI of *B. anthrac*is infection provided important insights into the pathogenesis and dissemination of the bacteria from three different routes of infection. In addition, this work highlights some of the differences in the limit of the detection of the bacteria and quenching of the light signals in different organs, which is important to take into account when interpreting data obtained using in vivo BLI.

3.6 Fungal Imaging

The use of in vivo BLI to study fungal infections is covered in Chapter 7.

3.7 Parasite Imaging

There have been multiple studies demonstrating that bioluminescent imaging can be used to study different types of infections caused by parasites (Table 3.2) [1, 2]. These have included the investigation of eukaryotic parasites such as *Trypanosoma cruzi* [51–53], which causes Chagas disease, as well as numerous prokaryotic parasites, such as *Toxoplasma* spp. [54, 55], *Leishmania* spp. [56–61], and *Plasmodium* spp. [62–68], which cause toxoplasmosis, leishmaniasis (cutaneous, mucocutaneous, and visceral), and malaria, respectively. For the most part, these bioluminescent parasites have been generated using firefly *luc* constructs that have used promoters that are either expressed ubiquitously or in certain stages of the specific life cycle of

Table 3.2 Bioluminescent parasites

Microorganism	Reporter	References
Entamoeba histolytica	*fluc*	[145]
Leishmania amazonensis	*fluc*	[58, 146]
Leishmania major	*fluc*	[57, 147–149]
Plasmodium berghei	*fluc*	[62, 63, 65, 66, 68, 150, 151]
Toxoplasma gondii	*fluc*	[54, 55, 152–154]
Trypanosoma brucei	*rluc*	[155, 156]
Trypanosoma cruzi	*fluc*	[51–53]

the parasites in conjunction with exogenous luciferin administration. In vivo BLI using these bioluminescent parasites has resulted in new insights about parasite dissemination and organ-specific localization during the acute and chronic infections, which relate to many of the findings observed in the disease pathogenesis in humans. The use of in vivo BLI to study parasitic infections is also covered in Chapter 7.

3.8 Viral Imaging

One of the first successful examples of using in vivo BLI to study the pathogenesis of viral infections was accomplished by Luker et al. in which a recombinant HSV-1 virus was generated to encode both *fluc* and *rluc* under an early gene promoter [69]. After systemic administration of firefly luciferin, bioluminescent signals from *fluc* could be readily detected in four different routes of infection and correlated with viral titers quantified by plaque assay [69]. In contrast, bioluminescent signals from *rluc* could not be detected after systemic administration of coelenterazine, but signals from an ocular HSV-1 infection could be detected after direct application of coelenterazine to the cornea [69]. These results suggest that *fluc* had superior detection compared with *rluc* during HSV-1 viral pathogenesis. As an alternative method, this same group later generated a transgenic mouse line that expressed the *fluc* construct under the control of the HSV-1 thymidine kinase promoter, which would result in bioluminescent signals only in cells that had active viral replication [70]. This reporter approach would allow the use of any clinical viral strain or mutant HSV-1 strain to be evaluated [70]. However, one caveat was that the bioluminescent signals were tenfold less sensitive than the *fluc* reporter virus, limiting its use to studying superficial HSV-1 infections such as in skin or ocular infections [2].

In addition to HSV-1, there have been numerous other bioluminescent viral strains that have been developed (Table 3.3) [1, 2, 71, 72]. For the most part, these have been easier for DNA viruses that have larger genomes, which thus can accommodate insertion of luciferase reporter constructs [1, 2, 71]. Some successes in studying viral pathogenesis have been made using viruses such as vaccinia [73–76], varicella zoster, murid herpesvirus-4 [77], and murine cytomegalovirus viruses [78]. For RNA viruses, a proof of concept for developing a viral bioluminescent strain was generated by Cook and Griffin with Sindbis virus as a representative alphavirus [79]. Using this strain, the investigators were able to monitor dissemination of the virus from the mouse foot pad to the CNS [79]. Of note, the reporter Sindbis viral strains were about 50% attenuated in mice [79], highlighting potential problems with inserting luciferase reporter constructs into RNA viruses. Other RNA bioluminescent viruses have been generated including *Chikungunya* [80] and Venezuelan equine encephalitis [81] viruses (Table 3.3).

As an alternative to generating bioluminescent virus strains for RNA viruses, fluorescent viral strains have been generated for influenza A virus, including a GFP-expressing viral strain [82]. However, due to the short wavelength of light and background autofluorescence, fluorescent signals from influenza-infected lungs could only be detected ex vivo [82]. The recent development of the very small, yet ultra-

Table 3.3 Bioluminescent viruses

Groups	Microorganism	Reporter	References
DNA viruses	Herpes simplex virus type I	*fluc*, *rluc*	[69, 70, 157–159]
	Koi herpes virus	*fluc*	[160, 161]
	Monkeypox virus	*fluc*	[162, 163]
	Murine cytomegalovirus	*gluc*	[78, 164]
	Murine gammaherpes virus	*fluc*	[165–167]
	Murine herpes virus 4	*fluc*	[77, 168]
	Vaccinia virus	*fluc*	[70, 73–76, 169]
	Varicella zoster virus	*fluc*	[170–172]
RNA viruses	Dengue virus	*rluc*, *fluc*	[173, 174]
	Ebola virus	*gluc*	[175]
	Equine encephalitis virus	*fluc*	[81, 176, 177]
	Infectious hematopoietic necrosis virus	*rluc*	[178]
	Influenza A virus	*fluc*	[82, 179, 180]
	Marburg virus	*gluc*	[175]
	Sendai virus	*fluc*	[181, 182]
	Sindbis virus	*fluc*	[79, 183, 184]

bright NanoLuc luciferase allowed Dr. Andrew Mehle to generate luciferase-engineered influenza virus that circumvented most of these issues [83]. Moreover, a transgenic mouse strain expressing *fluc* driven by the IFN-β promoter has been used to investigate type I interferon responses to influenza [84].

3.9 Translation to the Clinic

To date, optical imaging techniques have been confined extensively to study the pathogenesis of infectious diseases in preclinical models of infection, as fluorescent signals can only penetrate several millimeters to perhaps 1 cm through host tissues. However, advances in NIR fluorophores, lasers, CCD detection cameras, and photoacoustic imaging have allowed fluorescent signals to be detected much deeper into host tissues for the potential use in humans [85].

To date, the attempts to translate optical imaging in infectious diseases to humans have been primarily focused on diagnosing an infection [85]. Although there are no targeted fluorescent probes for infectious diseases currently used in clinical practice, this is perhaps one of the best first indications for fluorescence imaging in humans. Diagnosing an infection noninvasively using targeted fluorescent probes and imaging could provide important clinical information about the anatomical location of the infection and the causative pathogenic microorganism, allowing appropriate medical or surgical therapy to be administered more rapidly. In addition, fluorescent imaging could provide this critical information without the need for invasive sampling and microbiological techniques, which are associated with complications and could take days to determine the causative pathogenic organism

Table 3.4 Fluorescent probes

Probe type	Probe agent	Label	Animal model	Detected bacteria	References
Bacterial surface	Zn-DPA	Deep red/NIR	Mice	Gram +/−	[23, 24]
Bacterial surface	Concanavalin A	IR750	Mice	*S. aureus*	[89]
Antibiotic	Vancomycin	800CW	Mice	*S. aureus*	[90]
Bacteriophage/antibody	Phage M13/anti-*S. aureus* antibody	SWNTs	Mice	*E. coli*, *S. aureus*	[91, 92]
Metabolizable	Maltodextrin	IR786	Rats	*E. coli*	[93]
Metabolizable	Prothrombin	Alexa Fluor680	Mice	*S. aureus*	[94]
Activatable	Oligonucleotide	Cye5.5	Mice	*S. aureus*	[95]
Activatable	Beta-lactamase	Cy5 dyes	Mice	*M. tuberculosis*	[96]

and its antimicrobial sensitivity and resistance profile. Most importantly, diagnosis of an infection using fluorescent imaging would permit effective treatment to be administered sooner before extensive tissue damage or invasive spread of the infection, which would greatly improve patient outcomes [85]. This is particularly relevant as the incidence of infectious diseases is increasing due to the rising numbers of patients with immune dysfunction (diabetics, organ transplant patients, chemotherapy patients, and HIV/AIDS patients), the aging population, increasing use of medical devices and implants, and the widespread emergence of antibiotic resistance. It should be mentioned that fluorescent imaging has some advantages over PET and SPECT imaging, which use targeted radioisotope-based probes, as fluorescence imaging is rapid and highly sensitive with excellent anatomic resolution and it does not involve the exposure of patients to ionizing radiation [85].

The approaches outlined in the previous sections require genetic modification of the bacteria, which limits their ability to image wild-type strains and may also affect their virulence. However, there have been several fluorescent probes that have been developed to help diagnose an infection in preclinical animal models of infection, including probes targeted against bacterial surface components, antibiotics, bacteriophages, and antibodies as well as metabolizable and activatable fluorescent probes. Several representative studies using fluorescent probes are described below (Table 3.4).

3.9.1 Bacterial Surface Probes

As mentioned above, Zn-DPA, which binds to the negatively charged anionic surfaces of bacteria, can be conjugated to a NIR fluorophore and used to detect *S. aureus* bacteria in an in vivo mouse thigh infection model [23, 24]. More recent studies have shown that this probe can also detect Gram-negative bacteria such as

Salmonella enterica serovar typhimurium [86, 87]. Interestingly, a commercially available version of the Zn-DPA-based probe (PSVue®794) was also found to bind to phosphatidylserine on the surface of apoptotic neutrophils [88]. Thus, although the Zn-DPA imaging probe can bind to bacteria membranes, there might be detectable fluorescent signals from the probe binding to apoptotic neutrophils during the inflammatory response to infection that should be taken into account when interpreting results using Zn-DPA and in vivo FLI.

Another example is concanavalin A (Con A), which is a plant-derived lectin that binds with high affinity to mannose residues on the surface of bacteria. Tang et al. conjugated Con A with a nanoparticle carrier to an NIR fluorophore (IR750), which was administered by directly applying it to infected wounds or a *S. aureus*-infected catheters in mice [89]. After washing away the unbound probe with saline, the Con A-IR750 probe resulted in increased fluorescent signals in the infected wounds and catheters [89].

3.9.2 Antibiotic Probes

An alternative approach to provide targeted imaging of a bacterial infection is the use of fluorescently labeled antibiotics, which bind to or are taken up by specific bacteria. Such an approach was employed by van Oosten et al. in which the antibiotic vancomycin, which binds with high affinity to the D-Ala-D-Ala of the C-terminus of lipid II in the cell wall of Gram-positive bacteria, was labeled with the near-infrared (NIR) 800CW dye (vanco-800CW) [90]. After systemic administration of vanco-800CW, the NIR fluorescent signals accumulated at the site of an in vivo *S. aureus* thigh infection model in mice using in vivo FLI as well as at the site of a human postmortem leg that was surgically implanted with a plate infected with a biofilm of *S. epidermidis* [90]. The authors further demonstrated that vanco-800CW was specific for Gram-positive bacteria as the probe did not accumulate at the site of sterile inflammation (i.e., Cytodex beads) or at the site of a Gram-negative (i.e., *E. coli*) thigh infection model [90]. Taken together, these results provide important evidence that such an approach of using fluorescently labeled antibiotics can identify the anatomical localization of the site of an infection as well as providing important information (e.g., Gram positive vs. Gram negative) about the pathogenic bacteria causing the infection.

3.9.3 Bacteriophage and Antibody Probes

Bardhan et al. set out to use the filamentous, non-lytic bacteriophage M13 as a fluorescent target probe because it binds to F′-pili on certain bacteria and thus could potentially distinguish between F′-pili-positive and F′-pili-negative bacteria [91]. In addition, to allow deep fluorescent signals to be detected, the authors conjugated the M13 bacteriophage with single-walled carbon nanotubes (SWNTs), which are longer-wavelength (900–1400 nm range) NIR II fluorophores [92]. They demonstrated that the M13-SWNT probes in combination with in vivo FLI could accurately distinguish between F′-pili-positive and F′-pili-negative *E. coli* strains in an in vivo thigh infection model in mice. Furthermore, to expand the use of the probe to detect other bacteria that are F′-pili-negative, the M13-SWNT probe was modified by attaching a *S. aureus*-specific antibody via a streptavidin-biotin reaction, and the probe was then successfully able to detect *S. aureus* in a deep-tissue in vivo endocarditis model in mice [92]. These studies demonstrate the feasibility of using both a bacteriophage- and antibody-based probes to detect and discriminate in vivo bacterial infections. Moreover, since the SWNTs are long-wavelength NIR fluorophores, they have the added capability of allowing detection of invasive infections in deep tissues and organs.

3.9.4 Metabolizable Probes

An example of a metabolizable probe is the maltodextrin-based fluorescent imaging probe (MDP) developed by Ning et al. [93]. This probe takes advantage of the ability of bacteria, but not mammalian cells, to use maltohexaose as an energy source. The MDP is comprised of maltohexaose conjugated to either perylene or IR786 NIR fluorophores [93]. Bacteria express the maltodextrin transporter and were readily able to take up this probe through the transporter, whereas mutant bacteria that did not express the transporter were unable to take up the probe. The probe successfully was taken up by *E. coli*, *P. aeruginosa*, *B. subtilis*, and *S. aureus* but not mammalian cells, including macrophages [93]. In an in vivo thigh infection model in rats, MDP was able to specifically detect an *E. coli* infection with a sensitivity of 10^5 CFU [93]. In addition, the in vivo FLI signals were detected in an *E. coli* parent strain that expressed the maltodextrin transporter but not in a mutant *E. coli* strain that did not express the transporter [93]. Therefore, MDP represents a metabolizable probe that is highly specific for bacteria, but not for host cells, and could provide a novel approach to accurately detect the presence of a bacterial infection using in vivo FLI.

Another example of a probe that relies on activity of the bacteria at the site of an infection involves the *S. aureus*-secreted cofactor staphylocoagulase, which binds, activates, and forms complexes with prothrombin to promote clotting and virulence during *S. aureus* endocarditis infections. Panizzi et al. generated a probe comprised of an inactivated human prothrombin analog to Alexa Fluor 680 dye (AF680-ProT) to target *S. aureus* staphylocoagulase [94]. The AF680-ProT probe bound with high affinity to staphylocoagulase and was incorporated into staphylocoagulase-AF680-ProT complexes, as would normally occur with staphylocoagulase-prothrombin complexes [94]. After administration to an in vivo mouse model of *S. aureus* endocarditis, the AF680-ProT probe was able to detect *S. aureus* in endocarditic vegetations using in vivo FLI [94]. In addition, the AF680-ProT probes became deposited throughout early vegetations but only found in the periphery of mature vegetations, which is likely related to expression levels of staphylocoagulase [94]. Taken together, this study provides the proof of concept for targeting bacterial virulence factors for future diagnostic fluorescence-based imaging.

3.9.5 Activatable Probes

An activatable or "smart" probe is based on the concept of having the probe signal turned on once the probe encounters the target [85]. In fluorescence imaging, this can be accomplished by generating a fluorescent probe that includes the presence of both a fluorophore and a quenching molecule in a configuration in which the target can separate the fluorophore from the quencher to allow fluorescent signal activation [85]. Hernandez et al. developed an activatable probe that targeted a micrococcal nuclease (MN) of *S. aureus* that has robust DNase and RNase activities on both single- and double-stranded DNA substrates [95]. This was accomplished by using a "TT probe" consisting of a pair of deoxythymidines flanked by several 2′-*O*-methyl-modified nucleotides that was linked to a 5′ fluorophore (Cy5.5, excitation/emission, 685/706 nm) and 3′ quenchers (ZEN and Iowa Black RQ) [95]. Once this probe encountered the MN of *S. aureus*, the oligonucleotide was digested, and the fluorescent signal was no longer quenched, resulting in detectable fluorescent signals [95]. The authors demonstrated that this probe had specificity against *S. aureus* as it was activated in culture supernatants of *S. aureus* but not *S. epidermidis*, *P. aeruginosa*, *S. pneumoniae*, *A. baumannii*, and *K. pneumoniae* [95]. The TT probe was further evaluated in vivo in a *S. aureus* thigh muscle infection model, and the probe was found to be activated at the site of the *S. aureus* infection expressing the MN but not in mice infected with a MN-negative mutant strain [95].

Another example of an activatable probe was performed by Kong et al. and involved the targeting of β-lactamase (BlaC), an enzyme that is naturally expressed by *Mycobacterium tuberculosis* (Mtb) [96]. The authors developed several NIR fluorogenic substrates of BlaC (CNIR4 [Cy5] or CNIR5, CNIR9, and CNIR10 [Cy5.5]) and linked them to a quencher QSY21 or QSY22 on the 3′ end [96]. Upon exposure of the CNIR probes to Mtb expressing the BlaC reporter enzyme in vitro, fluorescence signals were emitted and detected with high sensitivity, especially for CNIR5 (detection limit in the 10^2 CFU range) [96]. The CNIR5 probe was evaluated in an in vivo model of pulmonary infection with bacillus Calmette-Guérin and Mtb, and the authors found that after systemic administration of the probe, fluorescent signals could be detected from the lungs using in vivo FLI (i.e., 3D fluorescence-mediated molecular tomography) with high sensitivity in the 10^4 CFU range [96]. Finally, the authors demonstrated that the CNIR5 probe could also be used to monitor the response to treatment as after administration of isoniazid and rifampin in vitro to bacteria or to infected mice, there was a significant decrease in fluorescent signals [96]. Taken together, these studies provide evidence that activatable probes can result in both high specificity of the particular bacterial species of interest and excellent sensitivity of detection with the potential of monitoring the response to treatment.

3.10 Photoacoustic Imaging

Photoacoustic imaging involves the use of laser excitation of a fluorophore that causes thermoelastic expansion of the surrounding tissue, leading to ultrasonic pressure waves that can be detected using ultrasound sensors [9–12]. These ultrasonic pressure waves can be detected up to 8 cm into tissue, which is substantially deeper penetration than traditional in vivo FLI and thus has the translational potential to detect fluorescent signals in deeper tissues and organs in humans [9–12]. Other tissues/organs can also produce photoacoustic signals after laser excitation such as hemoglobin in blood vessels, allowing these signals to also be detected. In addition, anatomical information can simultaneously be obtained as photoacoustic imaging can be performed in conjunction with traditional ultrasound imaging so that tissues, organs, and other anatomic structures can be visualized, providing 3D spatial resolution of the photoacoustic signals within the surrounding tissue/organ anatomy.

A promising application of photoacoustic imaging is to combine this imaging modality with NIR fluorescent pathogen-specific probes (such as the preclinical examples described in the previous section above) to detect the presence of an infection and/or monitor the response to treatment . We evaluated the capability of using fluorescently labeled teicoplanin, which is a glycopeptide semisynthetic antibiotic that binds to the cell wall of Gram-positive bacteria, as a bacteria-specific probe using photoacoustic imaging. Teicoplanin was conjugated to the NIR dye indocyanine green (ICG) (Teic-ICG) and was evaluated in a mouse model of a *S. aureus* orthopedic implant infection, involving the surgical placement of an orthopedic-grade titanium Kirschner-wire into the femurs of mice and inoculating *S. aureus* into the knee joints prior to closure [3, 39–42]. After laser light excitation of the Teic-ICG and detection of the photoacoustic signals (Vevo LAZR photoacoustic and microultrasound imaging system) (FUJIFILM VisualSonics, Toronto, Canada), Teic-ICG at the site of infection resulted in a greater photoacoustic signal than hemoglobin in the tissue (Figure 3.4a). In addition, the Teic-ICG (visualized in green) accumulated precisely at the site of the *S. aureus* infection in the postoperative knees of mice, and the signal could be discriminated from the photoacoustic signal of hemoglobin in a nearby blood vessel (visualized in purple) (Figure 3.4b) [97]. This study provides the proof of concept for using photoacoustic imaging with a NIR pathogen-specific probe to diagnose a clinically relevant infection. Future studies will undoubtedly continue to develop photoacoustic imaging for infectious

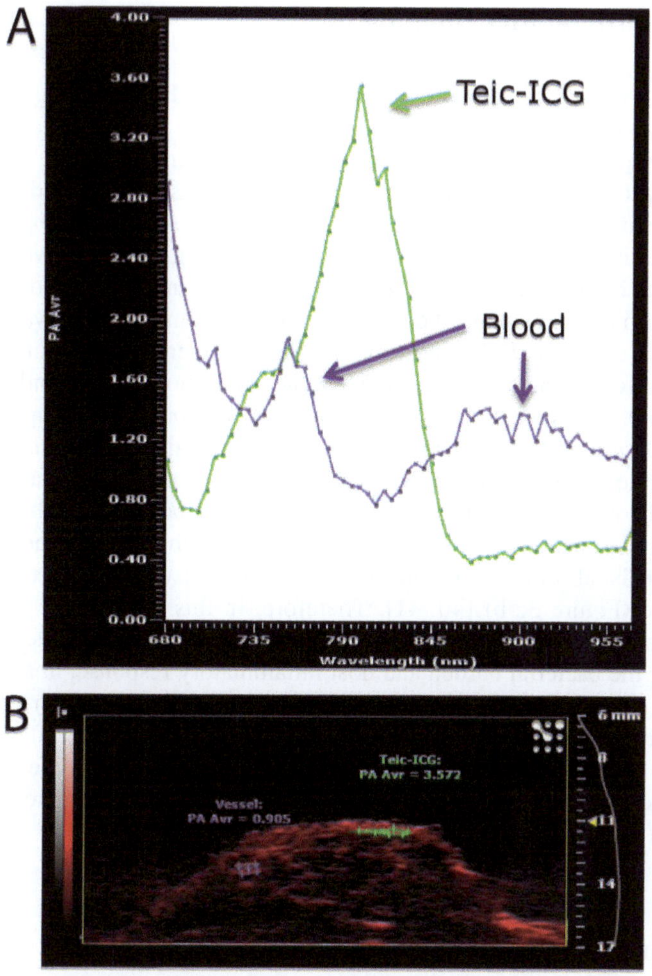

Figure 3.4 In vivo photoacoustic imaging of an antibiotic-based fluorescent imaging probe. An orthopedic infection model was used in which *S. aureus* was inoculated in the right knee joints of mice in the presence of a titanium K-wire implant extending from the femoral intramedullary canal. Teicoplanin conjugated to indocyanine green (Teic-ICG) was administered intravenously, and photoacoustic signals from the infected knee joints of mice were obtained 4 days after probe administration [97]. (**a**) Photoacoustic signals of Teic-ICG versus hemoglobin at the site of infection in the postsurgical *S. aureus*-infected knee joints of mice. (**b**) Photoacoustic signals of Teic-ICG (*green*) accumulated at the postsurgical *S. aureus*-infected knee joints of mice compared with the photoacoustic signal of hemoglobin in a nearby blood vessel (*purple*)

diseases as this modality combines all of the advantages of traditional in vivo FLI (rapid, highly sensitive, and excellent anatomic structure without using ionizing radiation) with substantially greater tissue penetration and the ability to co-localize the signals with anatomic information from simultaneous ultrasound imaging.

3.11 Multimodality Imaging

Multimodality imaging involves combining the use of different imaging modalities (e.g., in vivo BLI, in vivo FLI, X-ray, CT, MRI, PET, SPECT, ultrasound, photoacoustic imaging, etc.) to take advantage of the different imaging techniques to provide improved information of the biological processes being studied. With particular relevance to optical imaging, one of the most successful approaches is to combine in vivo BLI and/or in vivo FLI with μCT imaging, which would allow the detection of bioluminescent and fluorescent signals in a 3D anatomical context obtained with μCT imaging. There is currently one commercially available system that has this capacity (IVIS SpectrumCT, PerkinElmer). This system enables 3D data acquisition for both optical (luminescence and fluorescence) and μCT images (Figure 3.5a). As an example, we used our *S. aureus* orthopedic implant infection model (as described above), using a bioluminescent strain of *S. aureus* [3, 39–42] in LysEGFP mice (which possess EGFP-fluorescent neutrophils) [7], and 3D in vivo BLI and FLI in conjunction with μCT imaging were performed. This enabled the bacterial bioluminescent signals to be co-localized with the EGFP-neutrophil fluorescent signals, all in the anatomic context of the postsurgical infected knee joints of the mice (Figure 3.5b) [40, 41]. Therefore, in this example of multimodality imaging, the combination of optical and μCT imaging provided the capability of monitoring the bacterial burden and host inflammatory response, in addition to the pathologic changes in the bone, in the same mice longitudinally over time [40, 41]. Similar multimodality imaging studies can be performed in many different preclinical animal models of infection to provide new insights into the infectious disease pathogenesis, to evaluate pathogen-specific NIR probes, and to monitor the response to different antimicrobial therapies.

3.12 Photodynamic Therapy

Beyond diagnosing an infection, the use of pathogen-targeted fluorescent imaging probes could also be used to treat an infection by using photodynamic therapy (PDT) [14]. PDT was first described by Oscar Raab, a medical student in Munich, Germany, when he found that microorganisms incubated with certain dyes were killed when exposed to light [98]. It was later discovered that the mechanism by which PDT induced killing of the bacteria or mammalian cells involved the generation of reactive oxygen species (ROS) following the exposure of a photosensitizer molecule to light (typically with wavelengths ranging between 200 and 1000 nm) at the appropriate wavelength matched to the absorption of the photosensitizer [98]. The light absorbed by the photosensitizer induced a photochemical reaction, leading to production of ROS (e.g., superoxide, hydroxyl radicals, and singlet oxygen), which caused oxidative damage to cellular components (e.g., proteins, lipids, nucleic acids), and ensuing cytotoxicity of microorganisms and mammalian cells

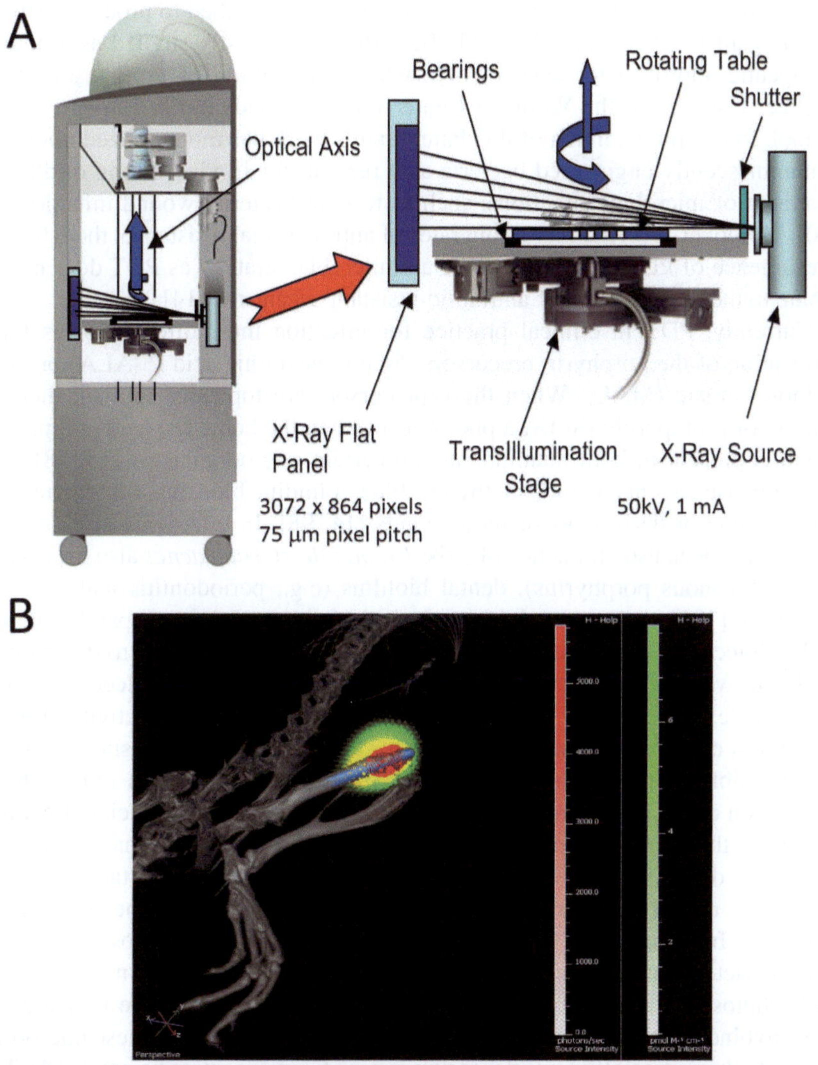

Figure 3.5 Multimodality in vivo BLI, FLI, and μCT imaging system. (**a**) Configuration of a commercially available in vivo imaging system (IVIS SpectrumCT, PerkinElmer) with integrated optical (luminescence and fluorescence) and μCT technology. This system has a horizontally rotating animal platform that allows the acquisition of CT data, in conjunction with full tomographic 3D optical imaging capabilities. (**b**) An orthopedic infection model was imaged as an example in which *S. aureus* was inoculated in the right knee joints of LysEGFP mice (possessing fluorescent neutrophils) in the presence of a titanium K-wire implant extending from the femoral intramedullary canal. The in vivo BLI of *S. aureus* (*red*), in vivo FLI of EGFP-neutrophil fluorescence (*green*), and merged bioluminescence and fluorescence signals (*yellow*) are shown in the right knee joint possessing the titanium implant (*blue*) in the anatomical context of the surrounding bone obtained with μCT imaging

[98]. Although the original description of PDT was described to promote killing of microorganisms, between 1970 and 2010, PDT was mostly studied as a potential therapeutic approach for cancer [14], with the exception of groups such as Dr. Michael Hamblin at the Wellman Center for Photomedicine at Harvard Medical School. Interestingly, much of this latter team's work has monopolized upon using bioluminescently engineered bacteria as a readout for in vivo killing during PDT treatment of microbial infections, such as to treat bacterial wound infections [99, 100]. Moreover, with the increasing rates of antimicrobial resistance, there has been a resurgence of PDT as an alternative antimicrobial strategy as PDT does not contribute to the development of antibiotic-resistant organisms [14].

Currently, PDT in clinical practice for infection most often involves topical application of the porphyrin precursors: 5-aminolevulinic acid (5-ALA) or methyl aminolevulinate (MAL). When these precursors are topically applied, there is a buildup of protoporphyrin IX, a photosensitizer in the heme biosynthesis pathway, which is present in both mammalian and certain microorganisms [14, 98]. Other clinically used agents include methylene blue, toluidine blue, neutral red, and polyethylenimine or derivatives of these agents [14, 98]. In infectious diseases, these agents have been used for acne vulgaris (*Propionibacterium acnes* also expresses its own endogenous porphyrins), dental biofilms (e.g., periodontitis and root canal infection) [101], cutaneous leishmaniasis lesions, and human papilloma virus (HPV) infections (e.g., warts, condyloma, and cervical HPV) and to decrease bioburden in wounds (burn, chronic leg wounds, and diabetic foot ulcers [102]) [14, 98]. Of note, in the case of leishmaniasis and viral infections, the activity of ALA is on the host cells and not the microorganisms themselves since parasites and viruses are incapable of porphyrin biosynthesis. Since these approaches require topical application of the photosensitizer, they are only suitable for superficial infections.

Due to the increasing rates of antimicrobial resistance, there has been intense interest in developing new photosensitizers that are specifically targeted against pathogenic microorganisms, especially Gram-positive and Gram-negative bacteria and fungi. In general, the photosensitizers that would have the most effectiveness against bacteria or fungi need to penetrate the cell wall of these microorganisms [14]. Photosensitizers that are cationic are more effective because they are more likely to bind to and penetrate the negatively charged cell walls of these microorganisms, which is especially important for targeting Gram-negative bacteria [14]. There have been multiple attempts to impart a positive charge to photosensitizers or using permeabilizing agents (e.g., polymyxin nonapeptide, EDTA, and various different nanoparticles) to facilitate penetration into bacteria and fungi [14]. In addition, photosensitizers with absorption wavelengths between 650 and 800 nm are generally more effective because they circumvent the absorption of the light by hemoglobin and other endogenous chromophores while also having enough energy for the photochemical reactions to generate ROS [14]. However, for infectious diseases, these newer photosensitizers have only been evaluated extensively in vitro or in preclinical animal models of infection, and their efficacy in large-scale human trials has not yet been determined [14].

3.13 Conclusions and Future Directions

In conclusion, in vivo optical imaging has become an extremely valuable approach to noninvasively and longitudinally monitor the pathogenic mechanisms of infectious diseases in live animals, including the ability to monitor host–pathogen interactions, immune responses, and response to antimicrobial therapies. This has been made possible by combining the use of engineered light-emitting pathogens with highly sensitive optical imaging instrumentation that can detect and quantify photons generated from either luminescence or fluorescence signals in vivo, providing spatial resolution (both 2D and 3D) of the dissemination of the infection in different tissues and organs in the same animals over time.

In vivo optical imaging was once thought to be limited to small preclinical animal models, due to poor penetration of the optical signal in deep tissue. However, refinements in longer-wavelength near-infrared fluorescent probe chemistries, as well as advances in photoacoustic imaging techniques, allow optical signals to be detected several centimeters into tissue, providing the opportunity to move optical imaging into the clinic for the detection of microbial infections. Notably, fluorescently labeled probes targeted against certain pathogenic microorganisms are under preclinical development to provide noninvasive diagnostic information about the causative pathogenic microorganism, as well as the response to treatment.

A potential future application of fluorescently labeled targeted probes would be to use them in image-guided surgery to help surgeons identify infected tissue during an operation. This would facilitate the more accurate determination of the extent of the infectious process for better debridement and potentially improved patient outcomes. In addition, multimodality imaging techniques that combine optical imaging with other imaging approaches (e.g., X-ray, CT, MRI, PET, SPECT, ultrasound, and photoacoustic imaging) provide the new capability of co-registering optical imaging signals with anatomical and structural information during an infection.

Finally, PDT uses light in conjunction with targeted photosensitizers as a novel approach to treat an infection without contributing to antibiotic resistance. It may even be possible to develop a targeted fluorescent imaging agent against a pathogenic microorganism that could be used to both diagnose the infection while also serving as photosensitizer to treat the same infection using PDT. Taken together, the future for optical imaging of infections is bright, and there will be many new and exciting opportunities to expand this technology into clinical practice.

3.14 Summary

The development of in vivo optical imaging techniques, including advances in related instrumentation, molecular biology (especially luciferases and fluorescent proteins), and probe chemistries, has revolutionized the study and treatment of infectious diseases. In particular, in vivo optical imaging has permitted the noninvasive and longitudinal monitoring of host–pathogen interactions, including the dynamics of infection burden and dissemination, host immune responses, and the effects of therapy, all measured in the same live animals over time. These approaches provide highly accurate information about microbial pathogenesis and treatment while also significantly reducing animal numbers and cost. Although optical imaging was once considered to be applicable only to preclinical animal research, new methodologies are advancing these techniques into clinical practice to monitor, diagnose, and treat infectious diseases.

References

1. Andreu, N., A. Zelmer, and S. Wiles, *Noninvasive biophotonic imaging for studies of infectious disease.* FEMS Microbiol.Rev., 2011. **35**(2): p. 360-394.
2. Hutchens, M. and G.D. Luker, *Applications of bioluminescence imaging to the study of infectious diseases.* Cell Microbiol., 2007. **9**(10): p. 2315-2322.
3. Bernthal, N.M., et al., *A mouse model of post-arthroplasty Staphylococcus aureus joint infection to evaluate in vivo the efficacy of antimicrobial implant coatings.* PLoS.ONE., 2010. **5**(9): p. e12580.
4. Cho, J.S., et al., *Neutrophil-derived IL-1beta is sufficient for abscess formation in immunity against Staphylococcus aureus in mice.* PLoS.Pathog., 2012. **8**(11): p. e1003047.
5. Miller, L.S., et al., *MyD88 mediates neutrophil recruitment initiated by IL-1R but not TLR2 activation in immunity against Staphylococcus aureus.* Immunity., 2006. **24**(1): p. 79-91.
6. Matsushima, H., et al., *Intravital imaging of IL-1beta production in skin.* J.Invest Dermatol., 2010. **130**(6): p. 1571-1580.
7. Faust, N., et al., *Insertion of enhanced green fluorescent protein into the lysozyme gene creates mice with green fluorescent granulocytes and macrophages.* Blood, 2000. **96**(2): p. 719-726.
8. van, O.M., et al., *Real-time in vivo imaging of invasive- and biomaterial-associated bacterial infections using fluorescently labelled vancomycin.* Nat.Commun., 2013. **4**: p. 2584.
9. Wang, L.V. and S. Hu, *Photoacoustic tomography: in vivo imaging from organelles to organs.* Science, 2012. **335**(6075): p. 1458-62.
10. Ntziachristos, V., et al., *Looking and listening to light: the evolution of whole-body photonic imaging.* Nat.Biotechnol., 2005. **23**(3): p. 313-320.
11. Ntziachristos, V. and D. Razansky, *Molecular imaging by means of multispectral optoacoustic tomography (MSOT).* Chem Rev, 2010. **110**(5): p. 2783-94.
12. Zackrisson, S., S.M. van de Ven, and S.S. Gambhir, *Light in and sound out: emerging translational strategies for photoacoustic imaging.* Cancer Res, 2014. **74**(4): p. 979-1004.
13. Silva, Z.S., Jr., et al., *Animal models for photodynamic therapy (PDT).* Biosci Rep, 2015. **35**(6).
14. Kharkwal, G.B., et al., *Photodynamic therapy for infections: clinical applications.* Lasers Surg Med, 2011. **43**(7): p. 755-67.
15. Sjollema, J., et al., *The potential for bio-optical imaging of biomaterial-associated infection in vivo.* Biomaterials, 2010. **31**(8): p. 1984-1995.
16. Badr, C.E. and B.A. Tannous, *Bioluminescence imaging: progress and applications.* Trends Biotechnol., 2011. **29**(12): p. 624-633.
17. Zhao, H., et al., *Emission spectra of bioluminescent reporters and interaction with mammalian tissue determine the sensitivity of detection in vivo.* J Biomed Opt, 2005. **10**(4): p. 41210.
18. Chang, M., et al., *Real-time bioluminescence imaging of mixed mycobacterial infections.* PLoS One, 2014. **9**(9): p. e108341.

19. Kadurugamuwa, J.L., et al., *Reduction of astrogliosis by early treatment of pneumococcal meningitis measured by simultaneous imaging, in vivo, of the pathogen and host response.* Infect Immun, 2005. **73**(12): p. 7836-43.
20. Shimomura, O., *The discovery of aequorin and green fluorescent protein.* J Microsc, 2005. **217**(Pt 1): p. 1-15.
21. Shaner, N.C., et al., *Improved monomeric red, orange and yellow fluorescent proteins derived from Discosoma sp. red fluorescent protein.* Nat Biotechnol, 2004. **22**(12): p. 1567-72.
22. Merzlyak, E.M., et al., *Bright monomeric red fluorescent protein with an extended fluorescence lifetime.* Nat Methods, 2007. **4**(7): p. 555-7.
23. Leevy, W.M., et al., *Noninvasive optical imaging of staphylococcus aureus bacterial infection in living mice using a Bis-dipicolylamine-Zinc(II) affinity group conjugated to a near-infrared fluorophore.* Bioconjug Chem, 2008. **19**(3): p. 686-92.
24. Leevy, W.M., et al., *Optical imaging of bacterial infection in living mice using a fluorescent near-infrared molecular probe.* J Am Chem Soc, 2006. **128**(51): p. 16476-7.
25. Kamila, S., et al., *Diagnostic and Therapeutic Applications of Quantum Dots in Nanomedicine.* Top Curr Chem, 2016. **370**: p. 203-24.
26. Contag, C.H., et al., *Photonic detection of bacterial pathogens in living hosts.* Mol Microbiol, 1995. **18**(4): p. 593-603.
27. Francis, K.P., et al., *Visualizing pneumococcal infections in the lungs of live mice using bioluminescent Streptococcus pneumoniae transformed with a novel gram-positive lux transposon.* Infect Immun, 2001. **69**(5): p. 3350-8.
28. Winson, M.K., et al., *Engineering the luxCDABE genes from Photorhabdus luminescens to provide a bioluminescent reporter for constitutive and promoter probe plasmids and mini-Tn5 constructs.* FEMS Microbiol Lett, 1998. **163**(2): p. 193-202.
29. Francis, K.P., et al., *Monitoring bioluminescent Staphylococcus aureus infections in living mice using a novel luxABCDE construct.* Infect Immun, 2000. **68**(6): p. 3594-600.
30. Park, H.S., et al., *Membranous cells in nasal-associated lymphoid tissue: a portal of entry for the respiratory mucosal pathogen group A streptococcus.* J Immunol, 2003. **171**(5): p. 2532-7.
31. Stavrakis, A.I., et al., *Combination Prophylactic Therapy with Rifampin Increases Efficacy against an Experimental Staphylococcus epidermidis Subcutaneous Implant-Related Infection.* Antimicrob.Agents Chemother., 2014. **58**(4): p. 2377-2386.
32. Vuong, C., et al., *Development of real-time in vivo imaging of device-related Staphylococcus epidermidis infection in mice and influence of animal immune status on susceptibility to infection.* J.Infect.Dis., 2008. **198**(2): p. 258-261.
33. Hardy, J., et al., *Extracellular replication of Listeria monocytogenes in the murine gall bladder.* Science, 2004. **303**(5659): p. 851-3.
34. Plaut, R.D., et al., *Stably luminescent Staphylococcus aureus clinical strains for use in bioluminescent imaging.* PLoS.ONE., 2013. **8**(3): p. e59232.
35. Close, D.M., et al., *Autonomous bioluminescent expression of the bacterial luciferase gene cassette (lux) in a mammalian cell line.* PLoS One, 2010. **5**(8): p. e12441.
36. Cho, J.S., et al., *IL-17 is essential for host defense against cutaneous Staphylococcus aureus infection in mice.* J.Clin.Invest, 2010. **120**(5): p. 1762-1773.
37. Miller, L.S., et al., *Inflammasome-mediated production of IL-1beta Is required for neutrophil recruitment against Staphylococcus aureus in vivo.* J.Immunol., 2007. **179**(10): p. 6933-6942.
38. Guo, Y., et al., *In Vivo Bioluminescence Imaging To Evaluate Systemic and Topical Antibiotics against Community-Acquired Methicillin-Resistant Staphylococcus aureus-Infected Skin Wounds in Mice.* Antimicrob.Agents Chemother., 2013. **57**(2): p. 855-863.
39. Bernthal, N.M., et al., *Protective role of IL-1beta against post-arthroplasty Staphylococcus aureus infection.* J.Orthop.Res., 2011. **29**(10): p. 1621-1626.
40. Niska, J.A., et al., *Monitoring bacterial burden, inflammation and bone damage longitudinally using optical and micro-CT imaging in an orthopaedic implant infection in mice.* PLoS. ONE., 2012. **7**(10): p. e47397.

41. Niska, J.A., et al., *Daptomycin and tigecycline have broader effective dose ranges than vancomycin as prophylaxis against a Staphylococcus aureus surgical implant infection in mice.* Antimicrob.Agents Chemother., 2012. **56**(5): p. 2590-2597.
42. Niska, J.A., et al., *Vancomycin-Rifampin Combination Therapy Has Enhanced Efficacy against an Experimental Staphylococcus aureus Prosthetic Joint Infection.* Antimicrob. Agents Chemother., 2013. **57**(10): p. 5080-5086.
43. Hardy, J., J.J. Margolis, and C.H. Contag, *Induced biliary excretion of Listeria monocytogenes.* Infect Immun, 2006. **74**(3): p. 1819-27.
44. Rajashekara, G., et al., *Unraveling Brucella genomics and pathogenesis in immunocompromised IRF-1-/- mice.* Am J Reprod Immunol, 2005. **54**(6): p. 358-68.
45. Rajashekara, G., et al., *Temporal analysis of pathogenic events in virulent and avirulent Brucella melitensis infections.* Cell Microbiol, 2005. **7**(10): p. 1459-73.
46. Wiles, S., et al., *Organ specificity, colonization and clearance dynamics in vivo following oral challenges with the murine pathogen Citrobacter rodentium.* Cell Microbiol, 2004. **6**(10): p. 963-72.
47. Wiles, S., G. Dougan, and G. Frankel, *Emergence of a 'hyperinfectious' bacterial state after passage of Citrobacter rodentium through the host gastrointestinal tract.* Cell Microbiol, 2005. **7**(8): p. 1163-72.
48. Glomski, I.J., et al., *Inhaled non-capsulated Bacillus anthracis in A/J mice: nasopharynx and alveolar space as dual portals of entry, delayed dissemination, and specific organ targeting.* Microbes Infect, 2008. **10**(12-13): p. 1398-404.
49. Glomski, I.J., et al., *Noncapsulated toxinogenic Bacillus anthracis presents a specific growth and dissemination pattern in naive and protective antigen-immune mice.* Infect Immun, 2007. **75**(10): p. 4754-61.
50. Glomski, I.J., et al., *Primary involvement of pharynx and peyer's patch in inhalational and intestinal anthrax.* PLoS Pathog, 2007. **3**(6): p. e76.
51. Lewis, M.D., et al., *Bioluminescence imaging of chronic Trypanosoma cruzi infections reveals tissue-specific parasite dynamics and heart disease in the absence of locally persistent infection.* Cell Microbiol, 2014. **16**(9): p. 1285-300.
52. Henriques, C., et al., *In vivo imaging of mice infected with bioluminescent Trypanosoma cruzi unveils novel sites of infection.* Parasit Vectors, 2014. **7**: p. 89.
53. Hyland, K.V., et al., *Bioluminescent imaging of Trypanosoma cruzi infection.* Int J Parasitol, 2008. **38**(12): p. 1391-400.
54. Dellacasa-Lindberg, I., N. Hitziger, and A. Barragan, *Localized recrudescence of Toxoplasma infections in the central nervous system of immunocompromised mice assessed by in vivo bioluminescence imaging.* Microbes Infect, 2007. **9**(11): p. 1291-8.
55. Saeij, J.P., et al., *Bioluminescence imaging of Toxoplasma gondii infection in living mice reveals dramatic differences between strains.* Infect Immun, 2005. **73**(2): p. 695-702.
56. Reimao, J.Q., et al., *Generation of luciferase-expressing Leishmania infantum chagasi and assessment of miltefosine efficacy in infected hamsters through bioimaging.* PLoS Negl Trop Dis, 2015. **9**(2): p. e0003556.
57. Taheri, T., et al., *Generation of stable L. major(+EGFP-LUC) and simultaneous comparison between EGFP and luciferase sensitivity.* Exp Parasitol, 2015. **150**: p. 44-55.
58. Reimao, J.Q., et al., *Parasite burden in Leishmania (Leishmania) amazonensis-infected mice: validation of luciferase as a quantitative tool.* J Microbiol Methods, 2013. **93**(2): p. 95-101.
59. Michel, G., et al., *Luciferase-expressing Leishmania infantum allows the monitoring of amastigote population size, in vivo, ex vivo and in vitro.* PLoS Negl Trop Dis, 2011. **5**(9): p. e1323.
60. de La Llave, E., et al., *A combined luciferase imaging and reverse transcription polymerase chain reaction assay for the study of Leishmania amastigote burden and correlated mouse tissue transcript fluctuations.* Cell Microbiol, 2011. **13**(1): p. 81-91.
61. Thalhofer, C.J., et al., *In vivo imaging of transgenic Leishmania parasites in a live host.* J Vis Exp, 2010(41).

62. De Niz, M., et al., *An ultrasensitive NanoLuc-based luminescence system for monitoring Plasmodium berghei throughout its life cycle.* Malar J, 2016. **15**(1): p. 232.
63. Matsuoka, H., et al., *Visualization of Malaria Parasites in the Skin Using the Luciferase Transgenic Parasite, Plasmodium berghei.* Trop Med Health, 2015. **43**(1): p. 53-61.
64. Azevedo, M.F., et al., *Plasmodium falciparum transfected with ultra bright NanoLuc luciferase offers high sensitivity detection for the screening of growth and cellular trafficking inhibitors.* PLoS One, 2014. **9**(11): p. e112571.
65. Annoura, T., et al., *Quantitative analysis of Plasmodium berghei liver stages by bioluminescence imaging.* Methods Mol Biol, 2013. **923**: p. 429-43.
66. Braks, J., et al., *Bioluminescence imaging of P. berghei Schizont sequestration in rodents.* Methods Mol Biol, 2013. **923**: p. 353-68.
67. Hasenkamp, S., E.H. Wong, and P. Horrocks, *An improved single-step lysis protocol to measure luciferase bioluminescence in Plasmodium falciparum.* Malar J, 2012. **11**: p. 42.
68. Franke-Fayard, B., A.P. Waters, and C.J. Janse, *Real-time in vivo imaging of transgenic bioluminescent blood stages of rodent malaria parasites in mice.* Nat Protoc, 2006. **1**(1): p. 476-85.
69. Luker, G.D., et al., *Noninvasive bioluminescence imaging of herpes simplex virus type 1 infection and therapy in living mice.* J Virol, 2002. **76**(23): p. 12149-61.
70. Luker, K.E., et al., *Transgenic reporter mouse for bioluminescence imaging of herpes simplex virus 1 infection in living mice.* Virology, 2006. **347**(2): p. 286-95.
71. Bocan, T.M., R.G. Panchal, and S. Bavari, *Applications of in vivo imaging in the evaluation of the pathophysiology of viral and bacterial infections and in development of countermeasures to BSL3/4 pathogens.* Mol Imaging Biol, 2015. **17**(1): p. 4-17.
72. Bray, M., et al., *Molecular imaging of influenza and other emerging respiratory viral infections.* J Infect Dis, 2011. **203**(10): p. 1348-59.
73. Liu, Q., et al., *Bioluminescent imaging of vaccinia virus infection in immunocompetent and immunodeficient rats as a model for human smallpox.* Sci Rep, 2015. **5**: p. 11397.
74. Zaitseva, M., S. Kapnick, and H. Golding, *Measurements of vaccinia virus dissemination using whole body imaging: approaches for predicting of lethality in challenge models and testing of vaccines and antiviral treatments.* Methods Mol Biol, 2012. **890**: p. 161-76.
75. Zaitseva, M., et al., *Application of bioluminescence imaging to the prediction of lethality in vaccinia virus-infected mice.* J Virol, 2009. **83**(20): p. 10437-47.
76. Luker, K.E., et al., *Bioluminescence imaging of vaccinia virus: effects of interferon on viral replication and spread.* Virology, 2005. **341**(2): p. 284-300.
77. Milho, R., et al., *In vivo imaging of murid herpesvirus-4 infection.* J Gen Virol, 2009. **90**(Pt 1): p. 21-32.
78. Yamada, S., et al., *In vivo imaging assay for the convenient evaluation of antiviral compounds against cytomegalovirus in mice.* Antiviral Res, 2010. **88**(1): p. 45-52.
79. Cook, S.H. and D.E. Griffin, *Luciferase imaging of a neurotropic viral infection in intact animals.* J Virol, 2003. **77**(9): p. 5333-8.
80. Ziegler, S.A., et al., *In vivo imaging of chikungunya virus in mice and Aedes mosquitoes using a Renilla luciferase clone.* Vector Borne Zoonotic Dis, 2011. **11**(11): p. 1471-7.
81. Patterson, M., et al., *Rapid, non-invasive imaging of alphaviral brain infection: reducing animal numbers and morbidity to identify efficacy of potential vaccines and antivirals.* Vaccine, 2011. **29**(50): p. 9345-51.
82. Kittel, C., et al., *Rescue of influenza virus expressing GFP from the NS1 reading frame.* Virology, 2004. **324**(1): p. 67-73.
83. Mehle, A., *Fiat Luc: Bioluminescence Imaging Reveals In Vivo Viral Replication Dynamics.* PLoS Pathog, 2015. **11**(9): p. e1005081.
84. Kallfass, C., et al., *Visualizing the beta interferon response in mice during infection with influenza A viruses expressing or lacking nonstructural protein 1.* J Virol, 2013. **87**(12): p. 6925-30.

85. van Oosten, M., et al., *Targeted imaging of bacterial infections: advances, hurdles and hopes.* FEMS Microbiol Rev, 2015. **39**(6): p. 892-916.
86. White, A.G., et al., *Deep-red fluorescent imaging probe for bacteria.* Bioorg Med Chem Lett, 2012. **22**(8): p. 2833-6.
87. White, A.G., et al., *Optical imaging of bacterial infection in living mice using deep-red fluorescent squaraine rotaxane probes.* Bioconjug Chem, 2010. **21**(7): p. 1297-304.
88. Thakur, M.L., et al., *Targeting apoptosis for optical imaging of infection.* Mol Imaging Biol, 2012. **14**(2): p. 163-71.
89. Tang, E.N., et al., *In vivo imaging of infection using a bacteria-targeting optical nanoprobe.* J Biomed Nanotechnol, 2014. **10**(5): p. 856-63.
90. van Oosten, M., et al., *Real-time in vivo imaging of invasive- and biomaterial-associated bacterial infections using fluorescently labelled vancomycin.* Nat Commun, 2013. **4**: p. 2584.
91. Bardhan, N.M., D. Ghosh, and A.M. Belcher, *Carbon nanotubes as in vivo bacterial probes.* Nat Commun, 2014. **5**: p. 4918.
92. Bardhan, N.M., D. Ghosh, and A.M. Belcher, *M13 virus based detection of bacterial infections in living hosts.* J Biophotonics, 2014. **7**(8): p. 617-23.
93. Ning, X., et al., *Maltodextrin-based imaging probes detect bacteria in vivo with high sensitivity and specificity.* Nat Mater, 2011. **10**(8): p. 602-7.
94. Panizzi, P., et al., *In vivo detection of Staphylococcus aureus endocarditis by targeting pathogen-specific prothrombin activation.* Nat Med, 2011. **17**(9): p. 1142-6.
95. Hernandez, F.J., et al., *Noninvasive imaging of Staphylococcus aureus infections with a nuclease-activated probe.* Nat Med, 2014. **20**(3): p. 301-6.
96. Kong, Y. and J.D. Cirillo, *Reporter enzyme fluorescence (REF) imaging and quantification of tuberculosis in live animals.* Virulence, 2010. **1**(6): p. 558-62.
97. Wang, Y., et al., *Preclinical evaluation of photoacoustic imaging as a novel noninvasive approach to detect an orthopaedic implant infection.*. J Am Acad Orthop Surg., 2017: epub ahead of print. https://www.ncbi.nlm.nih.gov/pubmed/27941556
98. Abrahamse, H. and M.R. Hamblin, *New photosensitizers for photodynamic therapy.* Biochem J, 2016. **473**(4): p. 347-64.
99. Gad, F., et al., *Targeted photodynamic therapy of established soft-tissue infections in mice.* Photochem Photobiol Sci, 2004. **3**(5): p. 451-8.
100. Demidova, T.N., et al., *Monitoring photodynamic therapy of localized infections by bioluminescence imaging of genetically engineered bacteria.* J Photochem Photobiol B, 2005. **81**(1): p. 15-25.
101. Kikuchi, T., et al., *Adjunctive Application of Antimicrobial Photodynamic Therapy in Nonsurgical Periodontal Treatment: A Review of Literature.* Int J Mol Sci, 2015. **16**(10): p. 24111-26.
102. Morley, S., et al., *Phase IIa randomized, placebo-controlled study of antimicrobial photodynamic therapy in bacterially colonized, chronic leg ulcers and diabetic foot ulcers: a new approach to antimicrobial therapy.* Br J Dermatol, 2013. **168**(3): p. 617-24.
103. Sanz, P., et al., *Detection of Bacillus anthracis spore germination in vivo by bioluminescence imaging.* Infect Immun, 2008. **76**(3): p. 1036-47.
104. Crawford, M.A., et al., *Antimicrobial effects of interferon-inducible CXC chemokines against Bacillus anthracis spores and bacilli.* Infect Immun, 2009. **77**(4): p. 1664-78.
105. Cronin, M., et al., *Development of a luciferase-based reporter system to monitor Bifidobacterium breve UCC2003 persistence in mice.* BMC Microbiol, 2008. **8**: p. 161.
106. Cronin, M., et al., *High resolution in vivo bioluminescent imaging for the study of bacterial tumour targeting.* PLoS One, 2012. **7**(1): p. e30940.
107. Riedel, C.U., et al., *Construction of p16Slux, a novel vector for improved bioluminescent labeling of gram-negative bacteria.* Appl Environ Microbiol, 2007. **73**(21): p. 7092-5.
108. Disson, O., et al., *Modeling human listeriosis in natural and genetically engineered animals.* Nat Protoc, 2009. **4**(6): p. 799-810.

109. Steinhuber, A., et al., *Bioluminescence imaging to study the promoter activity of hla of Staphylococcus aureus in vitro and in vivo.* Int J Med Microbiol, 2008. **298**(7-8): p. 599-605.
110. Cho, J.S., et al., *Noninvasive in vivo imaging to evaluate immune responses and antimicrobial therapy against Staphylococcus aureus and USA300 MRSA skin infections.* J Invest Dermatol, 2011. **131**(4): p. 907-15.
111. Pammi, M., et al., *Farnesol decreases biofilms of Staphylococcus epidermidis and exhibits synergy with nafcillin and vancomycin.* Pediatr Res, 2011. **70**(6): p. 578-83.
112. Mook-Kanamori, B.B., et al., *Daptomycin in experimental murine pneumococcal meningitis.* BMC Infect Dis, 2009. **9**: p. 50.
113. Alam, F.M., et al., *Non-invasive monitoring of Streptococcus pyogenes vaccine efficacy using biophotonic imaging.* PLoS One, 2013. **8**(11): p. e82123.
114. Zhang, Y., et al., *Potentiation of antimicrobial photodynamic inactivation mediated by a cationic fullerene by added iodide: in vitro and in vivo studies.* Nanomedicine (Lond), 2015. **10**(4): p. 603-14.
115. Zhang, Y., et al., *Antimicrobial blue light therapy for multidrug-resistant Acinetobacter baumannii infection in a mouse burn model: implications for prophylaxis and treatment of combat-related wound infections.* J Infect Dis, 2014. **209**(12): p. 1963-71.
116. Radhakrishnan, G.K., et al., *Brucella TIR Domain-containing Protein Mimics Properties of the Toll-like Receptor Adaptor Protein TIRAP.* J Biol Chem, 2009. **284**(15): p. 9892-8.
117. Owen, S.J., et al., *Nasal-associated lymphoid tissue and olfactory epithelium as portals of entry for Burkholderia pseudomallei in murine melioidosis.* J Infect Dis, 2009. **199**(12): p. 1761-70.
118. Warawa, J.M., et al., *Bioluminescent diagnostic imaging to characterize altered respiratory tract colonization by the burkholderia pseudomallei capsule mutant.* Front Microbiol, 2011. **2**: p. 133.
119. Collins, J.W., et al., *4D multimodality imaging of Citrobacter rodentium infections in mice.* J Vis Exp, 2013(78).
120. Wiles, S., et al., *In vivo bioluminescence imaging of the murine pathogen Citrobacter rodentium.* Infect Immun, 2006. **74**(9): p. 5391-6.
121. Gibson, D.L., et al., *Toll-like receptor 2 plays a critical role in maintaining mucosal integrity during Citrobacter rodentium-induced colitis.* Cell Microbiol, 2008. **10**(2): p. 388-403.
122. Karsi, A., S. Menanteau-Ledouble, and M.L. Lawrence, *Development of bioluminescent Edwardsiella ictaluri for noninvasive disease monitoring.* FEMS Microbiol Lett, 2006. **260**(2): p. 216-23.
123. Menanteau-Ledouble, S. and M.L. Lawrence, *Use of bioluminescence mutant screening for identification of Edwardsiella ictaluri genes involved in channel catfish (Ictalurus punctatus) skin colonization.* Vet Microbiol, 2013. **162**(2-4): p. 724-30.
124. Rocchetta, H.L., et al., *Validation of a noninvasive, real-time imaging technology using bioluminescent Escherichia coli in the neutropenic mouse thigh model of infection.* Antimicrob Agents Chemother, 2001. **45**(1): p. 129-37.
125. Jawhara, S. and S. Mordon, *Monitoring of bactericidal action of laser by in vivo imaging of bioluminescent E. coli in a cutaneous wound infection.* Lasers Med Sci, 2006. **21**(3): p. 153-9.
126. Foucault, M.L., et al., *In vivo bioluminescence imaging for the study of intestinal colonization by Escherichia coli in mice.* Appl Environ Microbiol, 2010. **76**(1): p. 264-74.
127. Wang, L., et al., *The Chlamydia muridarum Organisms Fail to Auto-Inoculate the Mouse Genital Tract after Colonization in the Gastrointestinal Tract for 70 days.* PLoS One, 2016. **11**(5): p. e0155880.
128. Mason, K.M., R.S. Munson, Jr., and L.O. Bakaletz, *Nontypeable Haemophilus influenzae gene expression induced in vivo in a chinchilla model of otitis media.* Infect Immun, 2003. **71**(6): p. 3454-62.

129. Bookwalter, J.E., et al., *A carcinoembryonic antigen-related cell adhesion molecule 1 homologue plays a pivotal role in nontypeable Haemophilus influenzae colonization of the chinchilla nasopharynx via the outer membrane protein P5-homologous adhesin.* Infect Immun, 2008. **76**(1): p. 48-55.
130. Ratet, G., et al., *Live imaging of bioluminescent leptospira interrogans in mice reveals renal colonization as a stealth escape from the blood defenses and antibiotics.* PLoS Negl Trop Dis, 2014. **8**(12): p. e3359.
131. Sjolinder, H. and A.B. Jonsson, *Imaging of disease dynamics during meningococcal sepsis.* PLoS One, 2007. **2**(2): p. e241.
132. Kadurugamuwa, J.L., et al., *Noninvasive biophotonic imaging for monitoring of catheter-associated urinary tract infections and therapy in mice.* Infect Immun, 2005. **73**(7): p. 3878-87.
133. Burkatovskaya, M., et al., *Use of chitosan bandage to prevent fatal infections developing from highly contaminated wounds in mice.* Biomaterials, 2006. **27**(22): p. 4157-64.
134. Hamrahi, V., et al., *Gram-negative bacterial infection in thigh abscess can migrate to distant burn depending on burn depth.* Interdiscip Perspect Infect Dis, 2012. **2012**: p. 567140.
135. BitMansour, A., et al., *Myeloid progenitors protect against invasive aspergillosis and Pseudomonas aeruginosa infection following hematopoietic stem cell transplantation.* Blood, 2002. **100**(13): p. 4660-7.
136. Ramphal, R., et al., *Control of Pseudomonas aeruginosa in the lung requires the recognition of either lipopolysaccharide or flagellin.* J Immunol, 2008. **181**(1): p. 586-92.
137. Munder, A., et al., *In vivo imaging of bioluminescent Pseudomonas aeruginosa in an acute murine airway infection model.* Pathog Dis, 2014. **72**(1): p. 74-7.
138. Sedgley, C., et al., *Real-time imaging and quantification of bioluminescent bacteria in root canals in vitro.* J Endod, 2004. **30**(12): p. 893-8.
139. Sedgley, C.M., et al., *Influence of irrigant needle depth in removing bioluminescent bacteria inoculated into instrumented root canals using real-time imaging in vitro.* Int Endod J, 2005. **38**(2): p. 97-104.
140. Brovko, L.Y., et al., *In vivo assessment of effect of fermented milk diet on course of infection in mice with bioluminescent Salmonella.* J Food Prot, 2003. **66**(11): p. 2160-3.
141. Heuts, F., et al., *Use of non-invasive bioluminescent imaging to assess mycobacterial dissemination in mice, treatment with bactericidal drugs and protective immunity.* Microbes Infect, 2009. **11**(14-15): p. 1114-21.
142. Andreu, N., et al., *Optimisation of bioluminescent reporters for use with mycobacteria.* PLoS One, 2010. **5**(5): p. e10777.
143. Andreu, N., et al., *Rapid in vivo assessment of drug efficacy against Mycobacterium tuberculosis using an improved firefly luciferase.* J Antimicrob Chemother, 2013. **68**(9): p. 2118-27.
144. Wager, B., et al., *BB0744 Affects Tissue Tropism and Spatial Distribution of Borrelia burgdorferi.* Infect Immun, 2015. **83**(9): p. 3693-703.
145. Asgharpour, A., et al., *Resistance to intestinal Entamoeba histolytica infection is conferred by innate immunity and Gr-1+ cells.* Infect Immun, 2005. **73**(8): p. 4522-9.
146. Lang, T., et al., *Bioluminescent Leishmania expressing luciferase for rapid and high throughput screening of drugs acting on amastigote-harbouring macrophages and for quantitative real-time monitoring of parasitism features in living mice.* Cell Microbiol, 2005. **7**(3): p. 383-92.
147. Giraud, E., et al., *A combined luciferase-expressing Leishmania imaging/RT-qPCR assay provides new insights into the sequential bilateral processes deployed in the ear pinna of C57BL/6 mice.* Parasitol Int, 2014. **63**(1): p. 245-53.
148. Lecoeur, H., et al., *Optimization of topical therapy for Leishmania major localized cutaneous leishmaniasis using a reliable C57BL/6 Model.* PLoS Negl Trop Dis, 2007. **1**(2): p. e34.
149. Lecoeur, H., et al., *Early curative applications of the aminoglycoside WR279396 on an experimental Leishmania major-loaded cutaneous site do not impair the acquisition of immunity.* Antimicrob Agents Chemother, 2010. **54**(3): p. 984-90.

150. Franke-Fayard, B., et al., *Murine malaria parasite sequestration: CD36 is the major receptor, but cerebral pathology is unlinked to sequestration.* Proc Natl Acad Sci U S A, 2005. **102**(32): p. 11468-73.
151. Spaccapelo, R., et al., *Plasmepsin 4-deficient Plasmodium berghei are virulence attenuated and induce protective immunity against experimental malaria.* Am J Pathol, 2010. **176**(1): p. 205-17.
152. Pittman, K.J., M.T. Aliota, and L.J. Knoll, *Dual transcriptional profiling of mice and Toxoplasma gondii during acute and chronic infection.* BMC Genomics, 2014. **15**: p. 806.
153. Hitziger, N., et al., *Dissemination of Toxoplasma gondii to immunoprivileged organs and role of Toll/interleukin-1 receptor signalling for host resistance assessed by in vivo bioluminescence imaging.* Cell Microbiol, 2005. **7**(6): p. 837-48.
154. Di Cristina, M., et al., *Temporal and spatial distribution of Toxoplasma gondii differentiation into Bradyzoites and tissue cyst formation in vivo.* Infect Immun, 2008. **76**(8): p. 3491-501.
155. Claes, F., et al., *Bioluminescent imaging of Trypanosoma brucei shows preferential testis dissemination which may hamper drug efficacy in sleeping sickness.* PLoS Negl Trop Dis, 2009. **3**(7): p. e486.
156. Vodnala, S.K., et al., *Preclinical assessment of the treatment of second-stage African trypanosomiasis with cordycepin and deoxycoformycin.* PLoS Negl Trop Dis, 2009. **3**(8): p. e495.
157. Summers, B.C. and D.A. Leib, *Herpes simplex virus type 1 origins of DNA replication play no role in the regulation of flanking promoters.* J Virol, 2002. **76**(14): p. 7020-9.
158. Pasieka, T.J., et al., *Bioluminescent imaging reveals divergent viral pathogenesis in two strains of Stat1-deficient mice, and in alphassgamma interferon receptor-deficient mice.* PLoS One, 2011. **6**(9): p. e24018.
159. Murphy, A.A., et al., *Synergistic control of herpes simplex virus pathogenesis by IRF-3, and IRF-7 revealed through non-invasive bioluminescence imaging.* Virology, 2013. **444**(1-2): p. 71-9.
160. Boutier, M., et al., *Rational development of an attenuated recombinant cyprinid herpesvirus 3 vaccine using prokaryotic mutagenesis and in vivo bioluminescent imaging.* PLoS Pathog, 2015. **11**(2): p. e1004690.
161. Costes, B., et al., *The major portal of entry of koi herpesvirus in Cyprinus carpio is the skin.* J Virol, 2009. **83**(7): p. 2819-30.
162. Falendysz, E.A., et al., *Evaluation of monkeypox virus infection of black-tailed prairie dogs (Cynomys ludovicianus) using in vivo bioluminescent imaging.* J Wildl Dis, 2014. **50**(3): p. 524-36.
163. Osorio, J.E., et al., *Comparison of monkeypox viruses pathogenesis in mice by in vivo imaging.* PLoS One, 2009. **4**(8): p. e6592.
164. Marquardt, A., et al., *Single cell detection of latent cytomegalovirus reactivation in host tissue.* J Gen Virol, 2011. **92**(Pt 6): p. 1279-91.
165. Hwang, S., et al., *Persistent gammaherpesvirus replication and dynamic interaction with the host in vivo.* J Virol, 2008. **82**(24): p. 12498-509.
166. Reese, T.A., et al., *Helminth infection reactivates latent gamma-herpesvirus via cytokine competition at a viral promoter.* Science, 2014. **345**(6196): p. 573-7.
167. Jia, Q., et al., *Induction of protective immunity against murine gammaherpesvirus 68 infection in the absence of viral latency.* J Virol, 2010. **84**(5): p. 2453-65.
168. Gill, M.B., et al., *Murid herpesvirus-4 lacking thymidine kinase reveals route-dependent requirements for host colonization.* J Gen Virol, 2009. **90**(Pt 6): p. 1461-70.
169. Rivera, R., et al., *Murine alveolar macrophages limit replication of vaccinia virus.* Virology, 2007. **363**(1): p. 48-58.
170. Zhang, Z., et al., *Genetic analysis of varicella-zoster virus ORF0 to ORF4 by use of a novel luciferase bacterial artificial chromosome system.* J Virol, 2007. **81**(17): p. 9024-33.
171. Zhang, Z., et al., *Genome-wide mutagenesis reveals that ORF7 is a novel VZV skin-tropic factor.* PLoS Pathog, 2010. **6**: p. e1000971.

172. Zhang, Z., Y. Huang, and H. Zhu, *A highly efficient protocol of generating and analyzing VZV ORF deletion mutants based on a newly developed luciferase VZV BAC system.* J Virol Methods, 2008. **148**(1-2): p. 197-204.
173. Li, X.F., et al., *Noninvasive bioluminescence imaging of dengue virus infection in the brain of A129 mice.* Appl Microbiol Biotechnol, 2013. **97**(10): p. 4589-96.
174. Schoggins, J.W., et al., *Dengue reporter viruses reveal viral dynamics in interferon receptor-deficient mice and sensitivity to interferon effectors in vitro.* Proc Natl Acad Sci U S A, 2012. **109**(36): p. 14610-5.
175. Uebelhoer, L.S., et al., *High-throughput, luciferase-based reverse genetics systems for identifying inhibitors of Marburg and Ebola viruses.* Antiviral Res, 2014. **106**: p. 86-94.
176. Phillips, A.T., et al., *Entry Sites of Venezuelan and Western Equine Encephalitis Viruses in the Mouse Central Nervous System following Peripheral Infection.* J Virol, 2016. **90**(12): p. 5785-96.
177. Gardner, C.L., et al., *Eastern and Venezuelan equine encephalitis viruses differ in their ability to infect dendritic cells and macrophages: impact of altered cell tropism on pathogenesis.* J Virol, 2008. **82**(21): p. 10634-46.
178. Harmache, A., et al., *Bioluminescence imaging of live infected salmonids reveals that the fin bases are the major portal of entry for Novirhabdovirus.* J Virol, 2006. **80**(7): p. 3655-9.
179. Heaton, N.S., et al., *In vivo bioluminescent imaging of influenza a virus infection and characterization of novel cross-protective monoclonal antibodies.* J Virol, 2013. **87**(15): p. 8272-81.
180. Tran, V., et al., *Highly sensitive real-time in vivo imaging of an influenza reporter virus reveals dynamics of replication and spread.* J Virol, 2013. **87**(24): p. 13321-9.
181. Burke, C.W., et al., *Relationships among dissemination of primary parainfluenza virus infection in the respiratory tract, mucosal and peripheral immune responses, and protection from reinfection: a noninvasive bioluminescence-imaging study.* J Virol, 2015. **89**(7): p. 3568-83.
182. Miyahira, A.K., et al., *TANK-binding kinase-1 plays an important role during in vitro and in vivo type I IFN responses to DNA virus infections.* J Immunol, 2009. **182**(4): p. 2248-57.
183. Stelter, L., et al., *Tumor-specific targeting with modified Sindbis viral vectors: evaluation with optical imaging and positron emission tomography in vivo.* Mol Imaging Biol, 2013. **15**(2): p. 166-74.
184. Tseng, J.C., et al., *Systemic tumor targeting and killing by Sindbis viral vectors.* Nat Biotechnol, 2004. **22**(1): p. 70-7.

Chapter 4
Radiochemistry

Thomas Ebenhan, Carl Wagener, Lauren E. Bambarger, Alvin S. Kalinda, and Jan Rijn Zeevaart

4.1 Introduction

Radiochemistry is the science that encompasses the production, separation, and purification of radionuclides, as well as the synthesis of radiolabeled compounds for biochemical or biological research. Commercial radiochemistry uses radionuclides in the synthesis of radiopharmaceuticals for clinical diagnostic studies or therapy. Inorganic chemistry, and especially coordination chemistry, is the basis for labeling methodologies to produce the metal-based radiopharmaceuticals such as those labeled with ^{99m}Tc, ^{64}Cu, ^{67}Ga, ^{68}Ga, and ^{111}In. Organic chemistry provides the foundation for the development of radiopharmaceuticals labeled with ^{123}I, ^{124}I, ^{18}F, ^{11}C, and others.

In contrast to "conventional" chemistry, radiochemical reactions are accomplished using very small amounts of the radionuclides. For instance, the concentration of ^{18}F-fluoride in a typical radiolabeling reaction is in the range of parts per trillion. Such a small number of atoms can alter the expected behavior of a reaction. There are also practical considerations when using very small amounts of radionuclides, such as the risk of having a significant proportion of a radionuclide sample adsorbed onto the reaction glassware. The successful application of radiochemical

T. Ebenhan
Department of Nuclear Medicine, Steve Biko Academic Hospital, University of Pretoria, Pretoria, South Africa

C. Wagener • J.R. Zeevaart (✉)
Radiochemistry Group, Department of Applied Chemistry, South African Nuclear Energy Corporation SOC Limited, Pelindaba, South Africa
e-mail: janrijn.zeevaart@necsa.co.za

L.E. Bambarger • A.S. Kalinda
Department of Pediatrics, Johns Hopkins University School of Medicine, Baltimore, MD, USA

Center for Infection and Inflammation Imaging Research, Johns Hopkins University School of Medicine, Baltimore, MD, USA

S.K. Jain (ed.), *Imaging Infections*, DOI 10.1007/978-3-319-54592-9_4

Table 4.1 Characteristics of selected SPECT and PET radionuclides

Radionuclide	Half-life (h)	Radiation	Abundance (%)	$Energy_{max}$ (keV)	Preferred production method(s)
^{99m}Tc	6.0	γ	86	140	$^{99}Mo/^{99m}Tc$ generator
^{123}I	13.2	γ	83	159	Cyclotron $^{124}Te(p, 2n)^{123}I$
^{111}In	67.3	γ	90, 94	173, 247	Cyclotron $^{111}Cd(p, n)^{111}In$
^{67}Ga	78.3	γ	3, 36, 20, 15, 5	91, 93, 185, 300, 393	Cyclotron $^{68}Zn(p, 2n)^{67}Ga$ $^{67}Zn(p, n)^{67}Ga$
^{125}I	1425.6	γ	7	35	Nuclear reactor $^{124}Xe(n,\gamma)\ ^{125}I$
^{11}C	0.34	β^+	100	961	Cyclotron $^{14}N(p,\alpha)^{11}C$
^{68}Ga	1.1	β^+	89, 1	1899, 822	$^{68}Ge/^{68}Ga$ generator
^{18}F	1.83	β^+	97	634	Cyclotron $^{18}O(p, n)^{18}F$
^{64}Cu	12.7	β^+	17	653	Cyclotron $^{64}Ni(p, n)^{64}Cu$
^{124}I	100.8	β^+	23	2100	Cyclotron $^{124}Te(d,2n)^{124}I$

techniques requires painstaking attention to detail and lots of practice. Furthermore, there is the need to comply with the regulations regarding the safe handling of radioactive material. In 2004, ^{18}F-2-fluoro-deoxy-D-glucose (^{18}F-FDG) was introduced to clinics in an era that coincided with regulatory efforts to achieve global good manufacturing practice (GMP) harmonization.

Nuclear studies employ two imaging modalities, namely, single photon emission computed tomography (SPECT) and positron emission tomography (PET). SPECT and PET utilize gamma-emitting radionuclides or positron-emitting radionuclides respectively for the generation of the signal that makes possible the imaging of physiological and pathological processes in the body. Both modalities are often combined with computed tomography (CT) or magnetic resonance imaging (MRI) for anatomic reference. The radionuclides commonly used for the synthesis of imaging agents are listed in Table 4.1.

4.2 Radionuclides

In order to label with a radionuclide, the chemical properties of the nuclide must be considered: a highly efficient radiolabeling method is needed, yielding a radiopharmaceutical that is chemically and radiochemically pure or can easily be purified.

The radiopharmaceutical must be sufficiently stable in vitro and in vivo, must be nontoxic at concentrations used, and must find the target as intended. Some of the radiolabeling chemistries that can be identified for the production of infection imaging agents are discussed below.

4.2.1 Iodine Radionuclides

Radioiodine has been called a cornerstone in nuclear medicine, as the free radionuclide was the first to be used in imaging and in therapy. As a result of their well-defined chemistry and availability, radioiodine nuclides have been employed often in the development of radiopharmaceuticals, even ones that ultimately do not use a radioiodine nuclide [1]. Iodine-123 (^{123}I) has a half-life of 13.2 h and commonly produced by the $^{124}Te(p, 2n)^{123}I$ reaction on highly enriched ^{124}Te [2].

Iodine-124 (^{124}I) has a half-life of 4.2 days and has usually been produced by the $^{124}Te(d,2n)^{124}I$ nuclear reaction scheme [3]. As low-energy proton cyclotrons became more available, the $^{124}Te(p,n)^{124}I$ reaction has gained ground because it also leads to the highest levels of ^{124}I purity. It is important that the ^{124}Te target is highly enriched to minimize the competing $^{124}Te(p,2n)^{123}I$ and $^{124}Te(d,n)^{125}I$ reactions. During irradiation of the target, the probability for the competing reactions is a function of the irradiation energy. The energy window must be carefully selected to minimize impurities, typically resulting in a trade-off between purity and yield. Iodine-125 (^{125}I) has a half-life of 59.4 days. ^{125}I is produced in nuclear reactors by the reaction $^{124}Xe(n,\gamma)^{125}I$. Both wet chemical and dry distillation methods are known to isolate the ^{125}I isotope [4]. The iodide anion can easily be oxidized to electrophilic iodine. Therefore electrophilic substitution reactions with high specific activity iodine are commonly used for radioiodine labeling. The C–I bond is weaker than the C–F bond and can be cleaved easier in vivo, which is a disadvantage of radioiodine compared with radiofluorine. Aromatic C–I bonds are stronger than aliphatic bonds and are preferred. Radioiodine is usually supplied in the iodide form and is then oxidized in situ by agents such as peracetic acid, chloroamine-T, and *N*-chlorosuccinimide. The electrophilic substitution reaction is mainly achieved by de-metalytion, such as de-stannalytion, which works well even for deactivated aromatic rings [1]. When the aromatic ring is activated, direct electrophilic substitution can be employed such as in the synthesis of ^{125}I-iodo-DPA-713 (Figure 4.1) [5]. Direct electrophilic substitution is also used to radiolabel proteins. Briefly, the radioiodine and the protein to be labeled are added to a mild oxidant, such as iodogen, and the reaction mixture is incubated for a few minutes after which purification is accomplished by HPLC [6]. It is also possible to directly label peptides with oxidized iodide, provided a tyrosine residue is present. For the labeling of small molecules, an isotope exchange reaction, a nucleophilic substitution reaction, can be performed as long as a high specific activity product is not required [1, 6]. Radiolabeling with iodine is done manually, and special care should be taken to avoid contamination and to protect against personal radiation exposure.

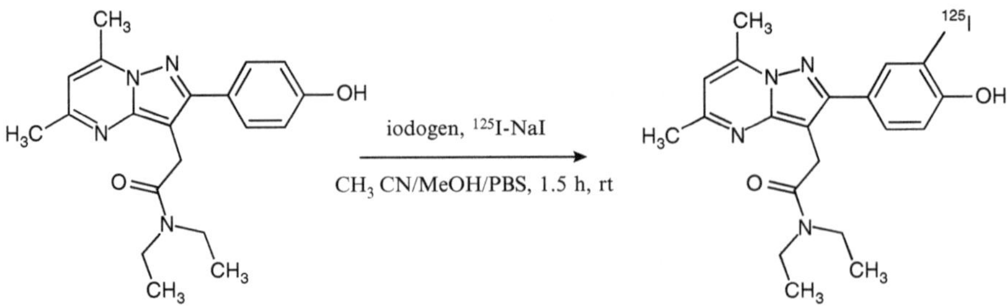

Figure 4.1 Labeling step of ^{125}I-iodo-DPA-713 synthesis [5]

4.2.2 Carbon-11 (C-11, ^{11}C)

C-11 is produced in a cyclotron target by the $^{14}N(p,\alpha)^{11}C$ reaction and has a half-life of 0.34 h. Depending on whether a trace of oxygen or a trace of hydrogen has been deliberately added to the target, $^{11}CO_2$ or $^{11}CH_4$ is then formed in situ [7]. These gases can already be used in labeling reactions, but it is more common to convert them to a large array of more reactive synthons such as $^{11}CH_3I$, $^{11}CH_3OTf$, ^{11}CO, $H^{11}CN$, or $^{11}COCl_2$ [8, 9]. The most common labeling reactions involve $^{11}CH_3I$ or $^{11}CH_3OTf$ in methylation reactions [10]. So, for example, $^{11}CH_3I$ or $H^{11}CN$ was used to radiolabel the frontline tuberculosis drugs rifampicin, isoniazid, and pyrazinamide in order to collect pharmacokinetic and drug distribution data in baboons [11]. As is shown with this example, a major advantage of ^{11}C chemistry is that radiopharmaceuticals can be produced that are identical to their "cold" counterparts. A disadvantage is the short half-life of ^{11}C which necessitate a cyclotron on the hospital site and quick labeling procedures. The short half-life of ^{11}C is also not always compatible with biological processes. More information on ^{11}C-radiochemistry has been reviewed by Scott et al. 2009 [8]. As an example, PET/CT imaging using ^{11}C-PK11195 ((R)-*N*-methyl-*N*-(1-methylpropyl)-1-(2-chlorophenyl)isoquinoline-3-carboxamide) has been successfully applied in a variety of neurological disorders including in patients with viral encephalitis [6].

4.2.3 Fluorine-18 (F-18, ^{18}F)

F-18 has a half-life of 109.8 min and there are more than 20 ways to produce ^{18}F. For ^{18}F-fluoride, the most effective method is to use the $^{18}O(p,n)^{18}F$ reaction on ^{18}O-enriched water and yields high specific activity ^{18}F. For electrophilic radiolabeling, $^{18}F\text{-}F_2$ is needed and either $^{18}O_2$ or ^{20}Ne gas targets can be used, with the $^{20}Ne(d,\alpha)^{18}F$ reaction considered to be the most practical, but only yields low specific activity radiofluorine. In both cases, the produced ^{18}F is adsorbed on the walls of the target and nonradioactive (cold) fluorine gas must be added so that $^{18}F\text{-}F_2$ can be recovered [12]. The chemistry of ^{18}F-fluoride has been reviewed often [13].

Typically, radiolabeling with ^{18}F-fluoride employs a metal/fluoride salt, typically K^+ ^{18}F-F^-, in nucleophilic substitution reactions. Electrophilic substitutions can also be carried out using ^{18}F-F_2 (^{18}F-^{19}F) [14]. Difluorine is a highly reactive gas making it difficult to selectively fluorinate a specific position on a precursor molecule. Because each ^{18}F-F_2 molecule contains a cold ^{19}F atom and cold ^{19}F-F_2 is added as a carrier to extract the ^{18}F-F_2 from the target, radiolabeling invariably leads to products with low specific activity. The development of less reactive equivalents of electrophilic ^{18}F-F_2, such as ^{18}F-Selectfluor and *N*-^{18}F-fluoro-benzenesulfonamide, can overcome the reactivity and selectivity drawbacks, but high specific activity products remain elusive. Nucleophilic substitution reactions are therefore preferred, although electrophilic reactions have certainly been of historical value and are still employed, for example, in the production of ^{18}F-L-dihydroxyphenylalanine (^{18}F-DOPA) [15].

The most common nucleophilic ^{18}F labeling procedure, called direct labeling, starts with receiving ^{18}F-fluoride dissolved in ^{18}O-enriched water from a cyclotron. The ^{18}F anions are then trapped on an ion exchange resin, usually using a solid phase extraction (SPE) cartridge. This step enables the isolation of the ^{18}F anion for later solubilization in an organic solvent, as the ^{18}O-enriched water and unwanted cations, including radioactive metals, are not retained by the resin [13]. Then, typically, the ^{18}F anion is eluted into a reactor by an aqueous weak base, such as potassium carbonate. An amino-polyether cryptand (Kryptofix 2.2.2) is usually delivered to the reactor by dissolving in the eluent. Thereafter, the reactor contents are thoroughly dried by adding the aprotic acetonitrile a number of times and removing the water by heating in an azeotropic distillation. The presence of any water or free protons will form the hydrogen fluoride species and renders the fluoride anion unreactive for nucleophilic substitution, hence the importance of introducing the base and the need to rigorously dry the reaction mixture. After drying, a solution of the precursor in the reaction solvent (typically between 1 and 5 mL of acetonitrile or DMSO) is added to the fluorine and chelator mixture. ^{18}F labeling reactions are accomplished non-stochiometrically with a huge excess (approximately 3000 fold) of the dissolved precursor, heated usually at >90 °C for about 10 min with ^{18}F-fluoride (in the picogram range). The huge excess of reagents, compared to the amount of ^{18}F-fluoride present, is necessary to ensure the shortest possible reaction time and compromises the chemical purity of the product. The impurities, consisting of reagents and by-products, must be removed, usually by a semi-preparative high-performance liquid chromatography (HPLC) separation, prior to use in biological or molecular imaging. Finally, the HPLC eluent must be removed, typically using solid phase extraction (SPE), before the product is reconstituted in a physiologically acceptable medium, such as 0.9% saline. It is sometimes possible to replace the HPLC purification with a simpler, cheaper, and faster SPE method usually involving a number of SPE cartridges. Distillation is also sometimes used to separate a volatile ^{18}F-labeled compound from the reaction mixture [13].

A classic example of direct labeling is the synthesis of ^{18}F-FDG, a radiopharmaceutical that is, inter alia, extensively used for infection imaging. Provided the precursor is fitted with a suitable leaving group, is not sensitive to base, and is thermally stable, the nucleophilic substitution reactions on aliphatic and heterocyclic

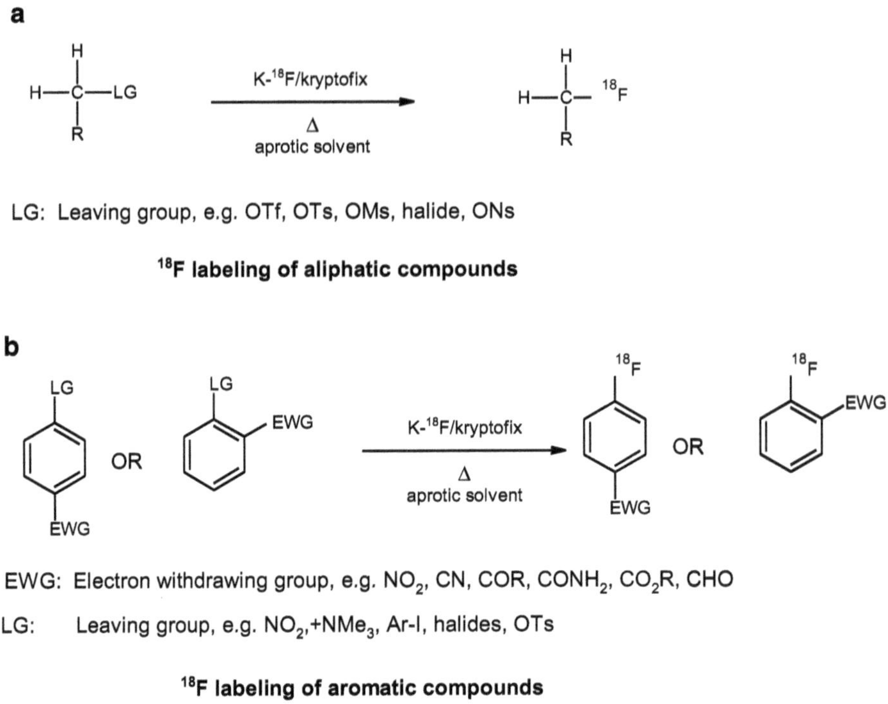

Figure 4.2 Scheme suggesting generic direct labeling procedures with ^{18}F of (**a**) aliphatic or (**b**) aromatic compounds [13]

small molecules proceed well (Figure 4.2a) [13]. The synthesis is more challenging if the ^{18}F radiolabel is needed on an aromatic ring. In this case, in addition to the aforementioned provisions, an electron withdrawing group is needed in the position para and/or ortho to the labeling position (Figure 4.2b). The radiolabeling of electron-rich arenes used to be difficult, if not impossible, to achieve using nucleophilic substitution reactions. To increase the scope of aromatic substitution reactions, the use of diaryliodonium salts as radiolabeling precursors was developed. In some instances, even electron-rich arenes could be radiolabeled [16]. More recently, palladium-assisted fluorinations were developed by effectively transforming ^{18}F-fluoride into an electrophilic reagent, enabling ^{18}F radiolabeling of electron-rich arenes [17]. A copper-mediated nucleophilic ^{18}F fluorination of aryl boronic esters that worked for both electron-poor and electron-rich arenes was also developed [18]. Starting with a precursor, there is often more than one reaction step necessary to yield the desired ^{18}F-labeled radiopharmaceutical. Another common practice is removing protecting groups in a post labeling step, as for the ^{18}F-Flutemetamol production [19]. The short half-life of ^{18}F and the demands of a high specific activity product dictate that the radiolabeling step must be as close as possible to the last step in a multistep procedure in order to achieve reasonable radio and chemical yields.

The high temperatures and basic conditions necessary for direct ^{18}F labeling on carbon usually lead to unwanted by-products. Direct radiolabeling is also not suitable for temperature and pH-sensitive biomolecule precursors, such as peptides. The presence of acidic groups on biomolecules, such as peptides, also renders ^{18}F-fluoride inactive for nucleophilic substitution on carbon [20]. The need for radiolabeled biomolecules is ever increasing, especially in the field of infection imaging, and indirect radiolabeling strategies must be employed to produce them effectively. In the *prosthetic group approach*, the radiolabel is attached using the direct methodology to a so-called prosthetic group, which is subsequently joined to a sensitive biomolecule [14]. The prosthetic group must have two reactive sites: one for the ^{18}F substitution and one for the subsequent coupling. This usually requires the protection of the second reactive site, which implies a subsequent deprotection step. After radiolabeling, the prosthetic group is purified before coupling to the biomolecule. The coupling can be achieved in numerous ways, such as acylation, oxime ligation, and thiol-alkylation; reviews by Kuhnast et al. [21] and Liu et al. [22] provide further detailed information on coupling. A specific example of the prosthetic group approach is the "click" chemistry approach which is often used to join the prosthetic group to the biomolecule [20, 23–27]. The Huisgen 1,3-dipolar cycloaddition of terminal alkynes and azides under Cu(I) catalysis is an often used procedure, as in the production of nanoparticles [28], which might become relevant for future infection imaging [29]. To avoid cytotoxic copper, metal-free reactions have also gained ground [23]. This is evidenced in the way the Staudinger ligation couples the ^{18}F labeled prosthetic group [30, 31]. A drawback of the prosthetic group method is that another reaction step, along with possible deprotection, is introduced after the initial ^{18}F radiolabeling step thereby increasing synthesis duration and equipment requirements.

Silicon, aluminum, and boron all form strong bonds with fluorine. For example, the bonding energy for the Si-F bond is 565 kJ mol^{-1} as compared to the 485 kJ mol^{-1} bonding energy of C-F [32]. The bonding energy for Al-F is 670 kJ mol^{-1} [33]. The high affinity of Si, Al, and B for F is at the heart of the so-called ^{18}F-fluoride acceptor chemistry. ^{18}F-Fluoride acceptor chemistry represents methodologies that have been developed to mitigate the drawbacks of the direct labeling method (i.e., high reaction temperatures) and the prosthetic group approach (i.e., multiple reaction steps). *Silicon-fluoride-acceptor (SiFA) procedures* rely on the strong Si-F bond and the more facile nucleophilic substitution at the silicon atom of organosilanes as compared to organo-carbons [32]. There are two distinct preparation methods as schematically shown using peptide radiolabeling in Figure 4.3. *Firstly*, isotope exchange may be used to displace ^{19}F with ^{18}F on a silicon atom. This procedure allows for direct labeling as the reaction proceeds under mild conditions (room temperature and below) in dipolar aprotic solvents (Figure 4.3a). As Si-F bond formation is fast compared to C-F bond formation, only microgram amounts of precursor are used to yield high specific activity products. As the precursor and product is chemically identical, and furthermore as there are no unwanted by-products courtesy of the mild reaction conditions, there is less of a need for exhaustive purification, with SPE purification being sufficient [32]. The SiFA procedure is also applied

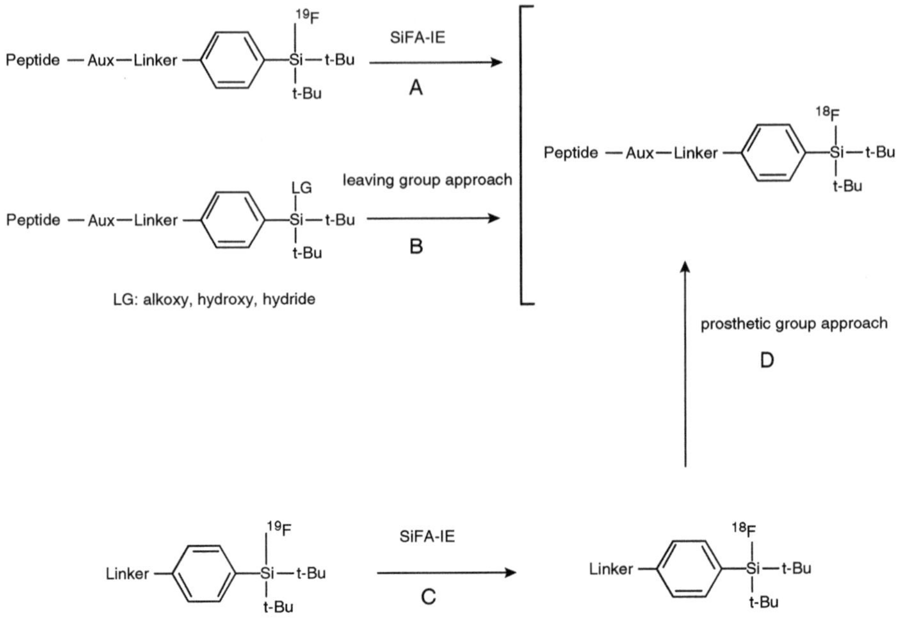

Figure 4.3 Scheme showing generic SiFA labeling procedures for peptides with (**a**) isotope exchange (IE), (**b**) leaving group (LG) approach, and (**c**) IE followed by (**d**) a prosthetic group approach

to label proteins and small molecules due to the mild reaction conditions. An example is the synthesis at room temperature of a SiFA-derivatized Tyr3-octreotate [34]. The quick production of cleaner and higher specific activity labeled Si compounds also allows for the joining of a prosthetic group after the SiFA-IE step (Figure 4.3c, d). For example, ^{18}F-SiFA-isothiocyanate was used to synthesize various radiolabeled model proteins such as rat serum albumin and apo-transferrin [35]. *Secondly*, a leaving group other than ^{19}F on the silicon atom is to be replaced by ^{18}F (Figure 4.3b). The approach was initially considered by groups such as Choudhry et al. in 2006 [36]. Currently, this method requires higher reaction temperatures leading to more impurities, making HPLC purification mandatory, and the elevated temperatures render it less attractive for the direct radiolabeling of biomolecules. To ensure the in vivo stability of the labeled SiFA molecules, it is a prerequisite that the Si is bonded to two bulky groups, such as the *t-Bu*-group, with the fourth position usually occupied by an aryl linker. Bulky groups increase the lipophilicity of the compound and may compromise the tracer pharmacokinetics during PET imaging. For this reason, lipophilicity-reducing auxiliaries are sometimes introduced between the linker and the biomolecule. To date, SiFA procedures have not been reported with a human clinical application [32]. Fluorine binds strongly to not only silicon but also to other metals, particular to aluminum; the *aluminum-fluoride* $(AlF)^{2+}$ *acceptor method* requires a crucial pH of 4; otherwise hydroxides (at higher pH) and HF (at lower pH) are dominant. Thus, $(Al^{18}F)^{2+}$ can be complexed to macrocyclic chelators

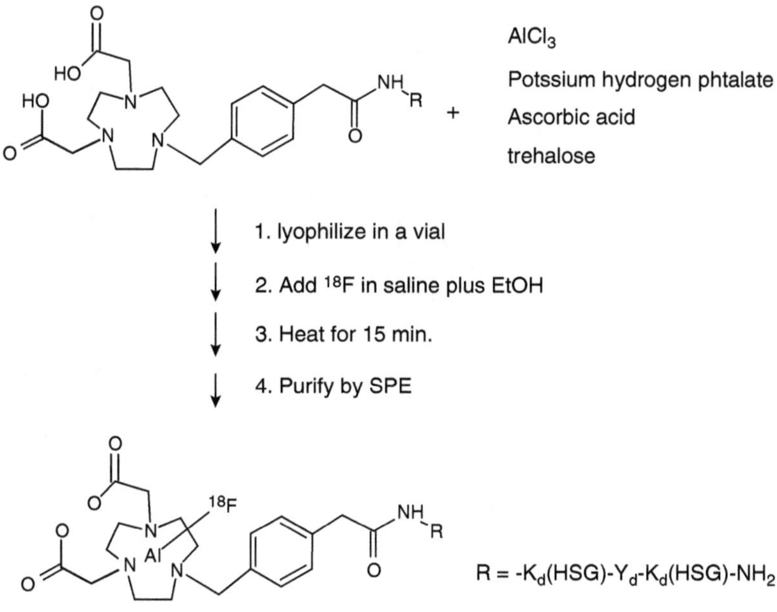

Figure 4.4 Example of a kit-like production for a NODA-MPAA-linked peptide [37]

linked to peptides and proteins. In this regard, McBride et al. have reviewed their work and those of others [33]. Initially using the 1,4,7-triazacyclononane-1,4,7-triacetic acid (NOTA) chelator and derivatives, peptides were successfully labeled by mixing acetate buffer, $AlCl_3$, purified aqueous ^{18}F-fluoride, and the chelator-functionalized peptide at 100 °C for 15 min. HPLC purification was not always necessary. The pentadentate 1,4,7-triazacyclononane-1,4-diacetate (NODA) chelator attached to a methyl phenylacetic acid group (MPAA) improved the $(Al^{18}F)^{2+}$ radiolabeling methodology. McBride et al. found that the NODA-MPAA-linked peptides could be formulated in a lyophilized kit and labeled at 100–110 °C in 15 min (Figure 4.4), followed by a rapid SPE purification step. Notable is the aqueous conditions, disposing of the need for rigorous ^{18}F-fluoride drying [37]. In areas where pharmaceutical grade ^{18}F-fluoride in saline for bone imaging is available, there is the advantage that the ^{18}F-fluoride can be used without further purification. A lyophilized kit was used to produce the integrin targeting ^{18}F-AlF^{2+}-NOTA-PRGD2 (^{18}F-alfatide) for PET evaluation studies in eight human patients with lung cancer and one patient with tuberculosis (TB) [38]. The high reaction temperatures needed for this direct radiolabeling procedure is unsuitable for the radiolabeling of many peptides and all proteins. McBride et al. also developed a two-step (prosthetic group) approach to radiolabel a protein [39].

The strong B-F bond and the relative ease of replacing nonradioactive fluorine with ^{18}F are exploited with the so-called Boron-fluoride-acceptor methodology [40]. An arylboronic ester or acid or a derivative thereof can be used to capture aqueous ^{18}F-fluoride in one step at room temperature. Biotinyl-ArB^{18}F-$^{19}F_2$ was synthesized

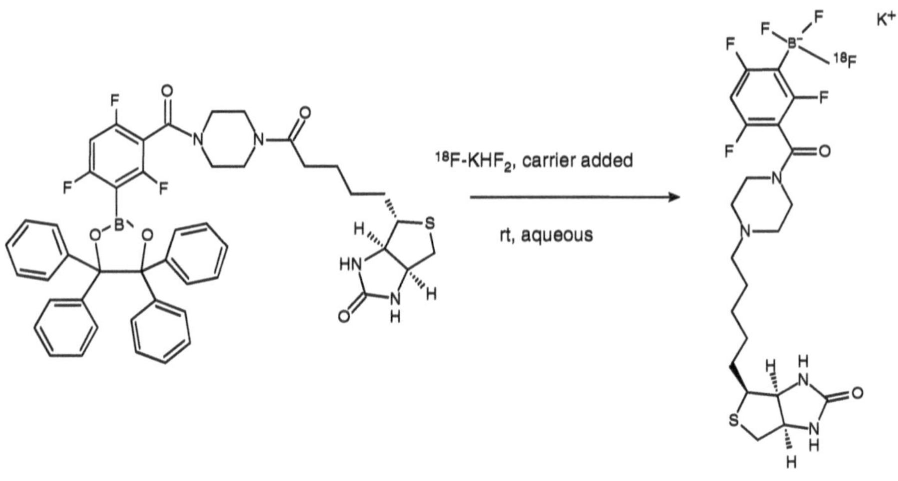

Figure 4.5 Preparation of biotinyl-ArB^{18}F-F$_2$ [40]

using this method (Figure 4.5). Alternatively, the conjugation can be done first with octreotate, as with the conjugation of ammoniomethyl-BF_3, followed by the addition of ^{18}F-fluoride in an isotope exchange reaction at 80 °C [41]. Advantages of the boron-fluoride approach are its suitability for aqueous media with nanomolar amounts of precursor, yielding a high specific activity product. The trifluoroborate anion is highly polar, and therefore hydrophilic, and reacts in the temperature range of 40–80 °C. Disadvantages are the acidic pH (2–3) needed (leading to biomolecule incompatibility) and the low reaction volumes (up to about 100 μL).

4.2.4 Technetium-99m (Tc-99m, ^{99m}Tc)

Tc-99m was discovered in 1938 as a medicinal radioisotope by Segré and Seaborg [42]. At present, ^{99m}Tc is without doubt one of the most utilized and valuable medical isotopes in modern nuclear medicine for two main reasons. Firstly, ^{99m}Tc has a half-life of approximately 6 h and decays almost exclusively (>98%) via the emission of 140 keV γ-rays that are readily detected by commercially available γ-cameras for SPECT applications. Secondly, because ^{99m}Tc is such a widely used isotope, it is affordable and accessible on a global scale [43]. The synthesis of ^{99m}Tc starts with the isolation of molybdenum-99 (^{99}Mo) [44]. ^{99}Mo is a fission product of the neutron bombardment of uranium-235 (^{235}U) fuel in a nuclear reactor and isolated in the form of the molybdate (MoO_4^{2-}) [45]. As ^{99}Mo decays, it yields the metastable clinical radioisotope, ^{99m}Tc [46]. Ion exchange chromatography is used to separate the MoO_4^{2-} from its decay product ^{99m}Tc pertechnetate ($^{99m}TcO_4^-$). During this process $^{99}MoO_4^{2-}$ is loaded onto an acidic (pH = 5) alumina (Al_2O_3) column contained in a shielded and mobile vessel called a "technetium cow." This allows for facile and rapid distribution of the radioisotope. As ^{99}Mo decays on the alumina column, $^{99m}TcO_4^-$ is produced. As a result of its singular charge, $^{99m}TcO_4^-$ has less affinity for the acidic alumina. Consequently, as the alumina column is eluted with saline solution, a process called "milking," $^{99m}TcO_4^-$ is washed off the column, while the $^{99}MoO_4^{2-}$ remains adhered to the alumina. The $^{99m}TcO_4^-$ is readily exchanged with the chloride ions (Cl^-) in a saline solution. Column elution yields of ^{99m}Tc range from 70 to 90% [47]. $^{99m}TcO_4^-$ is the most stable form of the radionuclide ^{99m}Tc in an aqueous medium. Even though $^{99m}TcO_4^-$ is a synthetic molecule that plays no role in any biological processes or pathways, it is capable of imitating the behavior of a true biological substrate as a result of its inherent physicochemical characteristics. For instance, its atomic radius and overall charge are very similar to that of iodide (I^-) [48]. Hence, minutes after intravenous injection of $^{99m}TcO_4^-$ into mice, it was observed that the radioactivity starts to concentrate in the thyroid gland, salivary glands, stomach, and bladder [49]. Although $^{99m}TcO_4^-$ possesses a marginally smaller ionic radius than I^-, it is transported more efficiently by the sodium/iodide symporter, the protein complex responsible for iodide transport .The original chemical formulations of technetium analogues synthesized for clinical use were ^{99m}Tc-sodium pertechnetate for use in brain and thyroid imaging and ^{99m}Tc-sulfur colloid which was used for liver, spleen, and bone marrow imaging [50]. New derivatives of ^{99m}Tc were developed for imaging other organs. To achieve this, it was necessary to prepare technetium-labeled compounds with technetium in various oxidation states [51]. Early analogues of ^{99m}Tc were synthesized by employing reducing agents to change the oxidation state of the metal. Radiolabeling yields were often inconsistent and a finishing purification step was frequently required to remove excess pertechnetate. The final solutions were then typically sterilized by membrane filtration or by autoclaving. The new formulations of ^{99m}Tc are prepared by the stepwise introduction of ligand, reducing agent, ^{99m}Tc pertechnetate, and adjuvant followed by pH or temperature adjustments if necessary. Sterile radiopharmaceutical kits are commercially available and have simplified the compounding procedure and increased the yields and purity of the technetium compounds without the need to remove uncomplexed pertechnetate. The typical technetium formulation kit consists of a reducing agent, a ligand for coordination, and adjuvants such as antioxidants, buffers, and ancillary chelating agents. Sn(II) as stannous chloride dihydrate, $SnCl_2{\cdot}2H_2O$, is the most common reducing agent utilized in ^{99m}Tc chemistry radiolabeling kits [52]. The vast majority of technetium radiolabeling occurs at a pH of ~6.8–7.3 with ample complexing agent to maintain the solubility of metal ions such as stannous and stannic ions and reduced ^{99m}Tc and ^{99}Tc [53]. To guarantee technetium complex formation and to minimize hydrolysis reactions (i.e., formation of tin hydroxides and technetium dioxide colloid), a large excess of coordinating ligand is added to the kits. To enhance chelation of metal ions, formulation kits may be supplemented with a chelating agent. The optimal formulation is unique to each kit [54]. The pH of the radiolabeling mixture is critical, and thus buffers are utilized to adjust the pH to ensure that reactions proceed efficiently. As soon as the technetium complex is synthesized, it will rapidly decompose via oxidation by inadvertent exposure to air. Degradation can also proceed through auto-radiolysis catalyzed by the presence of free radicals. Oxidative degradation can be attributed to OH• and reductive degradation to H•. Formulation kits vulnerable to auto-radiolysis may severely suppress technetium concentrations during radiolabeling reactions and may require free-radical scavengers, for example, ascorbic acid, gentisic acid, or para-aminobenzoic acid (PABA) [55]. In some instances air may be intentionally introduced into kits to minimize the generation of radiochemical impurities. Air, for example, is introduced to the ^{99m}Tc-MAG$_3$ kit to oxidize excess stannous ions, which may lower the oxidation state of the technetium in the desired complex. The introduction of air to a ^{99m}Tc-tetrofosmin kit also diminishes auto-radiolysis of the technetium complex by reducing the number of free radicals [56].

The central technetium metal can exist in a number of oxidation states. Sometimes the technetium core exists alone, or "naked," while in other cores it is associated with a functional group such as oxygen or nitrogen. The associated coordinating ligands of technetium play a major role in stabilizing the metal complexes. The reduction of Tc(VII), as pertechnetate, to Tc(I) yields a technetium atom bearing six extra electrons in a *d6* configuration that must be stabilized by π-acceptor ligands. π-acceptor ligands possess π-bonding orbitals devoid of electrons which can be occupied by the *d*-orbital electrons from the Tc(I) atom [57]. Tc(I) complexes are very stable when all six coordination sites are occupied by π-acceptor ligands resulting in the formation of an octahedral complex. Prime examples of the coordinating moieties that stabilize Tc(I) are the phosphines (P), diphosphines (P–P), isocyanides (CNR), and carbonyl (CO). The naked Tc^+ and the $Tc(CO)^{3+}$ complexes are the most explored technetium cores. The ligands in Tc(I) complexes can be readily functionalized to modify its chemical and biological properties, such as lipophilicity, without adverse effects on complex stability. The heart imaging agent ^{99m}Tc-sestamibi is a typical example of a Tc(I) core radiopharmaceutical. ^{99m}Tc-sestamibi is used to determine myocardial perfusion in ischemia and infarction. This Tc(I) core is very lipophilic with the Tc(I) atom coordinated by six monodentate 2-methoxy isobutyl isonitrile (MIBI) ligands, forming a stable octahedral complex. Because the MIBI ligands impart no charge on the sestamibi complex, the Tc^+ core retains a single positive charge. Due to the volatility of the MIBI ligands, they are complexed into a copper/boron fluoride complex to aid lyophilization [56]. In the first step of the preparation of ^{99m}Tc-sestamibi, both cysteine and stannous chloride act as reducing agents [58]. Initially, the citrate forms a complex with Tc(V) and Tc(IV) and also with Sn(II) and Sn(IV) with Sn(IV)-citrate, a more potent reducing agent, as well as a more stable complex than Sn(II)-citrate. In the following heating step of the radiolabeling process, the copper-MIBI bonds are broken liberating the MIBI ligands. In the concluding step of the synthesis, the MIBI ligands then displace the citrate adducts from the preformed ^{99m}Tc-citrate intermediate to yield ^{99m}Tc-sestamibi. After intravenous injection, the lipophilic ^{99m}Tc-sestamibi complex enters the heart via passive diffusion in proportion to myocardial blood flow [59]. Even though ^{99m}Tc-sestamibi remains as a cation, the Na-K ATPase membrane pumps do not efflux the complex. With a biological half-life of 6 h, ^{99m}Tc-sestamibi is retained in the myocytic mitochondria [60]. The *technetium tricarbonyl core* $^{99m}Tc(CO)_3^+$ is an instrumental raw material for the synthesis of a suite of radiopharmaceuticals. The versatility of the $^{99m}Tc(CO)_3^+$ core is realized by its ability to coordinate with multifunctional chelators possessing functional moieties that can be coupled with technetium to receptor-avid molecules. At present there is no US Food and Drug Administration (FDA)-approved target-specific radiotracer developed from the $^{99m}Tc(CO)_3^+$ core. However, the $^{99m}Tc(CO)_3^+$ core provides researchers with a potential scaffold for the synthesis of new radiopharmaceuticals. Radioactive molecules generated from the $^{99m}Tc(CO)_3^+$ core result in stable octahedral organometallic complexes of two distinct subtypes, *fac*-$Tc(CO)_3^+$ and $CpTc(CO)_3^+$. In the case of *fac*-$Tc(CO)_3^+$, the Tc^+ metal has sufficient space to associate with a variety of ligands, in addition to the three carbonyl ligands, to form an octahedral complex. In the instance of $CpTc(CO)_3^+$, besides the three carbonyl ligands, the Tc^+ metal is coordinated to a derivatized cyclopentadiene ligand that can then further bond to a directing molecule [61]. A versatile and robust precursor of *fac*-$Tc(CO)_3^+$ is the complex $[Tc(H_2O)_3(CO)_3]^+$. The $[Tc(H_2O)_3(CO)_3]^+$ complex is synthesized via direct hydride reduction of pertechnetate under a blanket of $CO_{(g)}$ at 75 °C [62]. This complex is stable throughout the pH range, and the labile water ligands can be displaced by donor ligands to yield highly derivatized radiopharmaceuticals. An alternative stable precursor, $[TcCl(H_2O)_2(CO)_3]$, has been routinely used to synthesize ^{99m}Tc-TROTEC-1, a neutral and lipophilic tropane containing analogue. ^{99m}Tc-TROTEC-1 has displayed high affinity for the dopamine transporter in the brain. Nonetheless, uptake in the brain is low. The salient advantages of the $CpTc(CO)_3^+$ core is its high degree of thermal stability, its lipophilicity, and the ease with which it can be functionalized with bioactive molecules or groups. The $CpTc(CO)_3^+$ core is a basic component of $Cp^{99m}Tc(CO)_3$-octreotide conjugate, which has displayed receptor mediated uptake in the adrenal glands and pancreas [63].

Unlike Tc(I), *the uncomplexed Tc(III) (Tc^{3+}) core* is typically coordinated to five, six, or even seven ligands. Furthermore, Tc(III) complexes are able to participate in redox reactions thereby establishing different oxidation states with different coordinating ligands. This is exemplified by the boronic acid adducts of technetium oxime (BATO compounds). Among the original Tc^{3+} compounds to be incorporated as a radiotracer in nuclear medicine is ^{99m}Tc-lidofenin, abbreviated as ^{99m}Tc-HIDA. Its analogues (^{99m}Tc-disofenin and ^{99m}Tc-mebrofenin) supersede ^{99m}Tc-HIDA in the hospital. Both are presently utilized for hepatobiliary imaging. Hepatocytes absorb ^{99m}Tc-disofenin or ^{99m}Tc-mebrofenin better at high plasma bilirubin than ^{99m}Tc-HIDA [64]. The hexa-coordinate complexes take the general form $[Tc\text{-}(HIDA)_2]$-resulting in the Tc(III) atom being stabilized by four oxygen and two nitrogen atoms forming two HIDA ligands. The overall charge of the complex is 1−. This is due to the four negatively charged oxygen atoms which offset the 3+ charge on Tc(III). Ligand exchange experiments with ^{99m}Tc-HIDA have shown that the complex is virtually kinetically inert in vivo [65]. When ^{99m}Tc-HIDA is incubated with EDTA at physiologic pH, no ^{99m}Tc-EDTA was detected. The in vivo stability of ^{99m}Tc-HIDA was confirmed by a study where reinjection of urinary and gall bladder contents of dogs previously injected with ^{99m}Tc-HIDA displayed an excretory pattern identical to the original molecule. Depending on a number of factors including the concentrations of pertechnetate, the Sn(II)/Sn(IV) ratio, as well as the pH, technetium forms as many as four distinct complexes (A-D) with 2,3-dimercaptosuccinic acid (DMSA or Succimer) [66]. Complexes A and B are formed at low pH, while complexes C and D are predominant at high pH. After intravenous introduction of complex A, it was revealed that the molecule quickly concentrated in bone and was expelled in urine with minimal kidney retention. Additional experiments found that complex A can be converted to complex B upon incubation with excess stannous ion. Unlike complex A, it was found that complex B concentrated primarily in the kidneys. The above studies proved that complex B was in fact Tc(III)-DMSA, an obvious product of the reduction of Tc(IV)-DMSA by excess stannous ion. Complexes C and D are formed by titration of Complexes A and B, respectively, to an alkaline pH. Complex Cs uptake was comparable to complex A as it localized almost entirely in the bone. Complex D, on the other hand, was found to accumulate in large quantities in the kidneys [67]. For example, ^{99m}Tc-teboroxime is a neutral, lipophilic complex comprising a boronic acid in the form of technetium dioxime (BATOs) and mainly used for myocardial perfusion imaging [68]. The synthesis of ^{99m}Tc-teboroxime follows an atypical path. The technetium metal ion provides the foundation on which a series of reactions are performed. In contrast to other ^{99m}Tc complexes, the synthesis of ^{99m}Tc-teboroxime stands alone in that the ligands are absent from the reaction vessel prior to the addition of pertechnetate. The ligand is instead constructed around technetium, which serves as the template atom. Due to ^{99m}Tc-teboroxime's undesirable in vivo myocardial kinetics after intravenous injection, the complex was subsequently withdrawn from the market. *The Tc(IV) core* is synthesized via the reduction of Tc(VII) and assumes a d^3 configuration. The Tc(IV) core is surprisingly common in a number of first generation technetium radiotracers. These radiotracers are typically synthesized in kits by the reduction of pertechnetate with $SnCl_2$ in the presence of coordinating ligands. Examples include technetium complexes containing pentetate (DTPA) and phosphonates (MDP, HDP), in addition to pyrophosphate (PPi). Even though these radiotracers are included in the class of Tc(IV) oxidation states, no study has decisively proven this to be true in each case. The only Tc(IV) molecule that is understood to exist in the Tc(IV) state is TcO_2. However, TcO_2 is considered a radio-impurity and is thus not utilized as a radiotracer. ^{99m}Tc-diethylenetriamine penta acetic acid (DTPA) is one of the original radiopharmaceuticals prepared in kit form with stannous chloride as reducing agent [69]. It is believed that the oxidation state of technetium in a DTPA synthesis kit starts as Tc(IV). It has been shown that, depending on the reaction conditions, a combination of both Tc(III) and Tc(IV) in ^{99m}Tc-DTPA can be obtained. The formation of ^{99m}Tc(III)-DTPA and ^{99m}Tc(IV)-DTPA is evident upon titration of a mixture of ^{99}Tc-pertechnetate and 0.4 M DTPA with stannous chloride under acidic conditions (pH 4). Under millimolar concentrations of ^{99}Tc-pertechnetate in excess of Sn(II), the electron transfer number is 3.5, suggesting that an equimolar solution of ^{99m}Tc(III)-DTPA and ^{99m}Tc(IV)-DTPA have been synthesized. Conversely, when the synthesis is conducted at a 6:1 molar ratio of Sn(II)/pertechnetate, the electron transfer number is 4, signifying that ^{99m}Tc(III)-DTPA is formed. The formation of Tc(III) is reported to occur in a rapid two-step reaction. Initially

Tc(VII) is reduced to Tc(V) followed by the reduction of Tc(V) to Tc(III). This suggests that ^{99m}Tc(III)-DTPA is synthesized predominantly in the radiopharmaceutical kits since the preparation of ^{99m}Tc-DTPA occurs with a molar excess of Sn(II) to pertechnetate. Nevertheless, there is limited experimental evidence to verify one particular oxidation state of technetium in ^{99m}Tc-DTPA. ^{99m}Tc-DTPA is most likely a six-coordinated complex coordinated to three nitrogen and three oxygen donor atoms. Shortly after intravenous injection, ^{99m}Tc-DTPA is rapidly removed from the bloodstream by glomerular filtration and is subsequently excreted unaltered into the urine. ^{99m}Tc-DTPA is commonly utilized to evaluate kidney function in a multitude of conditions and to measure the glomerular filtration rate [70].

4.2.5 Copper-64 (Cu-64, ^{64}Cu)

Cu-64 is a PET isotope with a long half-life (12.7 h) and emits a low-energy β^+ (190 keV with end point energy 579 keV) with a reasonable yield (17.4%). It is therefore comparable to ^{18}F in terms of the spatial resolution obtained with a PET camera, unlike other PET-emitting radiometals. It emits only one other gamma radiation (1345 keV) at low yield (0.47%) therefore contributing a minimal radiation dose to radiopharmacists during preparation, which is often a concern with other PET-emitting radiometals including ^{89}Zr. The only negative aspect is the co-emitted β^- (278 keV with end point energy 653 keV) resulting in an increased radiation dose to patients. This has no significant effect on the radiation dose to the radiopharmacists as this β^- is largely shielded by a glass vial.

Preparation of ^{64}Cu is either cyclotron or reactor produced, with the latter route resulting in either low specific activity (n,p) or high specific activity (n,p) products. At present, the most common production method for ^{64}Cu utilizes the ^{64}Ni(p,n)^{64}Cu reaction [71]. The target for producing ^{64}Cu is enriched ^{64}Ni (99.6%). The ^{64}Ni (typically 10–50 mg) is prepared and electroplated onto a gold disk. This results in high specific activities (Ci/mg) of ^{64}Cu because of the ease of separation from Ni. Alternatively, to save costs a ^{nat}Ni target, Zn targets, can be irradiated in a cyclotron [72]. The presence of nonradioactive Cu in the targets or separation equipment can lower the specific activity and care should be taken to minimize this [73]. The aqueous radiochemistry of Cu(II) is well understood, and the complexes of choice contain amine groups with a coordination number of four. A range of ligands have been investigated as complexing agents for ^{64}Cu ranging from DOTA (1,4,7,10-tetraazacyclododecane-1,4,7,10-tetraacetic acid) to the most commonly used TETA (1,4,8,11-tetraazacyclotetradecane-*N′*,*N″*,*N″*‘-tetraacetic acid). Often, the selection of the ligand is made based on the thermodynamic stability between the ligand and metal ion, which is important for the in vivo stability of the complexes to withstand competition by blood plasma ligands and metal ions. However, the kinetic stability of association and dissociation is just as important. For radiolabeling, a fast association is preferred, while for biomolecules with a long residence in vivo, the dissociation has to be slow or negligible [73]. Several new chelators have been proposed that meet this criteria such as SARAR (1-*N*-(4-aminobenzyl)-3, 6,10,13,16,19-hexaaza bicyclo[6.6.6] eicosane-1,8-diamine), NODAGA (2-(4,7-bis(carboxymethyl)-1,4,7-triazonan-1-yl)pentanedioic acid and CB-TE2A (a bridged version of TETA) to name a few [74].

^{64}Cu has not been exhaustively studied as a radionuclide used for infection imaging despite its theoretical promise as indicated above. In 2009, Bhargava et al. showed that direct labeling of white blood cells (WBC) with ^{64}Cu compared well with ^{111}In labeling of WBC and was superior to ^{18}F-FDG labeling of WBC [75]. This was in pursuit of a direct PET analogue for the routinely used ^{99m}Tc-labeling of WBC used in SPECT. This, however, did not take off perhaps due to the inherent problems of radiolabeling WBC such as risks associated with handling patient blood. ^{64}Cu-radiolabeled nanoparticles have been identified as possible infection imaging agents [29]. The experimental peptide ^{64}Cu-[cinnamoyl-Phe-D-Leu-Phe--D-Leu-Phe-Lys] [76] has been tested in mice to image bacterial lung infection [77]. In a similar fashion, Harper et al. successfully proved the hypothesis that TB granulomas are hypoxic using the well-known ^{64}Cu-ATSM diacetyl-bis (N4-methylthiosemicarbazone), hypoxia tracer [78]. Lastly ^{64}Cu-labeled NODAGA-LLP2A has been shown to be excellent imaging agents for melanoma and potentially other VLA-4–positive tumors [79]. Lately, this ^{64}Cu-labeled compound has been shown to be selective for T-cells in tuberculosis infection where its uptake in granulomas is being investigated [80]. Using ImmunoPET/MR, the murine antibody-based tracer ^{64}Cu-DOTA-JF5 was capable to discriminate bacterial lung infections from invasive pulmonary aspergillosis in a murine model [81].

4.2.6 Gallium-68 (Ga-68, ^{68}Ga)

Gallium has two natural stable isotopes, namely ^{69}Ga (60%) and ^{71}Ga (40%). Two trivalent gallium isotopes, ^{66}Ga ($t_{½}$ = 9.5 h) and ^{68}Ga ($t_{½}$ = 68 min), are suitable for PET imaging. ^{68}Ga (Q^{+} = 2.92 MeV; E_{max} = 1.89 MeV) disintegrates by positron emission (88.9%) and electron capture (11.1%) to the stable ^{68}Zn isotope. Besides the main transition, there are 13 weak gamma transitions from 5 excited levels in ^{68}Zn. ^{68}Ga-radiolabeling can be carried out via direct labeling or use of a chelating molecule. The direct labeling has limitations and applies mostly to proteins (e.g., lactoferrin, transferrin, ferritin) designed by nature for iron binding, thus utilizing the similar chemistry of Ga(III) and Fe(III) [82]. The direct ^{68}Ga-labeling and formation of low molecular weight complexes is commonly employed for the development of imaging agents for perfusion or for imaging of biological processes (i.e., Galligas, citrate, EDTA) where the agent uptake is defined by its charge, lipophilicity, and size [83, 84]. More commonly known is the chelator-mediated ^{68}Ga-labeling procedure. It requires first the conjugation of the targeting biomolecule with a chelating agent responsible for coordinating the Ga(III) ion. Structural modifications can be made by introducing various linker molecules (i.e., polyethylene glycol) if thermodynamic and kinetic stabilities are maintained. Geometry and lipophilicity of

Table 4.2 Selected chelator molecules suggested for ^{68}Ga (adapted from [93])

Open chain	
HBED	*N,N′*-Di(2-hydroxybenzyl)ethylenediamine-*N,N′*-diacetic acid
PLED	*N,N′*-Dipyridoxyethylenediamine-*N,N′*-diacetic acid
H_2dedpa	1,2-[[6-Carboxypyridin-2-yl]methylamino]ethane
CP256	Tris(hexadentate)3-hydroxy-4-pyridinone
BAPDMEN	*N,N′*-Bis(3-aminopropyl)-*N,N′*-dimethyl-ethylenediamine
Macrocyclic	
DTPA	Diethylenetriaminepentaacetic acid
DOTA	1,4,7,10-Tetraazacyclododecane-1,4,7,10-tetraacetic acid
PCTA	3,6,9,15-Tetraazabicyclo [9.3.1]pentadeca-1(15),11,13-triene-3,6,9-triacetic acid
NOTA	1,4,7-Triazacyclononane-triacetic acid
NODASA	1,4,7-Triazacyclononane-1-succinic acid-4,7-deacetic acid
NODAGA	1,4,7-Triazacyclononane-1-glutaric acid-4,7-diacetic acid
TACN-TM	1,4,7-Tris(2-mercaptoethyl)-1,4,7-triazacyclononane
TRAP	1,4,7-Triazacyclononane-phosphinic acid
NOPO	1,4,7-Triazacyclononane-1,4-bis[methylene(hydroxymethyl)phosphinic acid]-7-[methylene(2-carboxyethyl)phosphinic acid]
Macrobicyclic	
SarAr	1-*N*-(4-Aminobenzyl)-3, 6,10,13,16,19-hexaazabicyclo[6.6.6] eicosane-1,8-diamine

a chelator-metal ion complex are important parameters in the development of radiometal-based radiopharmaceuticals [85]. The chemical development of novel ^{68}Ga-based imaging agents depends on the critical evaluation of the aqueous chemistry of ^{68}Ga. The design of the chelator moiety and the functionalization of biomolecules for complexing of Ga (III) must not compromise the in vivo biodistribution of the conjugated biomolecules in their affinity for the target. The hard acid Ga(III) can form four-, five-, and six-coordinated complexes. The latter are the most stable with an octahedral coordination sphere. Oxygen, nitrogen, and sulfur donor atoms form stable coordinate bonds with Ga(III). There is a constant effort to develop new chelating agents. Table 4.2 shows a short overview of selected open-chain, macrocyclic, and macrobicyclic chelator molecules suggested for ^{68}Ga complexation [86–89]. Even though open-chain chelators serve the aim of rapid chelation at room temperature, they compete with the versatility of macrocyclic chelators such as DOTA, NOTA, or TRAP. Most of the commercially available chelating agents comprise esters, isothiocyanates, maleimides, hydrazides, and α-haloamides for reactions with nucleophilic functional groups ($-NH_2$, −SH, −OH) of biomolecules using solid-phase peptide synthesis. Milder reaction conditions could be carried out for the 6π-azaelectrocyclization using unsaturated (E)-ester aldehydes with 1,2-dihydropyridines [90] and Cu(I)-catalyzed azide-alkyne cycloaddition [91, 92]. Moreover, "click chemistry" using *N*-ε-azido derivatives of the peptides (mono-, di-, tetrameric cyclo(Arg-Gly-Asp-D-Phe-Lys)) allows high yields of their conjugated derivatives [91]. Detailed information are also provided by Velikyan [93].

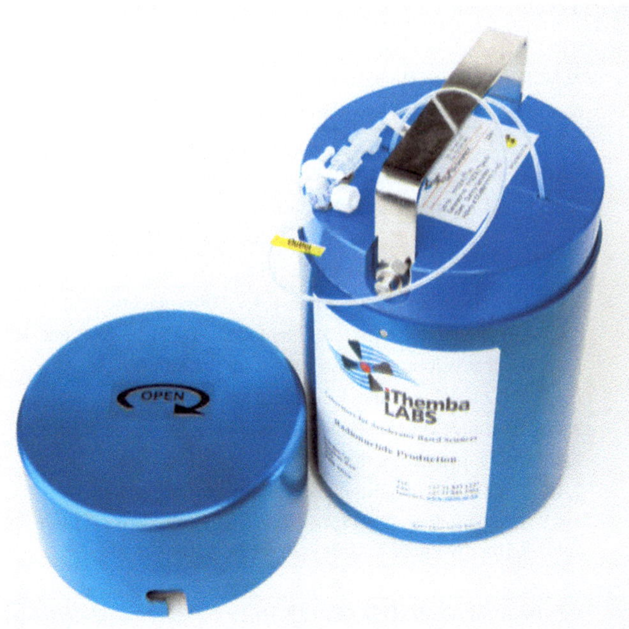

Figure 4.6 Example for $^{68}Ge/^{68}Ga$-generator (iThemba LABS, Somerset West, South Africa). The ^{68}Ga-activity can be eluted by elution with an acidic mobile phase (0.6 M HCl)

^{68}Ga is a generator-based radioisotope (Figure 4.6). The parent isotope is ^{68}Germanium (^{68}Ge) which is produced in an accelerator (p,2n) reaction on a Ga_2O_3 target. ^{68}Ge is considered the stationary material adsorbed on a column matrix inside the generator and naturally decays with a half-life of 270 days by electron capture, which enables a shelf life of the generator of up to a year. Gallium can be eluted from the generator on a daily basis by solvent extraction. Historically, the availability of ^{68}Ga as a PET radionuclide goes back to the time when ^{18}F tracers were not yet established. The first $^{68}Ge/^{68}Ga$ generator, the so-called positron cow, was developed by Gleason in 1960 [94]. A year later an improved generator was established employing an aluminum oxide (Al_2O_3)-based column matrix, and ^{68}Ga was extracted with a sodium ethylene diamine-*N,N,N′,N′*-tetraacetic acid (Na-EDTA) solution [95]. In 1974, the next generation of gallium generators was introduced by Kopecky and Mudrova, yielding $^{68}Ga^{3+}$ with acidic solvents from ion-exchange matrices [96]. This set the design of today's commercially available improved versions of these generators. The current generators are modified on metal oxides such as titanium dioxide (TiO_2), tin dioxide (SnO_2), Al_2O_3, and organic (pyrogallol-formaldehyde resins) or inorganic supports (silica based). The most commonly used commercially available $^{68}Ge/^{68}Ga$ generator is based on a TiO_2-solid support [97]. ^{68}Ga can be conveniently eluted with up to 10 mL diluted hydrochloric acid (0.1–0.6 N) as soluble $^{68}Ga^{3+}$ (i.e., $[^{68}Ga(H_2O)_6]^{3+}$ at a resulting pH of 0.5–1). Both, eluate fraction-

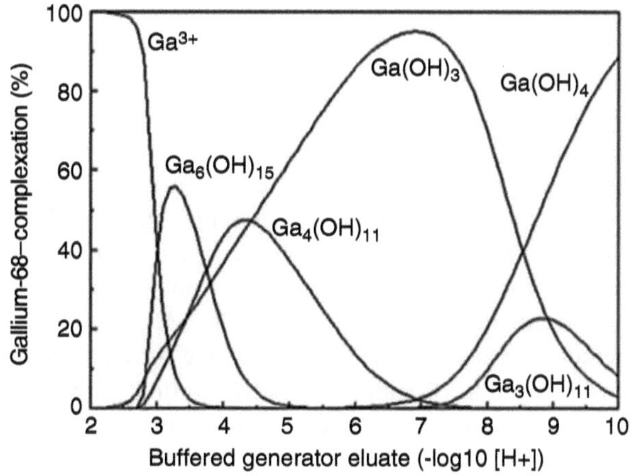

Figure 4.7 Simulated distribution of the Ga(III) ion into its free and hydroxylated species as a function of pH, with Ga(III) = 2 mmol*dm^{-3} (adopted from [258])

ation and pre-concentration methods use hydrochloric acid in the eluent and thus require buffers for the correct pH adjustment necessary for the complexation. $^{68}Ga^{3+}$ is only present within a narrow, low-pH range, whereas its various hydroxylated species have more presence toward physiological pH values. Hence, weak buffer complexation capability is also essential in order to act as a stabilizing agent and prevent ^{68}Ga(III) precipitation and colloid formation (Figure 4.7). A number of buffering systems such as HEPES, acetate, succinate, formate, tris, and glutamate were evaluated, and it was determined that HEPES, sodium acetate, and succinate buffers demonstrate very suitable characteristics [98].

Radiolabeling with ^{68}Ga has been done manually or through the use of automated modules [99]. Once eluted from the generator, the main limitations for direct use of ^{68}Ga to radiolabel for clinical PET applications are large volumes of generator eluate, a high H^+ concentration, ^{68}Ge breakthrough, and potential metallic impurities from Al, Sn, Ti, Cu, Zn, and Fe [100]. Therefore, efficient eluate pre-purification has been advised prior to the radiolabeling reaction step. Several approaches have been described using disposable cartridge units with anionic [101], cationic [97], combined cationic/anionic [102], and cationic/high Na^+Cl^+ concentration [103] ion exchange matrixes. The foremost advantage of the pre-purification step has been the concentrating effect for the ^{68}Ga-solution; small reaction volumes are desirable for high specific radioactivity and maximized radiolabeling yields. A simpler, but more conventional, procedure to overcome the crude volume is eluate fractionation, whereby the fraction with the highest volume activity (0.5–3 mL) is collected and buffered to an appropriate pH for radiolabeling [99, 104]. The disadvantage of this unpurified ^{68}Ga method has been indicated to result in a reduced specific activity of the final product [105]. Subsequently, a post-radiolabeling purification step becomes mandatory using solid phase extraction. However, this purification method has the potential to quantitatively separate the desired ^{68}Ga-labeled product from any uncomplexed ^{68}Ga or colloidal ^{68}Ga and simultaneously reduce the apparent breakthrough of the parent nuclide ^{68}Ge from the final product by 100- to 1000-fold [99]. The main manufacturers of the generators (Cyclotron Corp, Russia; Eckert and Ziegler, USA; iThemba Labs, South Africa; and Isotope Technologies Garching, Germany) have given the specification of the ^{68}Ge breakthrough to be at lower levels (0.01–0.001%) during the use of a new generator [106]. However, there are events where higher levels of ^{68}Ge breakthrough have been noted [107]. Contrary to ^{99}Mo/^{99m}Tc generators where the level of ^{99}Mo can be determined before preparation of kits, ^{68}Ge breakthrough can only [108] be determined retrospectively by measurement of ^{68}Ga after 1–2 days of decay of the eluate to ensure that any detected ^{68}Ga is a consequence of ^{68}Ge present in the eluate [89]. Although studies on absorption, distribution, and excretion of germanium were conducted in the 1950s, there does not appear to have been any recent studies to inform the establishment of an acceptable limit for ^{68}Ge breakthrough [93]. The limit to be set in the European Pharmacopoeia is 0.001% (10 ppm) ^{68}Ge relative to ^{68}Ga [109]. Other metals, particularly Fe(III), can compete in ^{68}Ga labeling reactions, as demonstrated by Velikyan et al., where the quantities of co-eluted metals increase with prolonged generator usage [108]. The use of hydrochloric acid solutions as the eluent may be harsh for microorganisms as compared to the saline solution used for ^{99}Mo/^{99m}Tc generators. However, the pre-purification and radiolabeling methods according to current procedures have been proven to deliver ^{68}Ga-labeled compounds in high radiochemical purity and specific activity. Even if the sterility of the generator eluate cannot be fully assured, the risk of incidental microbial contamination was found to be very low [110]. More detailed aspects of the production and application of ^{68}Ga-radiopharmaceuticals have been recently summarized by Velikyan et al. [111].

Given that ^{68}Ga can be acquired from parent/daughter designed ^{68}Ge/^{68}Ga generator, one could visualize a PET center, which utilizes a ^{68}Ge/^{68}Ga generator with several cold kits to perform a variety of clinical PET studies, in the same way that ^{99}Mo/^{99m}Tc generators are used with a range of cold kits to perform a variety of SPECT studies. Within the last 5 years, ^{68}Ga became a very promising radionuclide for molecular PET imaging, but its technical readiness, compared to ^{99m}Tc, was critically discussed by Balinger and Solanki [112], as follows: (1) ^{68}Ga generators are eluted with diluted hydrochloric acid (HCl), which is not suitable for direct injection and thus will need pharmaceutical preparation; (2) ^{68}Ga generators are considered not for human use, although manufactured under good manufacturing practice (GMP) conditions; (3) to date no licensed, commercial kit system is available for ^{68}Ga radiopharmaceutical; (4) routine ^{68}Ga radiolabeling procedures are manual and of concern for safe and radioprotective handling, as 511 keV annihilation gamma photons are ten times more penetrating than the 140 keV photons of ^{99m}Tc which makes an automated synthesis with manual intervention essential; and (5) multi-dosage design that ^{99m}Tc-labeled products can provide is challenging to ^{68}Ga-based productions, but the generator yield builds up rapidly (68 min half-life) which will allow for multiple generator elutions per day with parallel or consecutive radiolabeling procedures at intervals of 2–3 h.

4.2.7 *Gallium-67 (Ga-67, ^{67}Ga)*

Gallium-67 is produced in a cyclotron target by the ^{68}Zn (p,2n) ^{67}Ga reaction and has a half-life of 78.3 h. ^{67}Ga decays by electron capture to the stable ^{67}Zn isotope. A number of gamma photons of different energy are emitted (Table 4.1) [113]. Although ^{67}Ga salts have been used in clinical practice for many years, the amount of work on bioconjugate-derived radiopharmaceuticals based on ^{67}Ga is small compared to ^{68}Ga [114]. ^{67}Ga will display the same kind of coordination chemistry than ^{68}Ga described above [115].

4.2.8 *Indium-111 (In-111, ^{111}In)*

Indium-111 belongs to a group of low-energy gamma-emitting radiometals occurring in SPECT radiopharmaceuticals. The trivalent In^{3+} is the only stable aqueous oxidation state; due to its large size, the coordination number of $^{111}In^{3+}$ is 7–8. As a hard acid (pK_a 4.0), it allows conjugation with chelators having hard donor atoms. Thus, it forms stable metal complexes with DTPA, DOTA, or NOTA. Following ^{99m}Tc, ^{111}In is the next most common SPECT radioisotope used in bioconjugates. It decays by electron capture and emits gamma photons at 173 and 247 keV with a physical half-life of 67.3 h, which makes it a desired radioisotope for developing antibody-based radiopharmaceuticals (for so-called immuno-SPECT). It is produced in a cyclotron reaction by isolation from Ag or Cd solid target materials following coprecipitation with $La(OH)_3$ or $Fe(OH)_3$; ^{111}In(III) is purified from La(III) or Fe(III) by ion exchange chromatography [116]. The most common radiolabeling method is to attach ^{111}In to antibody fragments (mAb). A DTPA derivative with a *trans*-1,2-diaminocyclohexane backbone (CHX–A″–DTPA) is found to be the most desirable chelator for ^{111}In. It is also a procedure to conjugate proteins and allow for ^{111}In-labeling with high radiochemical yields by a simple addition of an $InCl_3$ solution to a suitable protein bioconjugate solution at ambient temperature. The specific activity is adjusted to about 4–6 mCi per mg of mAb, and the ratio of conjugation (chelate/mAb) should be around 1–2, which can be determined by a radiometric metal-binding assay [117]. Despite the high radiochemical labeling efficiency, there are a few limitations when using ^{111}In. The biggest challenge is the high nonspecific accumulation in the liver, kidneys, and spleen of a patient as ^{111}In is an iron mimic and can easily be taken up by transferrin. It is suggested that the liver uptake is not a result of the labeling process, but from metabolic liver processes toward the radiolabeled antibody. The introduction of suitable linker molecules, utilization of chelator alternatives, and route of administration are examples to overcome the limitation of the nonspecific organ accumulation of the radiotracer and may also result in reduction of renal uptake during SPECT imaging. Currently, ProstaScint, OncoScint, and Myoscint are commercially available oncologic SPECT radiodiagnostic agents, approved by the FDA for use in humans. WBCs labeled with ^{111}In-oxine (^{111}In-8-hydroxyquinoline, Table 4.3) have been successfully applied clinically in the field of infection/inflammation scintigraphy for many years.

4.3 Examples of Infection Imaging Agents

From a radiochemical point of view, the ideal infection molecular imaging agent should be easy and quick to manufacture, preferably at ambient temperatures. Simplified labeling from a kit allows for low-cost production and also aids in widening commercial availability. Also, a solvent-free radiolabeling approach is desirable as such agents are likely to cause adverse reactions or negatively influence the pharmacological behavior of the probe. Chemically, the desired imaging agent might be of neutral charge as charged molecules are likely to cause higher unspecific binding in vivo [118]. Technically, the production logistics may be a roadblock as certain radioisotopes such as ^{11}C, ^{13}N, or ^{15}O have extremely short half-lives and make it highly unlikely to be of wide use, unless manufactured and utilized on-site. There are also considerable radiation risks during production and during patient use. The commercial radiodiagnostic agents available for infection imaging are listed in Table 4.3. None of them are specific for infections.

Table 4.3 Commercial radiodiagnostic agents available for imaging of infection (adapted from [120])

Imaging procedure (trade name)	Final dose formulation	Indications
^{67}Ga-Citrate SPECT	Simple	May be useful as an aid in detecting some acute infections/inflammations
^{111}In-Oxine-leukocyte SPECT[a]	Simple[b]	Ex vivo radiolabeling of separated leukocytes and platelets, which are then reinjected
^{99m}Tc-HMPAO-leukocyte SPECT (CERETEC®)[c]	Simple[b]	Indicated for perfusion brain imaging but can also be used to label white blood cells ex vivo, which are then reinjected
^{18}F-FDG PET	Simple	Oncologic and cardiac indications but is also useful in detecting infection or inflammation
^{99m}Tc-(Sn-colloid) SPECT (Leukocyte®)[d]	Complex	Imaging of acute infection or inflammation
^{99m}Tc-MDP SPECT[e]	Simple	Skeletal infection imaging
^{99m}Tc-Besilesomab SPECT(Scintimun®)[f]	Complex	For locating infection or inflammation in peripheral bone in adults with suspected osteomyelitis
^{99m}Tc-Sulesomab SPECT (LeukoScan®)[g]	Simple	Locating infection or inflammation in peripheral bone in patients with suspected osteomyelitis, including patients with diabetic foot ulcers
^{99m}Tc-Sulfur-nano-colloids SPECT/CT (Nanocoll®)[h]	Simple	Suitable for detection of infection-associated inflammation (excluding abdominal inflammation)

[a]"Gold standard" radiolabeling procedure for white WBC
[b]Isolating and radiolabeling of white blood cells (WBC) is cumbersome and a multistep, complex procedure
[c]Kit vial preparation of ^{99m}Tc-Exametazime (i.e.,^{99m}Tc-hexamethylpropylene-amine-oxime)
[d]Kit vial preparation of ^{99m}Tc-leukocytes (i.e., ^{99m}Tc-Sn(O)F_2 colloids)
[e]Kit vial preparation of ^{99m}Tc-methylene-diphosphonate
[f]Kit vial preparation of ^{99m}Tc-anti-NCA-95 IgG, BW250/183
[g]Kit for the preparation of ^{99m}Tc-anti-NCA-90Fab' sulesomab
[h]Kit for the preparation of ^{99m}Tc-sulfur-nanocolloids

4.3.1 ^{67}Ga-Citrate SPECT

Biomedical studies with radiogallium started in the late 1940s, but by the mid-1950s, interest has waned; then in 1969, ^{67}Ga localization in soft tissue tumors was confirmed [119]. Regulatory approved ^{67}Ga-citrate has been available on several continents since the 1970s, and ^{67}Ga-citrate became an important SPECT agent with an estimated 250,000 diagnostic studies performed in 1977 alone at an estimated total radiopharmaceutical cost of ten million US dollars, approximately $40 per dose [120]. The half-life of ^{67}Ga of 78 h allows for delayed scintigraphy. ^{67}Ga-citrate is indicated for detecting certain cancers and acute inflammation and therefore non-specific. The ^{67}Ga-citrate injection is commercially available and still widely used, but the long-half-life and high-energy gamma emission poses risks in terms of radiation dose to the patient [121]. In addition, molecular imaging for infection is usually carried out 24–72 h after injection, requiring multiple visits to a nuclear medicine department [122, 123].

4.3.2 ^{111}In-Oxine-Leukocyte SPECT

Procedures were developed in the 1970s to label autologous leukocytes with ^{111}In. The most successful agent, that is still in use today, is ^{111}In-oxine [124]. Oxine (8-hydroxyquinoline) is a neutral lipophilic chelator, and the ^{111}In-oxine diffuses into cells, followed by intracellular binding of ^{111}In to macromolecules. Guidelines, aimed at Europe but generally useful taking into account the guidelines of the Society of Nuclear Medicine, the IAEA recommendations, and several national guidelines, were published for the preparation and quality control of ^{111}In-oxine labeled WBC [125]. To begin preparation of WBCs for radiolabeling, cell-free plasma is first isolated from a patient blood sample. ^{111}In-oxine cannot be used to radiolabel WBC in the presence of plasma. The cell-free plasma is used as the medium of re-suspension after radiolabeling. In a few steps, the mixed leukocytes are isolated in a pellet and this pellet is resuspended in saline for radiolabeling. The radiolabeling of mixed leukocytes is recommended, although a procedure for isolation of granulocytes is also given. Labeling with the ^{111}In-oxine (supplied by a vendor) is then done and involves centrifugation. The resuspended radiolabeled WBCs must be injected in the patient as soon as possible. For quality control, visual inspection and a radiolabeling efficiency determination of the final product are usually considered sufficient when in routine use. Periodic tests for cell viability are recommended due to the cell toxicity of ^{111}In. Periodic tests of post-release cell viability are also recommended. When initial validation is done, cell subset recovery tests and cell efflux of ^{111}In should be done. In vivo lung uptake must be monitored routinely to check for radiolabeled clumps of cells in the final product. Additional information is described previously in this chapter. The radiolabeling of the WBCs by ^{111}In is a laborious procedure with dangers of biohazard exposure to the operator and the patient. To do white blood cell labeling, a sterile area, centrifuge, and a Class A hood are required. The exact requirements vary from country to country. Legislation in about half of the countries in Europe prescribes that nuclear physicians, radiopharmacists, or pharmacists carry out the white blood cell labeling, and in most of the rest, at least well-trained operators are required [126]. The long preparation time, possible biohazard burden, high-level laboratory skills, and additional infrastructure required may pose challenges for some nuclear medicine departments.

4.3.3 ^{99m}Tc-HMPAO-Leukocyte-SPECT (CERETEC®)

^{99m}Tc-HMPAO came on the market in 1988. The ^{99m}Tc is conveniently eluted from a ^{99}Mo/^{99m}Tc isotope generator. It is used for perfusion brain imaging and is available as a simple kit preparation. Lipophilic ^{99m}Tc-HMPAO can also be used to radiolabel purified granulocytes or mixed leukocytes in an ex vivo procedure, but whole blood cannot be used [126]. Similar to ^{111}In-oxine, ^{99m}Tc-HMPAO enters the cell by diffusion [124]. A consensus protocol for radiolabeling of WBCs with ^{99m}Tc-HMPAO was published in 1998 [127], and similar to ^{111}In-oxine, updated guidelines were published in 2010 [126]. As with ^{111}In-oxine, the blood cell labeling is time-consuming lasting about 2 h and involves the collection of 30–40 mL of the patient's blood, the isolation of cell-free plasma for a radiolabeling medium, the isolation of mixed leukocytes, and, optionally, the isolation of the granulocytes. The ^{99m}Tc-HMPAO is then prepared. The WBCs must then be radiolabeled with ^{99m}Tc-HMPAO, immediately before administration to the patient. Occasional quality control is recommended for this step consisting of radiolabeling efficiency tests, visual inspection and periodic sterility, and Trypan blue exclusion tests. In vivo lung uptake must be performed routinely to monitor for radiolabeled clumps of cells in the injection product. During initial validation, cell subset recovery and cell efflux of ^{99m}Tc tests need to be performed [126]. ^{99m}Tc-HMPAO-labeled WBCs cannot distinguish between sterile inflammation and infection. More detailed descriptions of the radiolabeling and quality control procedures can be found in reference [127].

4.3.4 ^{18}F-FDG PET

^{18}F-FDG is the archetypal PET imaging agent. The synthesis in the early 1970s, by researchers at the University of Pennsylvania and at the National Institutes of Health, has shown that ^{14}C-deoxy-glucose (^{14}C-DG) can be used to map regional brain metabolism [128]. Syntheses and quality controls of ^{18}F-FDG have been extensively reviewed as exemplified in a review by Yu et al. in 2006 [129]. ^{18}F-FDG is a glucose analogue with the hydroxyl-group in the 2′ position replaced with ^{18}F. As with the ^{14}C-DG described above, sugar-avid cells take up the ^{18}F-FDG. ^{18}F-FDG is subsequently phosphorylated by hexokinase after which it cannot be metabolized further and is trapped within the cell. The synthesis of ^{18}F-FDG follows the classic direct radiolabeling route. The quality control requirements can differ among regulatory bodies but usually includes appearance, pH, radionuclidic identity (half-life) and purity (gamma spectroscopy), and radiochemical identity and purity (TLC or HPLC) based on the appropriate pharmacopeia regulation. The residual solvent test (GC) and a test for residual complexing agent (like Kryptofix 2.2.2) must be carried out. Furthermore, tests concerning the sterile filter integrity, the product osmolality and the presence of bacterial endotoxin (LAL) are usually required. The sterility of the batch also needs to be checked, but with the usual long time span of this test, batches are released without the sterility result. As far as ^{18}F radiopharmaceuticals are concerned, the ^{18}F-FDG process is the most optimized, and numerous vendors sell automated synthesis units, with the appropriate chemicals, in sterile "cassettes," for GMP production. The synthesis takes less than 30 min and the yield is >70%. The radiation danger of ^{18}F makes mandatory the use of expensive hot cells and just as expensive automated synthesis units. Sterility requirements dictate a Class A hot cell or similar, or at least a laminar flow cabinet for the final aseptic filtration; moreover an HPLC and GC apparatus for quality control is needed. Because it targets glucose metabolism, ^{18}F-FDG PET/CT is unable to readily distinguish malignancy from infection or sterile inflammation [130].

4.3.5 ^{99m}Tc-Sn-Colloid SPECT (Leukocyte®)

The leukocyte labeling kit used to prepare ^{99m}Tc-stannous fluoride colloid was introduced in clinics in the 1990s [120]. There are two vials in the kit: one containing an aqueous sodium fluoride solution and the other freeze-dried stannous fluoride. The contents of the two vials are mixed together and then filtered through a 0.22 μm filter. A portion of the filtrate is then added to diluted ^{99m}Tc-pertechnetate in saline. After an hour of rotating this mixture in a syringe, the ^{99m}Tc is consumed to form a ^{99m}Tc-stannous fluoride colloid. Quality control is done with TLC; the colloid stays at the baseline of the strip. The ^{99m}Tc-stannous fluoride colloid has a shelf life of up to 6 h [131]. The colloid is incubated with a heparinized patient whole blood sample, usually 15–20 mL, and rotated for about an hour in a syringe and then briefly centrifuged to separate cells from the plasma supernatant before the resuspended labeled blood cells are injected into the patient. It should be noted that ^{99m}Tc-stannous fluoride labeled blood cells cannot distinguish between sterile inflammation and infection [132]. Compared to the above ex vivo WBC procedures, leukocyte harvesting is not necessary, as only the leukocytes in the whole blood will engulf the colloid and be labeled which is less labor intensive and reduces costs. These advantages are offset by lower specificity and sensitivity [133].

4.3.6 ^{99m}Tc-MDP SPECT

Three-phase bone scintigraphy with ^{99m}Tc-MDP is the method of choice to diagnose osteomyelitis [121]. ^{99m}Tc-MDP scintigraphy is not specific for bone infection and for children up to 6 months old; the sensitivity of ^{99m}Tc-MDP for detecting osteomyelitis is low [133]. The mechanism of its action suggests that the accumulation of ^{99m}Tc-MDP is by both chemical adsorption onto the surface of the hydroxylapatite in the bone and incorporation into the crystalline structure of hydroxylapatite [134]. The ^{99m}Tc-MDP is available as a multi-dose kit reaction vial containing medronic acid, ascorbic acid, and stannous fluoride under nitrogen, which will react at a pH of 6.5, in 10 min with diluted ^{99m}Tc-sodium pertechnetate at room temperature. Quality control consists of a visual inspection and a radiochemical purity determination using a dual strip method [120]. The shelf life of the product is 6–8 h. Following injection, the excretion of ^{99m}Tc-MDP can be expected within 6 h, predominately via the renal route.

4.3.7 ^{99m}Tc-Besilesomab SPECT (Scintimun®)

The in vivo labeling of leukocytes was considered an appealing approach, and years ago already, radiolabeled monoclonal antibodies to target surface antigens of granulocytes were investigated [135]. Scintimun is a commercially available product that comes in a kit form with two vials, each containing a white powder. One vial contains the IgG1 murine monoclonal antibody BW 250/183 (besilesomab), together with sodium phosphate and sorbitol, under nitrogen. The second vial contains tetrasodium-1,1,3,3-propane-tetraphosphonate, stannous chloride, and sodium chloride under nitrogen. A simple reconstructive procedure with saline is applied to dissolve the contents of the tin-containing vial. One milliliter of this solution is added to the other vial, and dissolution is allowed to proceed for 1 min, without any shaking or inverting of the vial. To this solution is added the appropriate amount of ^{99m}Tc-pertechnetate. After 10 min, the solution is ready for injection. Still, no shaking or inverting of the vial is allowed. The shelf life of the multi-dose product is 3 h, and quality control is performed with a single strip developed in methyl ethyl ketone to determine radiochemical purity [120]. In adults, the recommended activity of technetium ^{99m}Tc-besilesomab should be between 400 and 800 MBq. This corresponds to the administration of 0.25–1 mg of besilesomab. SPECT imaging should start 3–6 h after administration. An additional acquisition 24 h after initial injection is recommended. Some disadvantages for the use of Scintimun are the possibility of the formation of human anti-mouse antibodies, the so-called HAMA response, which excludes repeated injections, the slow and low uptake at the infected site because of the high molecular mass of the antibody, and the high uptake in the liver and bone marrow [136]. ^{99m}Tc-Besilesomab-SPECT is not specific for infection.

4.3.8 ^{99m}Tc-Sulesomab SPECT (LeukoScan®)

To overcome the disadvantages of a HAMA response, including slow and low uptake at the infectious foci, slow blood clearance, and high liver and blood marrow uptake, lower molecular weight antibody fragments (Fab') were developed for labeling [137, 138]. One such commercially available product is LeukoScan®. It is a radiodiagnostic agent consisting of a murine monoclonal antibody Fab fragment, sulesomab, formulated to be labeled with ^{99m}Tc. The active component, sulesomab, is generated from a murine IgG1 monoclonal antibody (IMMU-MN3) produced in murine ascites. IMMU-MN3 is purified from the ascitic fluid and is digested with pepsin to produce F(ab′)2 fragments and is subsequently reduced to produce the 50 kDa sulesomab [139]. Each vial contains the nonradioactive materials necessary to prepare one patient dose. LeukoScan is a sterile, lyophilized formulation, containing 0.31 mg of sulesomab per vial and includes 0.22 mg stannous chloride dihydrate, 3.2 mg potassium sodium tartrate tetrahydrate, 7.4 mg sodium acetate trihydrate, 5.5 mg sodium chloride, glacial acetic acid (trace), hydrochloric acid (trace), and 37.8 mg sucrose under nitrogen (vacuum). The imaging agent, ^{99m}Tc-LeukoScan, is made in 10 min in a simple procedure at room temperature by reconstitution of the contents of the LeukoScan vial with 0.5 mL sodium chloride for injection (USP) followed by the addition of 1100 MBq of sodium pertechnetate-^{99m}Tc in 1 mL of saline for injection (USP) [140]. The resulting solution has a pH of 4.5–5.5. Quality control involves a radiochemical purity analysis that can be done by instant TLC using acetone as the solvent. The shelf life of the product is 4 h. When labeled with ^{99m}Tc, LeukoScan® is indicated for the detection of osteomyelitis in long bones and in the feet of patients with diabetic foot ulcers [141]. It was also used for the imaging of fever of unknown origin, endocarditis, and appendicitis [6]. Like Scintimun, the radiolabeled anti-granulocyte antibody localizes at infectious, inflammatory sites, mainly in a nonspecific way, due to locally enhanced vascular permeability, and in the main does not function by labeling leukocytes in vivo [13].

4.3.9 ^{99m}Tc-Sulfur-Nanocolloids SPECT (Nanocoll®)

Nanocoll is another commercially available kit, containing albumin-derived particles of 30–80 nm in diameter. When radiolabeled with ^{99m}Tc, it is used for bone marrow imaging [142]. It is also used in combination with radiolabeled WBCs to make a differential diagnosis of infection [136]. Seemingly, however, it is mostly used to exclude infection. Nevertheless, Nanocoll is a versatile radiodiagnostic; it can be administered for detection of inflammation of glands and vessels responsible for draining fluid caused by inflammation using a noninvasive whole body scintigraphic approach. ^{99m}Tc-albumin-nanocolloid accumulates at sites of inflammation due to increased vascular permeability. Blood clearance is rapid and an imaging study can be finished within an hour [6]. Reconstitution of the kit containing human albumin colloidal particles, stannous chloride, glucose, poloxamer, sodium phosphate, and sodium phytate under nitrogen is simple, and the quality control consists of a radiochemical purity determination using a single strip with methanol/water eluent. The quantity recommended to be administered for an adult ranges from 185 to 500 MBq. ^{99m}Tc-albumin-nanocolloid is inexpensive, but not specific for infection and unavailable in the USA [142].

4.4 Experimental Radiotracers for Infection Imaging

As mentioned in the sections above, having numerous options in radiochemistry to synthesize biomolecules, researchers have made tremendous progress in discovering novel bacteria-specific pathways and in developing novel tracers to detect bacteria or target the associated immune response. Various classes of tracers have been evaluated for bacteria-specific imaging including synthetics, antibiotics, autologous cells, and bacteria-specific tracers as well as macromolecules, antibodies, and small peptide fragments.

4.4.1 Synthetics and Biomimetics

N-Formyl-methionyl-leucyl-phenylalanine (fMLFK) is a chemotactic-acting peptide derivative, which has been labeled with ^{99m}Tc and ^{111}In via chelating agents such as DTPA or HYNIC. They are successful tracers for infection imaging by targeting polymorphonuclear neutrophils. ^{111}In-DTPA-fMLK was synthesized with a radiochemical purity (RCP) of 95% as explained above by 30 min incubation at room temperature followed by Sephadex-G10-based purification [143]. ^{99m}Tc-HYNIC-fMLFK was labeled for 30–60 min at ambient temperature followed by HPLC purification and formulation in sodium phosphate/saline buffer with a RCP of >96% [144].

Citrate (CIT) or buffered citrate solution (ACD-A) can be labeled with ^{68}Ga as a PET-mimic of ^{67}Ga-CIT-SPECT for clinical diagnosis of osteomyelitis, discitis [145], and tuberculosis [146]. The radiolabeling process is a simple reaction of ^{68}Ga(III) that is conveniently eluted from a generator and trapped on an anion exchange column and then washed off in a bolus of citric acid buffer solution in >98% yield [83]. Alternatively, single step kit preparations have been tested where the ^{68}Ga(III) is added and incubated for 20 min at ambient temperature and at pH > 5 [84, 147]. ITLC (methanol/glacial acidic acid 95/5 v/v) is used to characterize ^{68}Ga-CIT (Rf = 0.7–0.9) to decipher from ^{68}Ga (Rf = 0.0–0.15).

Siderophores are a synthetic group of catecholates, hydroxamates, and hydroxycarboxylates, which are specific for Fe(III). Since Ga(III) has similar chemistry to Fe(III), radiopharmaceutical chemistry to label molecules such as triacetylfusarinine C (TAFC) and ferrioxamine (FOXE) with ^{68}Ga has been exploited [148]. A RCP ≥ 95% for ^{68}Ga-TAFC and ^{68}Ga-FOXE was achieved in a solution of 1.1 M sodium acetate buffer by incubation at room temperature for 15–20 min at physiological pH.

Leukotriene (LT) B4 or 5,12-dihydroxyeicosa-6,8,10,14-tetraenoic acid is a molecule synthesized from arachidonic acid via the 5-lipoxygenase pathway. LTB4 is a secondary chemoattractant secreted early in the inflammatory process and also regulates neutrophil chemotaxis [149]. Agonistic and antagonistic ligands for LTB4 were radiolabeled to achieve the radiodiagnostic agent, ^{111}In-DTPA-LTB4 (i.e., DPC11870-11). The radiolabeling is performed at pH 5.5 in ammonium acetate buffer for 30 min at room temperature and HPLC purification; the RCP is greater than 95% and the resulting specific activity is 0.32 mCi/nmol [150]. ^{99m}Tc-HYNIC-LTB-4 (MB88), tricine buffer, isonicotinic acid, PBS, $SnSO_4$, pH 7 at 100 °C, 30 min HPLC purification, RCP > 95%, and ^{18}F-pFBA-LTB-4 (MB67) are labeled via reaction of the ^{18}F-fluorinated intermediate *p*-^{18}F-fluorobenzaldehyde (^{18}F-FB) (sodium acetate buffer, PBS, pH 4–7 at 50 °C, >30 min 65–85%, evaporation under argon atmosphere) [151].

^{68}Ga-Chloride PET imaging was successfully carried out in an osteomyelitis rat model [152] and in mice bearing genital infection [153]. The ^{68}Ga-chloride was collected from a generator and neutralized with 1.0 M sodium hydroxide before administration. Once injected intravenously, ^{68}Ga-chloride is trans-chelated to form ^{68}Ga-transferrin or ^{68}Ga-lactoferrin. ^{68}Ga-chloride has also been tested as “Gallgas” for homogeneities or abnormalities in lungs [154].

4.4.2 Antibiotics

Fluoroquinolones, a class of agents whose antimicrobial activity stems from their insertion between the DNA and the bacterial DNA gyrase and/or topoisomerase IV enzymes of dividing bacteria, have been labeled with ^{99m}Tc [155]. Among them are ^{99m}Tc-ciprofloxacin, ^{99m}Tc-enrofloxacin, and ^{99m}Tc-pefloxacin. ^{99m}Tc-ciprofloxacin is the most studied and was widely available as *Infecton* (Draximage Inc., Quebec, Canada). Showing great promise at first, also after an IAEA coordinated clinical trial, this compound has become somewhat controversial, as subsequent results showed that it is not as specific for infection as initially thought and *Infecton* was withdrawn from the market [156]. The familiar theme here is again that increased local blood supply, together with increased vascular permeability, expansion of the extracellular space, and probably an increase in leukocyte accumulation, may enhance accumulation of the ^{99m}Tc-ciprofloxacin at the inflammatory site [155]. For example, ^{99m}Tc-ciprofloxacin and ^{99m}Tc-enrofloxacin were made in exactly the same manner and tested and compared in vitro and in vivo in Wister rats infected with a fungus and cocci. No discrimination between infection and sterile inflammation was observed. In both instances, the fluoroquinolone was labeled with ^{99m}Tc by mixing 500 µg stannous tartrate with 400 MBq of freshly eluted sodium pertechnetate, adding 0.5 mL of a 4 mg/mL fluoroquinolone solution and heating at 60 °C for 10 min. A high radiochemical efficiency and purity were achieved by tracer

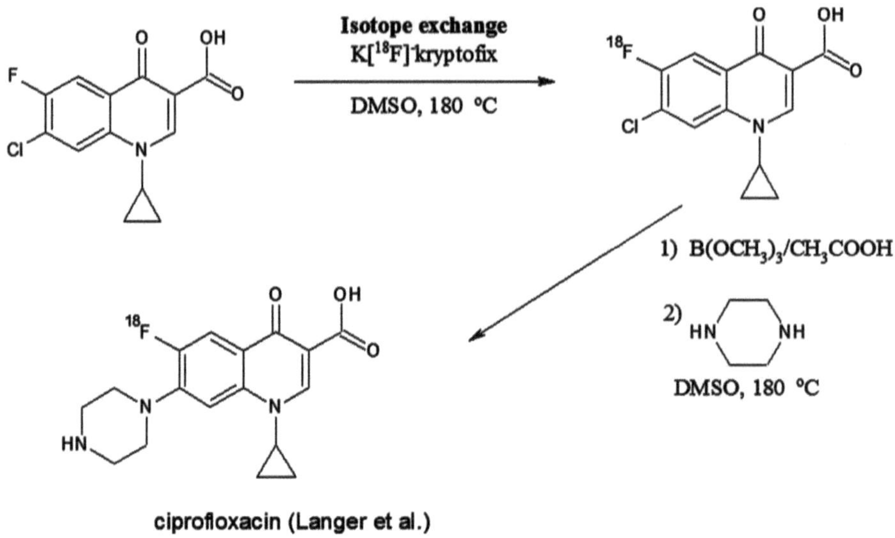

Figure 4.8 ^{18}F labeling of ciprofloxacin via isotope exchange [169]

purification using a tC2 light Sep-Pak cartridge [157]. As with all ^{99m}Tc labeled compounds, the exact structure of ^{99m}Tc-fluoroquinolones cannot be known. It was thought that structural (conformational) differences between the fluoroquinolone and the radiolabeled fluoroquinolone product and structural variety among the labeled products may help explain the occasional contradictory results. These results have not stopped interest in the radiolabeling of fluoroquinolones, however, and lomefloxacin and ofloxacin [158], sparfloxacin [159], moxifloxacin [160], norfloxacin [161], gemifloxacin [162], rufloxacin [163], clinafloxacin [164], garenoxacin [165], gatifloxacin [166], and levofloxacin [167] have all been radiolabeled with ^{99m}Tc. It is seemingly easy to radiolabel these compounds as the fluoroquinolone precursor is readily available, and provided a ^{99m}Tc-generator is available, the synthesis is simple. These compounds have mostly undergone preliminary testing in an infection animal model and were almost all reported to do better than ^{99m}Tc-ciprofloxacin in discriminating infection from sterile inflammation. Other work includes the ^{99m}Tc labeling of a number of fluoroquinolones using the *fac*-(^{99m}Tc-tricarbonyl) precursor. Again, some of these compounds were shown to perform better than ^{99m}Tc-ciprofloxacin in an animal model of infection [168]. As opposed to labeling with ^{99m}Tc, radiolabeling with ^{18}F of a fluoroquinolone in the 6-position is complicated. One success so far was to use isotope exchange to produce ^{18}F-ciprofloxacin in a two-step procedure, yielding a low-specific activity product (Figure 4.8) [169]. In a follow-up study, it was concluded that ^{18}F-ciprofloxacin is not suitable as a bacteria-specific infection imaging agent [170]. ^{18}F-fluoroquinolones that are not structurally identical to any commercial antibiotic have also been synthesized. An example is the synthesis of a number of N4′-^{18}F-fluoroalkylated ciprofloxacin analogues, one of which showed antibacterial activity in vitro [171].

Fluconazole is an antifungal agent, and not long after its discovery, it was already radiolabeled with ^{18}F. The labeling was done by substituting a diazonium group on the aromatic ring with ^{18}F to give a labeled product, chemically identical to fluconazole, in very low yield, as is typical for Schiemann ^{18}F labeling reactions. The ^{18}F-fluconazole was administered to rabbits infected with *C. albicans*. The aim of the study was not to find an infection imaging agent but to demonstrate that ^{18}F-PET can assist in determining the pharmacokinetics and dosimetry of the new fluconazole drug in humans and that was indeed what the researchers concluded [172]. Studies were then done in healthy human volunteers [173]. Later, fluconazole was radiolabeled with ^{99m}Tc to see if ^{99m}Tc-fluconazole imaging can distinguish between fungal and bacterial infections [174]. The radiolabeling was done as for peptides in a somewhat long procedure that included stirring for 2 h. The reaction mixture was analyzed by HPLC, and the radiolabeling yield and stability of the final product were determined by ITLC. Infected mice were injected with ^{99m}Tc-fluconazole and it was concluded that ^{99m}Tc-fluconazole distinguishes infections with *C. albicans* from bacterial infections and sterile inflammations.

Ceftizoxime is a third generation cephalosporin which binds to the bacterial wall, inhibits the synthesis of peptidoglycan and the synthesis of the bacterial wall [175]. Ceftizoxime was directly labeled with ^{99m}Tc by Gomes Baretto et al. [176]; later, a kit formulation for ceftizoxime radiolabeling was developed [177]. The lyophilized kit, containing 2.5 mg of ceftizoxime and 6.0 mg sodium dithionite (reducing agent), was hereby reconstituted with 1.0 mL of ^{99m}Tc-pertechnetate solution (370 MBq). The resulting solution was boiled for 10 min, cooled down, and filtered through a 0.22 μm cellulose filter in an overall simple procedure. Radiochemical purity was measured by ITLC. ^{99m}Tc-ceftizoxime was able to identify an *E. coli* infection site in rats [176].

Vancomycin is a glycopeptide that inactivates the peptidoglycan biosynthesis of the bacterial cell wall. Vancomycin was labeled with ^{99m}Tc by reacting it with ^{99m}Tc-pertechnetate using $SnCl_2{\cdot}2H_2O$ as the reducing agent in a simple procedure [178]. The radiochemical purity and stability of ^{99m}Tc-vancomycin was determined by thin layer chromatography. Biodistribution studies of ^{99m}Tc-vancomycin performed in a model of bacterial (*S. aureus*) infection in rats showed higher uptake at the sites of bacterial infection as compared to the sites of sterile inflammation [178].

Kanamycin is an aminoglycoside that is taken up intracellularly and interacts with the 30 S subunit of prokaryotic ribosomes and indirectly inhibits translocation during protein synthesis [120]. ^{99m}Tc-kanamycin was produced by reacting kanamycin with ^{99m}Tc-pertechnetate (370 MBq) for 30 min in the presence of $SnCl_2(H_2O)_2$ at pH 6–7 at room temperature in a simple procedure [179]. Radiolabeling efficiency and radiochemical purity were hereby measured by a combination of ascending paper chromatography and ITLC [142]. Imaging studies showed that ^{99m}Tc-kanamycin localized at the site of bacterial (*S. aureus*) infection in rats [179].

Cefoperazone is a third generation cephalosporin labeled with ^{99m}Tc by reacting it with ^{99m}Tc-pertechnetate (400 MBq) for 10 min using $SnCl_2(H_2O)_2$ at pH 8 at room temperature. Imaging studies showed that ^{99m}Tc-cefoperazone localized at the site of bacterial (*S. aureus*) infection in rats [180].

Cefuroxime axetil is a prodrug for the second generation cephalosporin cefuroxime. ^{99m}Tc-Cefuroxime axetil was achieved by reacting precursor in the presence of $SnCl_2$ with ^{99m}Tc-pertechnetate at room temperature, pH 3, for 20 min [181]. It was shown in vivo that ^{99m}Tc-cefuroxime axetil detects (*S. aureus*) infection in rats [182].

Novobiocin is an aminocoumarin and an inhibitor of bacterial DNA gyrase; its dithiocarbamate derivative was radiolabeled with a ^{99m}Tc-tricarbonyl in a high yield synthesis, without the need of final product purification, followed by a study with *S. aureus* infected rats indicating that ^{99m}Tc-labeled novobiocin might be specific for bacterial infection [183].

4.4.3 Radiolabeled Cells

^{111}In-Oxine-labeled autologous lymphocytes, granulocytes, and platelets have been administered to kidney graft patients to diagnose acute organ graft rejection [184] and to patients with inflammatory bowel disease [185]. These cells were isolated and radiolabeled with similar techniques described for ^{111}In-oxine-radiolabeling leukocytes. Doses ranging from 10 to 50 μCi/10^8 cells were utilized.

^{18}F-FDG-labeled autologous leukocyte preparation was reported by Bhattacharya et al. [186] and utilized to diagnose infected fluids related to pancreatitis. Briefly, 40 mL of venous blood was collected and kept upright in a stand at 37 °C for 60–70 min to separate the plasma followed by centrifugation at 450 *g* for 5 min. The white cell pellet was reconstituted and ca. 450 MBq ^{18}F-FDG were added to the suspension. This radiolabeled suspension was kept at 37 °C for 25–30 min, with gentle shaking every 5 min. After incubation, 12 mL of heparinized normal saline was added to the radiolabeled suspension, the tube was centrifuged at 450 *g* for 5 min, and the supernatant was removed. The radiolabeled white cell sediment was reconstituted with 4 mL of the patient's own cell-free plasma and reinjected intravenously. The Trypan blue-based viability test was conducted for the presence of any blue (nonviable) cells.

Dendritic cells (DC) have also been successfully radiolabeled using ^{111}In-oxine or ^{99m}Tc-HMPAO to further understand cellular and molecular mechanisms underlying infectious diseases or inflammation. A radiolabeling technique was reported by Blocklet et al. [187] in 2003 studying the influence of ^{111}In-oxime and ^{99m}Tc-HMPAO radiolabeling on the motility and actin content of antigen-loaded DCs in parallel with in vivo migration in humans. Therefore, human autologous monocyte-derived DCs were radiolabeled with ^{111}In (0.11–0.74 MBq/10^7 DCs) or ^{99m}Tc-HMPAO (18.5 or 185 MBq/10^7 DCs). ^{111}In labeling was much more stable than ^{99m}Tc-HMPAO labeling.

4.4.4 Bacteria-Specific Sugars

^{18}F-FDG-PET is presently the chief tracer for clinical imaging of bacterial infections, but despite high sensitivity, ^{18}F-FDG-PET lacks specificity, unable to distinguish between inflammation, cancer, and bacterial infection [188]. Recently, three prokaryotic-specific tracers have been developed for tomographic imaging bacterial infections [189–191].

2-^{18} F-fluorodeoxysorbitol (^{18} F-FDS); The *Enterobacteriaceae* bacteria family is the most common cause of gram-negative bacterial infections in humans including pathogens such as *E. coli*, *Yersinia* spp., and *Enterobacter* spp. The sorbitol analogue, 2-^{18}F-fluorodeoxysorbitol (^{18}F-FDS), has been shown to selectively target gram-negative bacteria allowing for more accurate infection diagnosis and treatment [189] . Not only is ^{18}F-FDS useful in targeting gram-negative bacterial infections, the tracer may be easily synthesized from commercial ^{18}F-FDG PET in 30 min as suggested in 2008 by Li et al. [192]. ^{18}F-FDS was synthesized by reduction of ^{18}F-FDG (12 mg, 0.066 mmol) using sodium borohydride ($NaBH_4$, 10 mg, 0.265 mmol) in 1 ml water, and the resulting mixture was stirred at 35 °C for 15 min. After quenching the reaction, the mixture was adjusted to a pH of 7.4 and filtered through an Alumina-N Sep-Pak cartridge.

6-^{18}F-Fluoromaltose makes use of the bacteria-specific maltodextrin pathway that enables bacteria to bind, transport, and utilize maltose and maltodextrin as energy sources [193]. 6-^{18}F-Fluoromaltose is taken up by multiple strains of pathogenic bacteria. It is not taken up by mammalian cancer cell lines and does not accumulate in inflamed tissue. The synthesis is published [190]. Briefly, 4-*O*-(α-D-glucopyranosyl)-6-deoxy-6-^{18}F-fluoro-D-glucopyranoside (6-^{18}F-fluoromaltose) was prepared by nucleophilic displacement of the nosylate group in a 1,2,3-tri-*O*-acetyl-4-*O*-(2′,3′,-di-*O*-aceteyl-4′,6′-benzylidene-α-D-glucopyranosyl)-6-deoxy-6-nosyl-D-glucopranosideprecursor by ^{18}F-fluoride ion in acetonitrile at 80 °C for 10 min. Initial purification was performed via a light C-18 Sep-Pak cartridge followed by passing the solution through a light neutral alumina Sep-Pak; deprotection was carried out first with 1 N HCl (110 °C, 10 min) followed by 2 N NaOH at room temperature for 4 min. After HPLC purification of the solution, 6-^{18}F-fluoromaltose was recovered in 5–8% radiochemical yield (decay corrected) with 95% radiochemical purity.

^{18}F-labeled maltohexaose (^{18}F-MH) is able to selectively differentiate bacterial infections from cancer or inflammation. Similar to the above mentioned sugar derivatives, MH has the advantage of mimicking food additives previously approved by the FDA. Sorbitol is a common "sugar-free" sweetener, maltose is frequently a component of various beverages and pastas, and maltodextrin is a food and beverage thickener. PET imaging has the potential to drastically improve diagnosis, and therefore treatment, of pathogenic bacterial infections through noninvasive, rapid means. Improving upon ^{18}F-FDG-PET, more bacteria-specific tracers are necessary to achieve a more precise diagnosis.

4.4.5 Macromolecules and Antibodies

Making up about 75% of the plasma antibodies, immunoglobulin G (IgG) is the most common form of antibody produced during a secondary immune response, triggered by repeated exposure to an antigen. The structure of IgG includes four peptide chains, two identical heavy chains and two identical light chains, arranged in a Y-shape. IgG binds to viruses, bacteria, and bacterially derived toxins in large enough quantities to neutralize the antigen by blocking its ability to bind the host. Along with the latter, the antigen-bound IgGs are able to destroy pathogens by binding to F_c receptors on macrophages and neutrophils, immune cells that destroy antigens via phagocytosis [194–196].

^{111}In-DTPA-IgG is an alternative for radiolabeled leukocytes which are not viable imaging agents for infectious disease imaging in neutropenic patients [197]. While attempting to develop tracers for imaging inflammation, nonspecific IgG was originally radiolabeled using the diethylenetriaminepentaacetic acid (DTPA) antibody chelate method, originally detailed by Krecjarek and Tucker and modified by Khaw et al. [198–200] Briefly, DTPA chelator is dissolved in water with triethylamine and subsequently lyophilized to yield an oily residue [200]. Isobutyl chloroformate is then added to a solution of pentatriethylammonium-DTPA in acetonitrile and is cooled to 0 °C in an ice bath. The reaction is then stirred for 30 min at 0 °C during which time triethylamine hydrochloride precipitates resulting in a mix of carboxycarbonic anhydride DTPA. Reacting polyclonal IgG with the DTPA-anhydride mixture forms a covalent bond between the amino group of an immunoglobulin and, typically, 2 DTPA molecules per IgG protein. This reaction yields a radiolabeling efficiency of greater than 98% [198]. To test this theory, a deep thigh ***E. coli*** rat infection model was used to compare tracer efficacy of ^{111}In-DTPA-IgG and ^{99m}Tc-HYNIC-IgG [201].

^{99m}Tc-HYNIC-IgG; Diffusion of radiolabeled IgG into expended protein space of inflammatory lesions is rapid; therefore, lesion imaging should be possible with high-count density images [202]. The limited photon flux associated with ^{111}In led to a search for more desirable radionuclides to label IgG, such as ^{99m}Tc. A study compared inflammatory imaging potential for ^{111}In-DTPA-IgG and ^{99m}Tc-HYNIC-IgG in human subjects and determined the preparations of IgG have similar biodistribution and imaging properties. However, based on the physical properties of ^{99m}Tc, there is a three-fold greater photon flux present at the lesion sites at 18 h post-injection when 20-fold more ^{99m}Tc-IgG is initially injected. The greater photon flux at earlier time points of ^{99m}Tc, as compared with ^{111}In, greatly enhances image quality [203]. Various methods for labeling IgG with ^{99m}Tc affect the quality of inflammation imaging results [203]. These methods include direct binding of technetium to donor atoms on IgG, labeling via bifunctional chelators, and conjugation of a preformed ^{99m}Tc-4,5-bis(thioacetanido)pentanoate active ester to protein amine groups (also known as the N_2S_2-method) [201]. Depending on the method, radiolabeled IgGs may clear more rapidly from circulation. The latter effect makes for better tissue-to-blood ratios; however, exposure of the labeled IgGs to the site of inflammation and/or infection may be compromised [203]. Direct ^{99m}Tc labeling can be achieved with a modification of the hinge region of IgG antibodies [120]. Reducing the disulfide bonds allows for ^{99m}Tc to coordinate directly with the free thiol groups. A kit formulation for direct labeling of ^{99m}Tc to hIgG has been available commercially for some time [120]. The direct labeling method was used a clinical study to evaluate the efficacy of ^{99m}Tc-hIgG as an imaging agent for localizing inflammatory bowel disease. When compared with ^{111}In-labeled granulocytes,

^{99m}Tc-hIgG proved to perform inferior and was therefore deemed unsuitable for inflammatory bowel disease PET imaging [120].

^{99m}Tc-Human Serum Albumin (HSA); Produced by the liver, albumin is the most abundant protein in plasma with a blood half-life of 19 days. HSA is secreted from liver cells into intravascular space at a rate of approximately 13–14 g/day. HSA levels can be detected in various human secretions such as milk, sweat, tears, and saliva. However, the highest concentrations of HSA lost are due to degradation in skin and muscle. Extravascular HSA is returned to vascular compartments via the lymphatic system. HSA functions to regulate plasma pH and colloidal blood pressure as well as a carrier of fatty acids, hormones, and drug transport protein in plasma [204]. Radiolabeled albumin is often used as an imaging agent for analyzing blood flow and lymphatic drainage. ^{99m}Tc-labeled macroaggregated albumin (MAA) is used to image lung perfusion, ^{18}F- and ^{68}Ga-albumin is a PET blood-pool marker, and ^{99m}Tc-HSA is used to monitor gastrointestinal bleeding. More recently in 2015, Fu et al. published an abstract claiming ^{99m}Tc-HSA to be a potential tracer in monitoring acute lung injury induced by lipopolysaccharide in rats [205].

^{99m}Tc-Infliximab; Infliximab, presently under the trade names Remicade, Remsima, and Inflectra is a chimeric IgG1 monoclonal antibody FDA-approved to treat autoimmune diseases such as Crohn's disease, pediatric Crohn's disease, ulcerative colitis, pediatric ulcerative colitis, rheumatoid arthritis, psoriatic arthritis, ankylosing spondylitis, and plaque psoriasis [206]. Most commonly and successfully, Infliximab is radiolabeled with ^{99m}Tc using a direct labeling method developed by Annovazzi et al. [207]. Briefly, disulfide bridges present in monoclonal antibodies are first reduced using 2-mercaptoethanol. Radiolabeling is then accomplished by using methylene diphosphonic acid as a weak competitive ligand. This direct labeling is highly efficient with labeling yields of greater than 97% [207, 208]. In 2005, a study utilized ^{99m}Tc-infliximab to assess the degree of TNF-α expression and monitor treatment for a patient suffering from inflammation at the knee joint. Initial assessment of TNF-α expression within the inflamed knee using ^{99m}Tc-infliximab showed intense accumulation within the affected knee joint, indicating a high density of TNF-α. TNF-α expression was monitored through intra-articular infliximab therapy with no uptake of ^{99m}Tc-infliximab detected after therapy [206, 208].

^{99m}Tc-hr-Interleukin 8 (IL-8); Also known as the neutrophil chemotactic factor, it is produced by macrophages and epithelial cells [209]. IL-8, stored within epithelial cell vesicles, binds with high affinity to neutrophil and monocytes receptors CXC1 and CXC2 to activate and recruit immune cells to the site of infection. Previous in vivo studies determined that uptake of IL-8 peaks 1–3 h postinjection [210]. IL-8 possesses various ideal qualities for use as an infection and inflammation image agent including rapid accumulation in target tissues as well as rapid clearance from blood and nontarget organs. IL-8 is mainly metabolized via the renal system, being superior to the hepatobiliary system because high activity in the liver and bowel would limit abdominal imaging capabilities [209]. In radiolabeling, IL-8 is first conjugated with the HYNIC chelator by adding succinimidyl-HYNIC in dry dimethyl sulfoxide dropwise to a solution of IL-8 and sodium bicarbonate (pH 8.2).

The reaction is quenched using excess glycine and diluted in phosphate-buffed saline. Reaction time as well as the ratio of protein concentration to succinimidyl-HYNIC is critical for sufficient labeling yields. The HYNIC-conjugated IL-8 is purified via dialysis and stored at −20 °C. When needed, the frozen conjugates are thawed and incubated with $^{99m}TcO_4^-$ with stannous sulfate at room temperature for 30 min. When using ideal conditions, a radiolabeling efficiency of up to 97% can be achieved [210]. Rennen et al. also utilized ^{99m}Tc-IL-8 to image *E. coli* infection and inflammation in a rabbit model and reported rapid visualization of infection within a few hours after injection as well as high target-to-background ratios.

^{99m}Tc-PEG-Liposomes; Liposomes are small, artificially made vesicles formed of phospholipids containing an aqueous core that may be used as a vehicle for drug delivery, genetic material, and cosmetics. Due to the advantage of the hydrophobic lipid tails and hydrophilic heads of the phospholipids, liposomes have the advantage of carrying both hydrophobic and hydrophilic compounds. Initial attempts to image infection using radiolabeled liposomes began unfavorably [211]. The initial approach of labeling liposomes aimed to entrap radionuclides within the liposome vesicle during the initial hydration of the lipids with aqueous phase; however, this approach led to low encapsulation yields of less than 30% for large, multi-lamellar liposomes and below 5% for small, unilamellar liposomes [212]. The labeled liposomes were rapidly removed from the blood via cells of the mononuclear phagocyte system (MPS), which compromised targeting of non-MPS tissues. Following encapsulation, further labeling attempts focused on surface labeling of the liposomes post-manufacture. Stannous chloride was used to reduce the oxidation state of ^{99m}Tc and was subsequently added to stannous chloride-treated liposomes. The ^{99m}Tc is added directly to the outer lipid surface of the liposome. This method yields variable results with reported radiolabeling efficiencies averaging 50% and typically has poor in vivo stability due to ^{99m}Tc dissociation and accumulation in the kidney and bladder. The next attempt at labeling aimed to incorporate a chelator, such as DTPA, covalently bound to an amphiphile incorporated in the lipid bilayer. Although the use of chelators in radiolabeling is fairly common and successful, the use of DTPA chelator in labeling liposomes requires precise amounts of tin in order to maintain the reduced state of the ^{99m}Tc while at the same time preventing the formation of colloidal tin. Owing to the sensitive nature of this preparation, there are large variations in synthesis yields and labeling efficacy. Adding to the latter, a similar approach encapsulates an already ^{99m}Tc chelated-HMPAO complex by using liposomes manufactured to encapsulate glutathione. The method of labeling is hypothesized to be the lipophilic HMPAO that carries the ^{99m}Tc into the liposome where it interacts with the encapsulated glutathione thereby converting it to a hydrophilic chelation complex and trapping the radionuclide within the liposome. Labeling efficiencies using this method range from 85 to 98% and stability is maintained as shown through its activity within the heart, liver, and spleen with no activity in the kidney or bladder. Therefore, a surface modification of the liposomes was necessary to promote long circulation of the tracer. Adding a synthetic lipid derivative, specifically polyethylene glycol (PEG), resulted in decreased recognition of

the liposomes by MPS, thereby increasing circulation time and blood residence time [211, 212].

^{99m}Tc-HYNIC-C5adR; A protein fragment of complement component C5a is a 74-amino acid glycoprotein produced from the activation of the complement system. The complement component C5 is cleaved into its components C5a and C5b by the protease C5-convertase. C5b is crucial to the complement cascade while C5a holds various roles as a mediator of inflammation both in vitro and in vivo. C5a induces smooth muscle contraction, promotes margination, causes chemotaxis and degranulation of neutrophils, increases vascular permeability, and stimulates the release of cytokines from macrophages [213]. C5a has relatively high receptor binding affinity compared with its C5adR metabolite; however, the spasmogenic and anaphylactic nature of C5a renders it unsuitable as a clinical imaging agent. C5adR, on the other hand, does not possess these same biological undesirables, but showed much lower uptake in the rabbit thigh *E. coli* abscess, most likely due to a lower binding affinity than C5a [214]. Using a radiolabeling synthesis similar to ^{99m}Tc-HYNIC-IL-8, Rennen et al. examined and compared C5a and C5adR as potential imaging agents. The leukocyte receptor binding proteins were labeled with ^{99m}Tc using the hydrazinonicotinamide (HYNIC) coupling agent and tested in an *E. coli* rabbit infection model. In this study, human C5adR were produced using *E. coli* cells. To synthesize the HYNIC-C5adR chelator complex, an excess of HYNIC, in dry DMSO, is added dropwise to a buffered solution (pH 8.2) of purified human C5adR. After 5 minutes of incubation at room temperature, an excess of glycine, in phosphate buffered saline (PBS), is added to quench the reaction. The excess HYNIC in solution was removed via dialysis. To radiolabel, the HYNIC-C5adR chelator complex is incubated in a PBS solution of tricine and tin(II) sulfate with $^{99m}TcO_4^-$ for 30 min at room temperature. The radiochemical purify was determined to be greater than 95% after gel filtration with 50% labeling efficiency of the HYNIC-C5adR [214].

Antibodies Radiolabeled with $^{123/125}$I-iodine; A murine Mab of the IgG_1 subclass was radiolabeled with ^{125}I via the iodogen method [1]. It was possible to detect the sites of soft tissue infection using a rat model of Fisher immunotype 1 *Pseudomonas aeruginosa* [215]. The anti-granulocyte antibody Mab47 was radiolabeled with ^{123}I using the iodogen method (^{123}I-Granuloscint) and was used over a number of years to image infections in human patients [216]. This radiopharmaceutical never achieved widespread usage possibly because of the disadvantages of biological compounds produced with hybridoma techniques [217, 218]. More recently, ^{123}I-hr-IL-1α &-1β radiolabeling was achieved with the aforementioned procedures. The chemokine interleukin 1 (IL-1) binds to various leukocytes with high affinity, making IL-1 a potential imaging agent to localize inflammatory tissue [219]. IL-1 is associated with both acute and chronic inflammation as well as a pro-inflammatory role in the nonspecific innate response to infection. The two subtypes IL-1α and IL-1β are 17-kDa proteins released by mononuclear phagocytes in response to an inflammation that stimulates T cells to liberate and produce more interleukin 2 (IL-2). Along with high binding affinity, IL-1 administered intravenously has been shown to rapidly clear from the blood of mice with a half-life of approximately 5–10 min [220]. The interleukin-1α subtype is synthesized by primary cells including keratinocytes, thymic epithelium, hepatocytes, endothelial cells, fibroblasts, and epithelial cells of mucous membranes. IL-1α was radiolabeled using $Na^{123}I$, according to the iodogen method, most effectively [220]. Briefly, a known concentration of human recombinant IL-1α and $Na^{123}I$ is incubated in phosphate buffer (pH 7.2) in glass tubing pre-coated with 3α,6α-diphenylglucoril for 10 min at room temperature. The latter method yields a specific activity of 216–270 µCi/µmol, indicative of an average of 1–2 ^{123}I atoms associated with each IL-1 molecule and a radiochemical purity of greater than 98%. Using this radioiodination method, van der Laken et al. also reported the imaging potential of iodinated IL-1 in a *S. aureus* mouse calf muscle infection model. ^{123}I -IL-1α was significantly concentrated in the infection abscess with an abscess-to-muscle ratio of 44:1 at 48 h postinjection [220]. *Interleukin-1β subtype* is also synthesized by various immune cells including monocytes, macrophages, dendritic cells, B-lymphocytes, and natural killer cells. IL-1β aids in the inflammatory response by enhancing T-cell activation and recognition of the antigen by developing and/or differentiating T-helper 17 cells that release IFNγ and prostaglandins at the site of inflammation. Regardless of the two IL-1 subtypes being divergent gene products, both subtypes recognize the same surface receptors as well as similar biological activities [120, 220]. Alternatively, the *Bolton-Hunter* method (BH) is a common radio-iodination method for radiolabeling both subtypes of IL-1 and the IL-1 receptor antagonist (IL-1ra), though this method produces much lower labeling efficiencies of 25–35% [221]. The BH method of radiolabeling was used as the preferred method maintaining the binding capacity of IL-1ra. Briefly, the commercially available BH reagent (*N*-succinimidyl 3-(4-hydroxy-5-phenyl) propionate) is incubated in methanol for 10 min at room temperature with ^{123}I and *N*-chlorosuccinimide. Then, IL-1 is incubated with the radiolabeled BH reagent in an aqueous bicarbonate buffer (pH 8.2) for 30 min at 0 °C. The radioiodinated BH reagent reacts with the terminal amino group of interleukin 1 as a way of indirectly radioiodinating, as opposed to directly binding iodine to the protein. This method produces low labeling efficiencies (25–35%); however, receptor binding efficiency was maintained and radiochemical purity exceeds 95%. In the same study, such radiolabeled IL-1α, IL-1β, IL-1ra, and the synthetic chemotactic peptide *N*-formyl-methionyl-leucyl-phenylalanyl-lysine (fMLFK) were compared as potential imaging agents for biodistribution and infection-localizing properties in an *E. coli* thigh infection model in rabbits [221].

^{68}Ga-Apo-Transferrin; Transferrins are a class of blood plasma glycoproteins able to bind iron with high affinity, thereby mediating the level of free iron in biological fluids. When not bound to free iron, transferrin is known as apo-transferrin. Since iron is crucial for bacterial growth, transferrin aids in maintaining low concentrations (10^{-12} µM) in body fluids creating undesirable growth environments for pathogenic bacteria. To overcome this, bacteria, including *S. aureus*, have been known to produce and release siderophores and transferrin-binding protein (TBP) that assimilate free iron from human transferrin-bound iron [222]. Transferrins are able to

chelate Ga^{3+} utilizing a mechanism similar to iron binding. Therefore, Kumar et al. aimed to prepare a $^{68}Ga^{3+}$-transferrin complex for rapid PET imaging of *S. aureus* infection in vivo [82]. The ^{68}Ga-labeled transferrins were synthesized by incubating the post-processed $^{68}GaCl_3$ with a sodium carbonate (0.1 M, pH 7.0) solution of transferrin in a 40 °C water bath for 1 h. For this method, radiochemical purity and yield were determined to be greater than 99%, and stability tests in carbonate solution determined the radiolabeled complex remained intact for 6 h after synthesis. The preclinical application of radiolabeled apo-transferrin (^{68}Ga-TF), uptake in a rat thigh infection model was also published in the same article [82].

4.4.6 Small Peptide Fragments

Peptides can be conveniently synthesized using solid phase peptide synthesizers and can be almost custom designed as very specific probes [223]. Chemically they are preferred as they show greater chemical stability and versatility over proteins or other compounds. Some peptide-based bioconjugates have been reported for infection imaging [224].

Ubiquicidin (UBI29-41) has been reported as one of more clinically advanced peptide radiodiagnostics for imaging bacterial presence in vivo. It is a 13mer, antimicrobial, cation-rich fragment (OH-Tyr-Gly-Arg-Ala-Lys-Arg-Arg-Met-Gln-Tyr--Asn-Arg-Arg-NH_2) which was initially radiolabeled with ^{99m}Tc in 2000 by Welling et al. [225]. Briefly, the peptide was added to an aseptic mixture of stannous chloride and sodium pyrophosphate in saline and mixed with a solution of potassium borohydrate in sodium hydroxide. Ca. 200 MBq ^{99m}Tc-sodium pertechnetate was added to this mixture, and the solution was then ready for use within 10 min incubation at room temperature. The purity and radioactive yield-of ^{99m}Tc-UBI29-41 was determined by HPLC and ITLC, respectively. Nowadays, a kit solution for the preparation of ^{99m}Tc-UBI29-41 has become available for use in humans. The kit lysophylate comprises 400 μg of UBI29-41 in acetic acid along with stannous ions from a standard pyrophosphate kit, sodium borohydrate in 0.1 N NaOH; and is maintained at a physiological pH. The preparation takes 10–15 min for incubation followed by formulation in saline and can be used within 6 h of reconstitution. More recently, the UBI29-41 was functionalized with NOTA using a method by Guerin et al. [226], characterized and successfully radiolabeled [227] to allow for PET imaging in a rabbit infection model [228]. ^{68}Ga was eluted from a generator and buffered with a sodium acetate solution to yield a pH of 3.5 for ^{68}Ga-complexation, which was achieved after adding 10–30 nmol NOTA-UBI2-41 and incubation for 10 min at 90 °C. Following purification using solid phase extraction, ^{68}Ga-NOTA-UBI29-41was qualified by radio-HPLC/UV analysis.

Human neutrophil peptide 1 (HNP-1) antimicrobial peptides of the defensin family [229] is one of the best studied peptides and was exploited for infection imaging [230]. Therefore, HNP-1 was purified from human neutrophils and radiolabeled with ^{99m}Tc [231]. Briefly, 10 μL of a solution of 1 mg/mL HNP-1 in 10 mmol/L sodium phosphate buffer (Na-PB), pH 7.4, was added to 2 μL of an aseptic solution containing 0.5 mg/mL stannous pyrophosphate. Immediately, 4 μL of a solution containing 10 mg/mL crystalline KBH_4 in 0.1 mol/L NaOH was added. After the addition of 200 MBq ^{99m}Tc-sodium pertechnetate, the mixture was gently stirred for 30 min at room temperature. To remove excess reactants, the mixture was purified by a Sep-Pak C18 cartridge-based procedure before ^{99m}Tc-HNP-1 was formulated in 100 μL Na-PB. The recovery of HNP-1 was 96% with a radiolabeling yield of 95%.

The human-beta-defensin (HDB) fragment HBD-3 was labeled through the cationic aqua complex $[^{99m}Tc\ (H_2O)_3(CO)_3]^+$, based on direct reduction of $^{99m}TcO_4^-$ with sodium borohydride in aqueous solution in the presence of carbon monoxide [232]. Briefly, 1 mL of water containing $^{99m}TcO_4^-$ (salt) was added to the Isolink vial, and the reaction mixture was heated at 100 °C for 20 min to synthesize the intermediate $[^{99m}Tc\ (H_2O)_3(CO)_3]^+$ followed by cooling to room temperature. At pH 8.0, 20–40 μg of peptide was added to the vial, and the mixture was left to react at room temperature for 60 min. The labeled HBD-3 was liberated from salts and inorganic ^{99m}Tc by gel chromatography through a Sephadex G-25 disposable column (PD-10) equilibrated and eluted in physiologic saline.

Lactoferrin-derived peptide (hLF) corresponds to amino acids residues 1–11 of hLF (GRRRRSVQWCA). The radiolabeling of hLF(1–11) with ^{99m}Tc was reported by Welling et al. [225] using the aforementioned method for ^{99m}Tc-UBI29-41.

Neutrophil-specific peptide targeting the formyl peptide receptor (FPR) on leukocytes was reported by Locke et al. (2009) [233]. The peptide cinnamoyl-F-(D) L-F-(D)L-FK (cFLFLF) was sequentially conjugated with a bifunctional polyethylene glycol moiety (PEG, 3.4 kD), and DOTA was conjugated to cFLFLF through a lysine spacer. The peptide radiolabeling was accomplished by adding $^{64}CuCl_2$ to 5–20 μg of DOTA-PEG-KFLFLFc in 0.1 N ammonium acetate (pH 5.5) buffer, and the mixture was incubated at 40 °C for 30 min followed by reverse phase (HPLC) purification. The radiochemical yield was >95% with a specific activity of 1.1×10^6 MBq/mmol (yield: 90%) ^{64}Cu-DOTA-PEG-KFLFLFc.

Vascular adhesion protein-1 (VAP-1) is induced at the sites of inflammation where extravasation of leukocytes from blood to the peripheral tissue occurs. It can be targeted by ^{68}Ga-DOTA-VAP-P1 (9mer linear peptide) or ^{68}Ga (cyclic 17mer peptide) which was yielded by conjugating DOTA via an 8-amino-3,6-diooxaoctanoyl linker (polyethylene glycol, PEG derivative) [234]. Radiolabeling was carried out using sodium acetate-buffered ^{68}Ga (pH ~5.5) in the presence of 30 nmol DOTA-peptide; the reaction mixture was incubated at 100 °C for 20 min and no further purification was needed. Radiochemical purity was determined by reversed-phase HPLC [235]. The same research group recently exploited a bioconjugate of DOTA and the sialic acid-binding immunoglobulin-like lectin 9 (Siglec-9) motif containing peptide (^{68}Ga-DOTA-Siglec-9) for PET imaging targeting inflammatory response due to *staphylococcal* peri-implant infection [236].

Integrins are universal targets with different expressions related to different diseases, and various radiolabeled antagonists have been introduced for integrin imaging [237]. The most studied compound for nuclear medical imaging is a tripeptide sequence consisting of Arg-Gly-Asp (RGD), which binds to a variety of integrins, including αvβ3. In particular, multi-meric RGD-motif containing bioconjugates can be considered for targeting inflammation. Dijkgraaf et al. synthesized ^{68}Ga-DOTA-E-[c(RGDfK)]$_2$ by reacting DOTA-E-[c(RGDfK)]$_2$ with ^{68}Ga in an ammonium acetate buffer (pH ~5.5) at 95 °C for 20 min. Radiochemical purity was ~98% as determined by high-performance liquid chromatography. The maximum specific activity was 11.2 MBq/nmol (0.3 mCi/nmol). ^{68}Ga-DOTA-E-[c(RGDfK)]$_2$ was stable in phosphate-buffered saline and human serum at 37 °C for 2 h [238].

Duramycin is a 19mer polypeptide produced by *Streptoverticillium cinnamoneus* targeting phosphatidylethanolamine. It is mainly reported in preclinical imaging studies targeting apoptotic tissue [239], but it was also related to targeting viral infection [240], for example, sporogonic stages of plasmodium [241]. HYNIC-conjugated duramycin was labeled with ^{99m}Tc using the tricine–phosphine coligand system by mixing 15 mg of HYNIC-conjugated duramycin with 40 mg of tricine, 1 mg of trisodium triphenylphosphine-3,3,3-trisulfonate (TPPTS), and 20 mg of $SnCl_2$ at pH 5.3. The labeling was initiated with the addition of about 37 MBq of ^{99m}Tc, reacting for 40 min at room temperature. ^{99m}Tc-duramycin was than analyzed and purified using HPLC [242]. A kit formulation for ^{99m}Tc-duramycin preparation became recently available; 150 μg of HYNIC-duramycin, 300 mg tricine, and 95 mg TPPTS were added, with 62.5 μg of $SnCl_2$ in a final volume of 5 mL to allow labeling with 30 mCi of ^{99m}Tc-pertechnetate [243]. Duramycin was also conjugated to yield *N*-(2-[^{18}F]fluoropropionyl)duramycin ([^{18}F]FP-Duramycin) which was prepared from the reaction of duramycin with 4-nitrophenyl 2-^{18}F-fluoropropionate (^{18}F-NFP) [244].

Depsipeptides were considered for infection and inflammation imaging, for example, TBIA-101. Following peptide synthesis and DOTA conjugation, ^{68}Ga radiolabeling was reported by Mokaleng et al. in 2015 using an adapted labeling protocol published for DOTATATE [245]. Briefly, 40 nmol DOTA-TBIA-101 was incubated for 15–20 min at pH 3.5 in the presence of sodium acetate buffered ^{68}Ga, followed by solid phase extraction, yielding ^{68}Ga-DOTA-TBIA-101 in >98% purity with radiolabeling yields of 69–98%.

4.4.7 Other Agents

Biotin is necessary for cell growth, fatty acid production, and metabolism of fats and amino acids. It also is used as a growth factor by certain bacteria. ^{111}In-Biotin-SPECT has been used clinically for diagnosing spinal infections [205, 246]. ^{111}In-labeled biotin derivatives were initially prepared by Virzi et al. [247]. Syntheses were done using DTPA and ethylene diamine tetraacetic acid (EDTA) derivatives of biotin, and labeling was carried out with sodium acetate buffered ^{111}In (pH 5.5–6.0); DTPA-biotin was mixed with radioactive indium chloride (^{111}In-$InCl_3$), and the mixture was incubated at room temperature for 15 min. Labeling efficiency of the reaction was reported to be >98% as determined with instant thin-layer chromatography.

Synthesis of two ^{18}F-labeled biotin derivatives was also attempted using a noncarrier-added approach [248].

Radiolabeled acycloguanosine and thymidine derivatives have been studied for in vitro imaging of the herpes simplex virus thymidine kinase 1 reporter gene system both in small animals and in humans. It was also utilized for targeting viral infection and inflammation.

9-(4-^{18}F-Fluoro-3-hydroxymethylbutyl)guanine (^{18}F-FHBG) is a side chain ^{18}F-labeled analogue of penciclovir. Penciclovir (9-(4-hydroxy-3-hydroxymethylbutyl)-guanine) was converted to the methoxy-trityl derivative followed by tosylation. The tosylate was reacted with either tetrabutylammonium ^{18}F-fluoride or ^{18}F-KF in the presence of Kryptofix 2.2.2, followed by acidic hydrolysis to produce ^{18}F-FHBG which was subsequently purified by HPLC. The radiochemical yield amounted up to >20% maximum (corrected for decay). Synthesis time was ca. 100 min, including HPLC purification with radiochemical purity >99% (specific activity of 11.8 GBq/mmol) [249]. An automated synthesis was reported to provide 10–15% yield within 60 min [250].

1-(2′-Deoxy-2′-fluoro-beta-D-arabinofuranosyl)-5-124I iodouracil (124I-FIAU) is able to detect bacterial infection including mycobacterium tuberculosis in vivo and allows for PET/CT imaging. 2′-Fluoro-2′-deoxy-1-beta-d-arabinofuranosyluracil (FAU) was generally labeled by direct radioiodination such as with ^{124}I-NaI to form ^{124}I-FIAU. ^{124}I-FIAU was isolated by HPLC purification with a radiochemical yield of 51–55% and with radiochemical purity of >97%. A higher radiochemical yield (>85%) can be achieved by utilizing 5-trimethylstannyl-1-(2′-fluoro-2′deoxy-1-beta-d-arabinofuranosyl)uracil (FTAU) to react with ^{124}I-NaI to form ^{124}I-FIAU [251]. The radiochemical yield was in the range of 85–95% with radiochemical purity of >98% [252]. A ^{18}F-labeled FAU radiodiagnostic agent (^{18}F-FFAU) is also reported by reaction of the triflate (2-deoxy-2-trifluoromethanesulfonyl-1,3,5-tri-*O*-benzoyl-α-D-ribofuranose) with tetrabutylammonium ^{18}F-fluoride. This reaction produced 2-^{18}F-fluoro-1,3,5-tri-*O*-benzoyl-α-D-arabinofuranose, which was converted to its 1-bromo derivative by treatment with hydrogen bromide in acetic acid (HBr/AcOH). After coupling with protected 5-fluorouracil, the resulting product was hydrolyzed (in base) and purified using HPLC [253].

Radioligands of the translocator protein (TSPO), formerly known as the peripheral benzodiazepine receptor, is overexpressed under pathological conditions. PK11195 is the prototype ligand for TSPO [254–256] and was subsequently labeled with ^{11}C [257] to detect macrophage-associated inflammation with PET imaging. However, the short half-life of ^{11}C limits the use; therefore the same article reported ^{18}F-DPA-714, whereas the labeling for ^{125}I-iodoDPA-713 was achieved by Wang et al. [5] as follows: to a solution of *N,N*-diethyl-2-(2-(4-hydroxyphenyl)-5,7-dimethyl-pyrazolo(1,5-*a*)pyrimidin-3-yl)-acetamide, 200 μg iodogen (1,3,4,6-tetrachloro-3α,6α-diphenyl-glycouril) and 74 MBq (2 mCi) ^{125}I-NaI was added. The mixture was incubated for 90 min at room temperature. *N,N*-diethyl-2-(2-(4-hydroxy-^{125}I-iodophenyl)-5,7-dimethyl-pyrazolo(1,5-*a*)pyrimidin-3-yl)-acetamide was purified with HPLC to provide a 47% radiochemical yield. *N,N*-diethyl-2-(2-(4-hydroxy-^{125}I-iodophenyl)-5,7-dimethyl-pyrazolo(1,5-*a*) pyrimidin-3-yl)-acetamide was *O*-methylated with CH_3I in the presence of K_2CO_3 to form ^{125}I-iodoDPA-713 with a radiochemical yield of 86%. The ^{125}I-iodoDPA-713 exhibited a radiochemical purity (as determined with HPLC) of >99% with a specific activity of 51.8 GBq/μmol (1.4 Ci/μmol).

4.5 Summary

We have described the radiochemical methods to produce radiopharmaceuticals for SPECT and PET and also discussed the synthesis of several agents used for infection imaging. Translation of new agents to the clinic requires excellent preclinical validation, robust synthetic schemes, and compliance with manufacturing guidelines such as the GMP regulations enforced by the FDA. The specialized equipment (e.g., cyclotron) required to produce radiopharmaceuticals can be a challenge. However, central radiopharmacies, now a common phenomenon throughout the world, and distribution networks have partially solved this problem. However, the use of on-site generators, such as those used to produce ^{68}Ga radiopharmaceuticals can greatly enhance the availably of radiopharmaceuticals, and kit formulations for ^{68}Ga labeling are eagerly anticipated. Finally, the discovery of novel targets for pathogen-specific imaging as well as their specific ligands is very exciting, and robust radiolabeling techniques could expedite the development of future rapid and specific, whole-body detection and monitoring of infections such as TB.

References

1. Adam, M.J. and D.S. Wilbur, *Radiohalogens for imaging and therapy.* Chemical Society Reviews, 2005. **34**: p. 153-163.
2. IAEA. *Cyclotron Produced Radionuclides : Physical Characteristics and Production Methods.* 2009.
3. Koehler, L., et al., *Iodine-124: A Promising Positron Emitter for Organic PET Chemistry.* Molecules, 2010. **15**: p. 2686-2718.
4. IAEA. *TECDOC-1512 Production techniques and quality control of sealed radioactive sources of palladium-103, iodine-125, iridium-192 and ytterbium-169.* 2006.
5. Wang, H., et al., *Synthesis of [125I]iodoDPA-713: A new probe for imaging inflammation.* Biochemical and Biophysical Research Communications, 2009. **389**: p. 80-83.
6. Signore, A., et al., *Molecular Imaging of Inflammation / Infection : Nuclear Medicine and Optical Imaging Agents and Methods.* Chemical Reviews, 2010. **110**: p. 3112-3145.
7. Clark, J.C. and P.D. Buckingham, *The preparation and storage of carbon-11 labelled gases for clinical use.* The International Journal of Applied Radiation and Isotopes, 1971. **22**(11): p. 639-646.
8. Scott, P.J., *Methods for the incorporation of carbon-11 to generate radiopharmaceuticals for PET imaging.* Angewandte Chemie International Edition, 2009. **48**(33): p. 6001-6004.
9. Tochon-Danguy, H.J., et al., *Positron emission tomography: radioisotope and radiopharmaceutical production.* Australasian Physical and Engineering Science in Medicine, 1999. **22**(4): p. 136-144.

10. Wuest, F., M. Berndt, and T. Kniess, *Carbon-11 labeling chemistry based upon [11C]methyl iodide.* Ernst Schering Research Foundation Workshop, 2007(62): p. 183-213.
11. Liu, L., et al., *Radiosynthesis and bioimaging of the tuberculosis chemotherapeutics isoniazid, rifampicin and pyrazinamide in baboons.* Journal of Medicinal Chemistry, 2010. **53**(7): p. 2882-2891.
12. Coenen, H.H., *Fluorine-18 Labeling Methods: Features and Possibilities of Basic Reactions.* Ernst Schering Research Foundation Workshop, 2007(62): p. 15-50.
13. Cai, L., S. Lu, and V.W. Pike, *Chemistry with [18F]fluoride ion.* European Journal of Organic Chemistry, 2008: p. 2853-2873.
14. Ermert, J., *18 F-Labelled Intermediates for Radiosynthesis by Modular Build-Up Reactions: Newer Developments.* BioMed Research International, 2014.
15. Kao, C.H.K., et al., *GMP production of [18F]FDOPA and issues concerning its quality analyses as in USP "fluorodopa F 18 Injection".* Annals of Nuclear Medicine, 2011. **25**: p. 309-316.
16. Ross, T.L., et al., *Nucleophilic 18F-Fluorination of Heteroaromatic Iodonium Salts with No-Carrier-Added [18F]Fluoride.* Journal of the American Chemical Society, 2007. **129**: p. 8018-8025.
17. Kamlet, A.S., et al., *Application of Palladium-Mediated 18F-Fluorination to PET Radiotracer Development: Overcoming Hurdles to Translation.* PLoS ONE, 2013. **8**: p. e59187.
18. Tredwell, M., et al., *A General Copper-Mediated Nucleophilic 18 F Fluorination of Arenes.* Angewandte Chemie International Edition, 2014. **53**: p. 7751-7755.
19. Mason, N.S., C.A. Mathis, and W.E. Klunk, *Positron emission tomography radioligands for in vivo imaging of Aβ plaques.* Journal of Labelled Compounds and Radiopharmaceuticals, 2013. **56**: p. 89-95.
20. Richter, S. and F. Wuest, *18F-Labeled Peptides: The Future Is Bright.* Molecules, 2014. **19**: p. 20536-20556.
21. Kuhnast, B. and F. Dolle, *The Challenge of Labeling Macromolecules with Fluorine-18: Three Decades of Research.* Current Radiopharmaceuticals, 2010. **3**: p. 174-201.
22. Liu, S., et al., *Recent Progress in Radiofluorination of Peptides for PET Molecular Imaging.* Current Organic Synthesis, 2011. **8**: p. 584-592.
23. Kettenbach, K., H. Schieferstein, and T.L. Ross, *18F-Labeling Using Click Cycloadditions.* BioMed Research International, 2014. **2014**: p. 1-16.
24. Schieferstein, H. and T.L. Ross, *A polar 18F-labeled amino acid derivative for click labeling of biomolecules.* European Journal of Organic Chemistry, 2014. **2014**: p. 3546-3550.
25. Zlatopolskiy, B.D., et al., *Synthesis of 18F-labelled β-lactams by using the Kinugasa reaction.* Chemistry - A European Journal, 2014. **20**: p. 4697-4703.
26. Bunschoten, A., et al., *Development and prospects of dedicated tracers for the molecular imaging of bacterial infections.* Bioconjugate Chemistry, 2013. **24**: p. 1971-1989.
27. Li, X.-G., M. Haaparanta, and O. Solin, *Oxime formation for fluorine-18 labeling of peptides and proteins for positron emission tomography (PET) imaging: A review.* Journal of Fluorine Chemistry, 2012. **143**: p. 49-56.
28. Goins, B.A., *Radiolabeled lipid nanoparticles for diagnostic imaging.* Expert Opinion on Medical Diagnostics, 2008. **2**: p. 853-873.
29. Loudos, G., G.C. Kagadis, and D. Psimadas, *Current status and future perspectives of in vivo small animal imaging using radiolabeled nanoparticles.* European Journal of Radiology, 2011. **78**: p. 287-295.
30. Pretze, M., et al., *The traceless Staudinger ligation with fluorine-18: A novel and versatile labeling technique for the synthesis of PET-radiotracers.* Tetrahedron Letters, 2010. **51**: p. 6410-6414.
31. Carroll, L., et al., *The traceless Staudinger ligation for indirect 18F-radiolabelling.* Organic & biomolecular chemistry, 2011. **9**: p. 136-140.
32. Bernard-Gauthier, V., et al., *18 F-Labeled Silicon-Based Fluoride Acceptors: Potential Opportunities for Novel Positron Emitting Radiopharmaceuticals.* BioMed Research International, 2014. **2014**: p. 1-20.

33. McBride, W.J., R.M. Sharkey, and D.M. Goldenberg, *Radiofluorination using aluminum-fluoride (Al18F).* European Journal of Nuclear Medicine and Molecular Imaging Research, 2013. **3**: p. 36.
34. Schirrmacher, R., et al., *18F-Labeling of Peptides by means of an Organosilicon-Based Fluoride Acceptor.* Angewandte Chemie International Edition, 2006. **45**: p. 6047-6050.
35. Rosa-Neto, P., et al., *[18 F]SiFA-isothiocyanate: A New Highly Effective Radioactive Labeling Agent for Lysine-Containing Proteins.* ChemBioChem, 2009. **10**: p. 1321-1324.
36. Choudhry, U., et al., *Alkoxysilane groups for instant labeling of biomolecules with 18F,.* Nuclear Medicine Communications, 2006. **27**(3): p. 27.
37. McBride, W.J., et al., *New lyophilized kit for rapid radiofluorination of peptides.* Bioconjugate Chemistry, 2012. **23**: p. 538-547.
38. Wan, W., et al., *First Experience of 18F-Alfatide in Lung Cancer Patients Using a New Lyophilized Kit for Rapid Radiofluorination.* Journal of Nuclear Medicine, 2013. **54**: p. 691-698.
39. McBride, W.J., et al., *The radiolabeling of proteins by the [18F]AlF method.* Applied Radiation and Isotopes, 2012. **70**: p. 200-204.
40. Ting, R., et al., *Toward [18 F] -Labeled Aryltrifluoroborate Radiotracers : In Vivo Positron Emission Tomography Imaging of Stable Aryltrifluoroborate Clearance in Mice.* Journal of the American Chemical Society, 2008. **130**: p. 12045-12055.
41. Liu, Z., et al., *Preclinical Evaluation of a High-Affinity 18F-Trifluoroborate Octreotate Derivative for Somatostatin Receptor Imaging.* Journal of Nuclear Medicine, 2014. **55**: p. 1499-1505.
42. Segrè, E.A. and G.T. Seaborg, *Nuclear Isomerism in Element 43.* Physical Review, 1938. **54**(9): p. 772.
43. Banerjee, S., M.R. Pillai, and N. Ramamoorthy, *Evolution of Tc-99m in diagnostic radiopharmaceuticals.* Seminars in Nuclear Medicine, 2001. **31**(4): p. 260-77.
44. Green, C.H., *Technetium-99m production issues in the United Kingdom.* Journal of Medical Physics, 2012. **37**: p. 66–71.
45. Pillai, M.R.A., et al. , *Sustained Availability of 99mTc: Possible Paths Forward,.* Journal of Nuclear Medicine, 2013. **54**: p. 313-323.
46. Seaborg, G.R., and E. Segrè, *Nuclear isomerism of element 43.* Physics Reviews, 1939. **55**: p. 808-814.
47. Richards, P., *Nuclide generators.* Radioactive Pharmaceuticals, 1965: p. 155-163.
48. Wang, C.H., et al., *99mTcO4- Scintigraphic detection of follicular thyroid cancer and multiple metastaic lesions: A case report.* Oncology Letters, 2013. **6**: p. 1729–1732.
49. Harper, P.V., et al., *Pharmacodynamics of some technetium-99m preparations.* Radioactive Pharmaceuticals, 1965: p. 335-358.
50. Taskeav E., et al., *Extraction generation for [99mTc]sodium pertechnetate production.* Applied Radiation and Isotopes, 1995. **46**: p. 13–16.
51. Liu, Y., et al., *A brief review of chelators for radiolabeling oligomers.* Materials, 2010. **3**: p. 3204-3217.
52. Liu, S., *6-Hydrazinonicotinamide Derivatives as Bifunctional Coupling Agents for 99mTc-Labeling of Small Biomolecules.* Topics in Current Chemistry, 2005. **252**: p. 117–153.
53. Richards, P., *Chemistry of technetium as applied to radiopharmaceuticals.* Radiopharmaceuticals, 1975: p. 23-35.
54. Srivastava, S.C., et al., *Problems associated with stannous 99mTc-radiopharmaceuticals,.* International Journal of Applied Radiation and Isotopes, 1977. **28**: p. 83-95.
55. Tofe, A.J. and M.D. Francis, *In vitro stabilization of a low-tin bone imaging agent (Tc-99m-Sn-HEDP) by ascorbic acid.* Journal of Nuclear Medicine, 1976. **17**: p. 820-825.
56. Burke, J., *Advances in 99mTc Radiopharmaceutical Chemistry.* Paper presented at the 148th Annual Meeting of the American Pharmaceutical Association, 2001.
57. Mazzi, U., et al., *Technetium coordination chemistry: development of new backbones for 99mTc radiopharmaceuticals.* Technetium and Rhenium in Chemistry and Nuclear Medicine p. 39-50.

58. Johannsen, B., et al., *Chemical and biological characterization of different Tc complexes of cysteine and cysteine derivatives.* Journal of Nuclear Medicine, 1978. **19**: p. 816-824.
59. Meerdink D.J. and J.A. Leppo, *Comparison of hypoxia and ouabain effects on the myocardial uptake kinetics of technetium-99m hexakis 2-methoxyisobutyl isonitrile and thallium-201.* Journal of Nuclear Medicine, 1989. **30**: p. 1500-1506.
60. Carvalho, P.A., et al., *Subcellular distribution and analysis of technetium-99m-MIBI in isolated perfused rat hearts.* Journal of Nuclear Medicine, 1992. **33**: p. 1516-1521.
61. Jurisson S.S. and J.D. Lydon, *Potential technetium small molecule radiopharmaceuticals.* Chemical Reviews, 1999. **99**: p. 2205-2218.
62. Alberto, R., et al., *A novel organometallic aquo complex of technetium for the labeling of biomolecules: Synthesis of [Tc(H2O)3(CO)3]+ from 99mTcO4- in aqueous solution and its reaction with a bifunctional ligand.* Journal of the American Chemical Society, 1998. **120**: p. 7987-7988.
63. Spradau, T.W., et al., *Synthesis and biological evaluation of Tc-99m cyclopentdienyltricarbonyltechnetium-labeled octreotide.* Nuclear Medicine and Biology, 1999. **26**: p. 1-7.
64. Kowalsky, R.J., *Radiopharmaceuticals in Nuclear Pharmacy and Nuclear Medicine, 2nd ed.* Washington, DC: American Pharmacists Association, 2004.
65. Loberg M.D. and A.T. Fields, *Stability of 99mTc-labeled N-substituted iminodiacetic acids: Ligand exchange reaction between 99mTc-HIDA and EDTA.* International Journal of Applied Radiation and Isotopes, 1977. **28**: p. 687-692.
66. Ikeda, I., et al., *Chemical and biological studies on Tc-99m DMS-II: Effect of Sn(II) on the formation of various Tc-DMS complexes.* International Journal of Applied Radiation and Isotopes, 1976. **27**: p. 681-688.
67. Ikeda, I., et al., *Preparation of various Tc-99m dimercaptosuccinate complexes and their evaluation as radiotracers.* Journal of Nuclear Medicine, 1977. **18**: p. 1222-1229.
68. Treher, E.N., et al., *Monocapped tris (dioxime) complexes of technetium(III): Synthesis and structural characterization of TcX(dioxime)3 B-R (x = Cl, Br; dioxime = dimethylglyoxime, cyclohexanedione dioxime; R = CH3, C4H9.* Inorganic Chemistry, 1989. **28**: p. 3411-3416.
69. Eckelman W. and P. Richards, *Instant Tc-99m DTPA.* Journal of Nuclear Medicine, 1970. **11**: p. 761.
70. Arnold, R.W., et al., *Comparison of Tc-99m complexes for renal imaging.* Journal of Nuclear Medicine., 1975. **16**: p. 357-367.
71. McCarthy, D.W., et al., *Efficient production of high specific activity 64Cu using a biomedical cyclotron.* Nuclear Medicine and Biology, 1997. **24**: p. 35-43.
72. Szűcs, Z., S. Takács, and B. Alirezapour, *Development of cost effective method for production of 64Cu from natNi.* Journal of Radioanalytical and Nuclear Chemistry, 2014. **302**: p. 1035-1038.
73. Jurisson, S., C. Cutler, and S.V. Smith, *Radiometal complexes: Characterization and relevant in vitro studies.* Quarterly Journal of Nuclear Medicine and Molecular Imaging, 2008. **52**: p. 222-234.
74. Stigers, D.J., et al., *A new phosphonate pendant-armed cross-bridged tetraaminechelator accelerates copper(ii) binding for radiopharmaceutical applications.* Dalton Transactions., 2010. **39**: p. 1699-1701.
75. Bhargava, K.K., et al., *In vitro human leukocyte labeling with 64Cu: an intraindividual comparison with 111In-oxine and 18F-FDG.* Nuclear Medicine and Biology, 2009. **36**: p. 545-549.
76. Chopra, A. and D. Pan, *cFLFLFK-PEG-64Cu.* Molecular Imaging and Contrast Agent Database.
77. Zhang, Y., et al., *Synthesis of novel neutrophil-specific imaging agents for Positron Emission Tomography (PET) imaging.* Bioorganic and Medicinal Chemistry Letters, 2007. **17**(24): p. 6876-8.
78. Harper, J., et al., *Mouse Model of Necrotic Tuberculosis Granulomas Develops Hypoxic Lesions.* Journal of Infectious Diseases, 2012. **205**: p. 595-602.

79. Beaino, W. and C.J. Anderson, *PET Imaging of Very Late Antigen-4 in Melanoma: Comparison of 68Ga- and 64Cu-Labeled NODAGA and CB-TE1A1P-LLP2A Conjugates.* Journal of Nuclear Medicine, 2014. **55**: p. 1856-1863.
80. Beaino, W., et al., *PET imaging of immune cells in a macaque tuberculosis model.* Journal of Nuclear Medicine, 2015. **56**: p. 651.
81. Rolle, A.M., et al., *ImmunoPET/MR imaging allows specific detection of Aspergillus fumigatus lung infection in vivo.* Proceedings of the National Academy of Sciences of the USA, 2016. **113**(8): p. E1026-33.
82. Kumar, V., et al., *Potential use of 68Ga-apo-transferrin as a PET imaging agent for detecting Staphylococcus aureus infection.* Nuclear Medicine and Biology, 2011. **38**: p. 393-398.
83. Rizzello, A., et al., *Synthesis and quality control of 68Ga citrate for routine clinical PET.* Nuclear Medicine Communications, 2009. **30**: p. 542-545.
84. Vorster, M., et al., *A modified technique for efficient radiolabeling of 68Ga-citrate from a SnO2-based 68Ge/68Ga generator for better infection imaging.* Hellenic Journal of Nuclear medicine, 2013. **16**: p. 193-198.
85. Varasteh, Z., et al., *The Effect of Mini-PEG-Based Spacer Length on Binding and Pharmacokinetic Properties of a 68Ga-Labeled NOTA-Conjugated Antagonistic Analog of Bombesin.* Molecules, 2014. **19**: p. 10455-10472.
86. Notni, J., K. Pohle, and H.-J. Wester, *Comparative gallium-68 labeling of TRAP-, NOTA-, and DOTA-peptides: practical consequences for the future of gallium-68-PET.* European Journal of Nuclear Medicine and Molecular Imaging Research, 2012. **2**: p. 28.
87. Kubíček, V.C., et al., *Gallium(III) Complexes of DOTA and DOTA−Monoamide: Kinetic and Thermodynamic Studies.* Inorganic Chemistry, 2010. **49**: p. 10960-10969.
88. de Sá, A., et al., *Gallium labeled NOTA-based conjugates for peptide receptor-mediated medical imaging.* Bioorganic & Medicinal Chemistry Letters, 2010. **20**: p. 7345-7348.
89. De León-Rodriguez, L.M., et al., *Solid-Phase Synthesis of DOTA–Peptides.* Chemistry - A European Journal, 2004. **10**: p. 1149-1155.
90. Tanaka, K., et al., *A Submicrogram-Scale Protocol for Biomolecule-Based PET Imaging by Rapid 6π-Azaelectrocyclization: Visualization of Sialic Acid Dependent Circulatory Residence of Glycoproteins.* Angewandte Chemie International Edition, 2008. **47**: p. 102-105.
91. Dijkgraaf, I., et al., *Synthesis of DOTA-conjugated multivalent cyclic-RGD peptide dendrimers via 1,3-dipolar cycloaddition and their biological evaluation: implications for tumor targeting and tumor imaging purposes.* Organic & Biomolecular Chemistry, 2007. **5**: p. 935-944.
92. Knör, S., et al., *Synthesis of Novel 1,4,7,10-Tetraazacyclodecane-1,4,7,10-Tetraacetic Acid (DOTA) Derivatives for Chemoselective Attachment to Unprotected Polyfunctionalized Compounds.* Chemistry - A European Journal, 2007. **13**: p. 6082-6090.
93. Velikyan, I., *Positron Emitting [68Ga]Ga-Based Imaging Agents: Chemistry and Diversity.* Medicinal Chemistry, 2011. **7**: p. 345-379.
94. Gleason, G.I., *A positron cow.* The International Journal of Applied Radiation and Isotopes, 1960. **8**: p. 90-94.
95. Greene, M. and W. Tucker, *An Improved Gallium-68 Cow.* The international journal of Applied Radiation and Isotopes, 1961. **12**: p. 62-63.
96. Kopecky, P. and B. Mudrova, *68Ge - 68Ga Generator for the Production of 68Ga in an Ionic Form.* The international Journal of Applied Radiation and Isotopes, 1974. **25**: p. 263-268.
97. Konstantin, P., et al., *Processing of Generator-Produced 68Ga for Medical Application.* The Journal of Nuclear Medicine, 2007. **48**: p. 1741-1748.
98. Bauwens, M., et al., *Optimal buffer choice of the radiosynthesis of (68)Ga-Dotatoc for clinical application.* Nuclear medicine communications, 2010. **31**: p. 753-758.
99. Decristoforo, C., et al., *A fully automated synthesis for the preparation of 68Ga-labelled peptides.* Nuclear Medicine Communications, 2007. **28**: p. 870-875.

100. de Blois, E., et al., *Characteristics of SnO2-based 68Ge/68Ga generator and aspects of radiolabelling DOTA-peptides.* Applied Radiation and Isotopes, 2011. **69**: p. 308-315.
101. Meyer, G.-J., et al., *68Ga-labelled DOTA-derivatised peptide ligands.* European Journal of Nuclear Medicine and Molecular Imaging, 2004. **31**: p. 1097-1104.
102. Loktionova, N.S., et al., *Improved column-based radiochemical processing of the generator produced 68Ga.* Applied Radiation and Isotopes, 2011. **69**: p. 942-946.
103. Mueller, D., et al., *Simplified NaCl Based 68 Ga Concentration and Labeling Procedure for Rapid Synthesis of 68 Ga Radiopharmaceuticals in High Radiochemical Purity.* Bioconjugate Chemistry, 2012. **23**: p. 1712-1717.
104. Rossouw, D.D. and W.A.P. Breeman, *Scaled-up radiolabelling of DOTATATE with 68Ga eluted from a SnO2-based 68Ge/68Ga generator.* Applied Radiation and Isotopes, 2012. **70**: p. 171-175.
105. Breeman, W.A.P., et al., *Radiolabelling DOTA-peptides with 68Ga.* European Journal of Nuclear Medicine and Molecular Imaging, 2005. **32**: p. 478-485.
106. Decristoforo, C., R.D. Pickett, and A. Verbruggen, *Feasibility and availability of 68Ga-labelled peptides.* European Journal of Nuclear Medicine and Molecular Imaging, 2012. **39**: p. 31-40.
107. Chakravarty, R., et al., *Development of a nano-zirconia based 68Ge/68Ga generator for biomedical applications.* Nuclear Medicine and Biology, 2011. **38**: p. 575-583.
108. Velikyan, I., et al., *The importance of high specific radioactivity in the performance of 68Ga-labeled peptide.* Nuclear Medicine and Biology, 2008. **35**: p. 529-536.
109. Roesch, F., *68Ge/68Ga Generators and 68Ga Radiopharmaceutical Chemistry on Their Way into a New Century.* Journal of Postgraduate Medicine Education and Research, 2013. **47**: p. 18-25.
110. Petrik, M., et al., *Microbial challenge tests on nonradioactive TiO2-based 68Ge/68Ga generator columns.* Nuclear Medicine Communications, 2012. **33**: p. 819-823.
111. Velikyan, I., *68Ga-Based Radiopharmaceuticals: Production and Application Relationship.* Molecules, 2015. **20**: p. 12913-12943.
112. Ballinger, J.R. and K.K. Solanki, *What will be required to bring 68Ga-labelled peptides into routine clinical use?* Nuclear Medicine Communications, 2011. **32**: p. 1109-1112.
113. Hupf, H.B. and J.E. Beaver, *Cyclotron production of carrier-free gallium-67.* The International Journal of Applied Radiation and Isotopes, 1970. **21**(2): p. 75-79.
114. El-Azony, K.M., K. Ferieg, and Z.A. Saleh, *Direct separation of 67Ga citrate from zinc and copper target materials by anion exchange.* Applied Radiation and Isotopes, 2003. **59**(5-6): p. 329-331.
115. Bartholoma, M.D., et al., *Technetium and gallium derived radiopharmaceuticals: comparing and contrasting the chemistry of two important radiometals for the molecular imaging era.* Chemical Reviews, 2010. **110**(5): p. 2903-2920.
116. Tarkanyi, F., et al., *Cross sections of proton induced nuclear reactions on enriched 111Cd and 112Cd for the production of 111In for use in nuclear medicine.* Applied Radiation and Isotopes, 1994. **45**: p. 239-249.
117. Arano, Y., et al., *Radiolabeled Metabolites of Proteins Play a Critical Role in Radioactivity Elimination from the Liver.* Nuclear Medicine and Biology, 1995. **22**: p. 555-564.
118. Boswell, C.A., et al., *Effects of Charge on Antibody Tissue Distribution and Pharmacokinetics.* Bioconjugate Chemistry, 2010. **21**: p. 2153-2163.
119. Hayes, R.L., *The medical use of gallium radionuclides: a brief history with some comments.* Seminars in Nuclear Medicine, 1978. **8**: p. 183-191.
120. Tsopelas, C., *Radiotracers Used for the Scintigraphic Detection of Infection and Inflammation.* The Scientific World Journal, 2015. **2015**: p. 1-33.
121. Signore, A. and A.W.J.M. Glaudemans, *The molecular imaging approach to image infections and inflammation by nuclear medicine techniques.* Annals of Nuclear Medicine, 2011. **25**: p. 681-700.
122. Palestro, C.J., *FDG-PET in musculoskeletal infections.* Seminars in Nuclear Medicine, 2013. **43**: p. 367-376.

123. Palestro, C.J., *The current role of gallium imaging in infection.* Seminars in Nuclear Medicine, 1994. **24**: p. 128-141.
124. Ballinger, J.R. and G. Gnanasegaran, *Radiolabelled leukocytes for imaging inflammation: how radiochemistry affects clinical use.* The Quarterly Journal of Nuclear Medicine and Molecular Imaging, 2005. **49**: p. 308-318.
125. Roca, M., et al., *Guidelines for the labelling of leucocytes with (111)In-oxine. Inflammation/Infection Taskgroup of the European Association of Nuclear Medicine.* European Journal of Nuclear Medicine and Molecular Imaging, 2010. **37**: p. 835-841.
126. De Vries, E.F.J., et al., *Guidelines for the labelling of leucocytes with 99mTc-HMPAO.* European Journal of Nuclear Medicine and Molecular Imaging, 2010. **37**: p. 842-848.
127. Roca, M., et al., *A consensus protocol for white blood cells labelling with technetium-99m hexamethylpropylene amine oxime.* European Journal of Nuclear Medicine and Molecular Imaging, 1998. **25**: p. 797-799.
128. Kennedy, C., et al., *Mapping of functional neural pathways by autoradiographic survey of local metabolic rate with (14C)deoxyglucose.* Science, 1975. **187**: p. 850-853.
129. Yu, S., *Review of 18F-FDG synthesis and quality control.* Biomedical Imaging and Intervention Journal, 2006. **2**: p. e57.
130. Glaudemans, A.W.J.M., et al., *The Use of 18F-FDG-PET/CT for Diagnosis and Treatment Monitoring of Inflammatory and Infectious Diseases.* Clinical and Developmental Immunology, 2013. **2013**: p. 1-14.
131. Kumar, V., *Radiolabeled white blood cells and direct targeting of micro-organisms for infection imaging.* The Quarterly Journal of Nuclear Medicine and Molecular Imaging, 2005. **49**: p. 325-338.
132. Tsopelas, C., *The radiopharmaceutical chemistry of 99mTc-tin fluoride colloid-labeled-leukocytes.* The Quarterly Journal of Nuclear Medicine and Molecular Imaging, 2005. **49**: p. 319-324.
133. Hughes, D.K., *Nuclear Medicine and Infection Detection: The Relative Effectiveness of Imaging with 99m Tc-Stannous Fluoride Colloid – Labeled.* Journal of Nuclear Medicine Technology, 2003. **31**: p. 196-201.
134. Kanishi, D., *99mTc-MDP accumulation mechanisms in bone.* Oral Surgery, Oral Medicine, Oral Pathology, 1993. **75**: p. 239-246.
135. Boerman, O.C., et al., *Radiopharmaceuticals for scintigraphic imaging of infection and inflammation.* Inflammation Research, 2001. **50**: p. 55-64.
136. Glaudemans, A.W.J.M., et al., *Leukocyte and bacteria imaging in prosthetic joint infection.* European Cells and Materials, 2012. **25**: p. 61-77.
137. Jimenez Heffernan, A., P.I. Contreras Puertas, and A.C. Rebollo Aguirre, *[99mTc-labelled antigranulocyte anibody fragment Fab scintigraphy (sulesomab, leukoscan) and three-phase bone scintigraphy in the study of painful hip and knee prosthesis].* Spanish Journal of Nuclear Medicine and Molecular Imaging, 2002. **21**(4): p. 286-93.
138. Rubello, D., *Timing for evaluating "specific" binding of 99mTc-sulesomab in peripheral bone infection.* Journal of Nuclear Medicine, 2005. **46**(2): p. 382-383.
139. Rubello, D., et al., *Role of anti-granulocyte Fab' fragment antibody scintigraphy (LeukoScan) in evaluating bone infection: acquisition protocol, interpretation criteria and clinical results.* Nuclear Medicine Communications, 2004. **25**(1): p. 39-47.
140. Schroeter, S. and L. Greiner-Bechert, *LeukoScan protocol.* Nuclear Medicine Communications, 2001. **22**(7): p. 841.
141. Delcourt, A., et al., *Comparison between Leukoscan (Sulesomab) and Gallium-67 for the diagnosis of osteomyelitis in the diabetic foot.* Diabetes and Metabolism, 2005. **31**(2): p. 125-33.
142. Palestro, C.J., *Radionuclide imaging of infection: in search of the grail.* Journal of Nuclear Medicine, 2009. **50**: p. 671-673.
143. Fischman, A.J., et al., *Imaging focal sites of bacterial infection in rats with indium-111-labeled chemotactic peptide analogs.* Journal of Nuclear Medicine, 1991. **32**: p. 483-491.

144. van der Laken, C.J., et al., *Technetium-99m-Labeled Chemotactic Peptides in Acute Infection and Sterile Inflammation.* Journal of Nuclear Medicine, 2015. **38**: p. 1310-1315.
145. Nanni, C., et al., *68Ga-citrate PET/CT for evaluating patients with infections of the bone: preliminary results.* Journal of Nuclear Medicine, 2010. **51**: p. 1932-1936.
146. Vorster, M., et al., *68Ga-citrate PET/CT in Tuberculosis: A pilot study.* The Quarterly Journal of Nuclear Medicine and Molecular Imaging, 2014 (**Epub** 2014).
147. Jensen, S.B., et al., *Fast and simple one-step preparation of 68Ga citrate for routine clinical PET.* Nuclear Medicine Communications, 2013. **34**: p. 806-812.
148. Petrik, M., et al., *Preclinical evaluation of two 68Ga-siderophores as potential radiopharmaceuticals for Aspergillus fumigatus infection imaging.* European Journal of Nuclear Medicine and Molecular Imaging, 2012. **39**: p. 1175-1183.
149. Afonso, P.V., et al., *LTB4 Is a Signal-Relay Molecule during Neutrophil Chemotaxis.* Developmental Cell, 2012. **22**: p. 1079-1091.
150. van Eerd, J.E., et al., *Scintigraphic Detection of Pulmonary Aspergillosis in Rabbits with a Radiolabeled Leukotriene B4 Antagonist.* Journal of Nuclear Medicine, 2004. **45**: p. 1747-1753.
151. Rennen, H.J.J.M., et al., *PET imaging of infection with a HYNIC-conjugated LTB4 antagonist labeled with F-18 via hydrazone formation.* Nuclear Medicine and Biology, 2007. **34**: p. 691-695.
152. Mäkinen, T.J., et al., *Comparison of 18F-FDG and 68Ga PET imaging in the assessment of experimental osteomyelitis due to Staphylococcus aureus.* European Journal of Nuclear Medicine and Molecular Imaging, 2005. **32**: p. 1259-68.
153. Nanni, C., et al., *Small animal PET for the evaluation of an animal model of genital infection.* Clinical Physiology and Functional Imaging, 2009. **29**: p. 187-192.
154. Borges, J.B., et al., *Ventilation distribution studies comparing Technegas and "Gallgas" using 68GaCl3 as the label.* Journal of Nuclear Medicine, 2011. **52**: p. 206-9.
155. Gemmel, F., N. Dumarey, and M. Welling, *Future Diagnostic Agents.* Seminars in Nuclear Medicine, 2009. **39**: p. 11-26.
156. Eggleston, H. and P. Panizzi, *Molecular Imaging of Bacterial Infections in vivo: The Discrimination between Infection and Inflammation.* Informatics, 2014. **1**: p. 72-99.
157. Siaens, R.H., et al., *Synthesis and Comparison of 99mTc-Enrofloxacin and 99mTc-Ciprofloxacin.* Journal of Nuclear Medicine, 2004. **45**: p. 2088.
158. Motaleb, M.A., *Preparation and biodistribution of 99mTc-lomefloxacin and 99mTc-ofloxacin complexes.* Journal of Radioanalytical and Nuclear Chemistry, 2007. **272**: p. 95-99.
159. Motaleb, M.A., *Preparation, quality control and stability of 99mTc-sparafloxacin complex, a novel agent for detecting sites of infection.* Journal of Labelled Compounds and Radiopharmaceuticals, 2009. **52**: p. 415-418.
160. Chattopadhyay, S., et al., *Synthesis and evaluation of 99mTc-moxifloxacin, a potential infection specific imaging agent.* Applied Radiation and Isotopes, 2010. **68**: p. 314-316.
161. Ibrahim, I.T., M.A. Motaleb, and K.M. Attalah, *Synthesis and biological distribution of 99mTc–norfloxacin complex, a novel agent for detecting sites of infection.* Journal of Radioanalytical and Nuclear Chemistry, 2010. **285**: p. 431-436.
162. Shah, S.Q. and M.R. Khan, *Radiolabeling of gemifloxacin with technetium-99m and biological evaluation in artificially Streptococcus pneumoniae infected rats.* Journal of Radioanalytical and Nuclear Chemistry, 2011. **288**: p. 307-312.
163. Shah, S.Q. and M.R. Khan, *Radiocharacterization of the 99mTc-rufloxacin complex and biological evaluation in Staphylococcus aureus infected rat model.* Journal of Radioanalytical and Nuclear Chemistry, 2011. **288**: p. 373-378.
164. Shah, S. and M. Khan, *Synthesis of 99m TcN-clinafloxacin dithiocarbamate complex and comparative radiobiological evaluation in staphylococcus aureus infected mice.* World Journal of Nuclear Medicine, 2014. **13**: p. 154-158.
165. Shah, S.Q., A.U. Khan, and M.R. Khan, *Radiosynthesis and biodistribution of 99mTcN-Garenoxacin dithiocarbamate complex a potential infection imaging agent.* Journal of Radioanalytical and Nuclear Chemistry, 2011. **288**: p. 59-64.

166. Motaleb, M.A., et al., *Study on the preparation and biological evaluation of 99mTc–gatifloxacin and 99mTc–cefepime complexes.* Journal of Radioanalytical and Nuclear Chemistry, 2011. **289**: p. 57-65.
167. Ali, S., et al., *Tc labeled levofloxacin as an infection imaging agent : a novel method for labeling levofloxacin using cysteine · HCl as co-ligand and in vivo study.* Turkish Journal of Chemistry, 2012. **36**: p. 267-277.
168. Nayak, D.K., et al., *Evaluation of 99mTc(I)-tricarbonyl complexes of fluoroquinolones for targeting bacterial infection.* Metallomics, 2012. **4**: p. 1197-1208.
169. Langer, O., et al., *Synthesis of fluorine-18-labeled ciprofloxacin for PET studies in humans.* Nuclear Medicine and Biology, 2003. **30**: p. 285-291.
170. Langer, O., et al., *In vitro and in vivo evaluation of [18F]ciprofloxacin for the imaging of bacterial infections with PET.* European Journal of Nuclear Medicine and Molecular Imaging, 2005. **32**: p. 143-150.
171. Sachin, K., et al., *Synthesis of N4'-[18F]fluoroalkylated ciprofloxacin as a potential bacterial infection imaging agent for PET study.* Bioconjugate chemistry, 2010. **21**: p. 2282-2288.
172. Fischman, A.J., et al., *Pharmacokinetics of 18F-labeled fluconazole in rabbits with candidal infections studied with positron emission tomography.* The Journal of pharmacology and experimental therapeutics, 1991. **259**: p. 1351-1359.
173. Fischman, A.J., et al., *Pharmacokinetics of 18F-Labeled Fluconazole in Healthy Human Subjects by Positron Emission Tomography.* Antimicrobial Agents and Chemotherapy, 1993. **37**: p. 1270-1277.
174. Lupetti, A., et al., *Technetium-99m labelled fluconazole and antimicrobial peptides for imaging of Candida albicans and Aspergillus fumigatus infections.* European Journal of Nuclear Medicine, 2002. **29**: p. 674-679.
175. Diniz, S.O.F., et al., *Scintigraphic imaging using technetium-99m-labeled ceftizoxime in an experimental model of acute osteomyelitis in rats.* Nuclear Medicine Communications, 2008. **29**: p. 830-836.
176. Gomes Baretto, V., et al., *Labelling of ceftizoxime with 99m Tc.* Spanish Journal of Nuclear Medicine and Molecular Imaging, 2014. **19**: p. 479-483.
177. Odília, S., et al., *Technetium-99m Ceftizoxime Kit Preparation.* Brazilian Archives of Biology and Technology, 2005. **48**: p. 89-96.
178. Roohi, S., A. Mushtaq, and S.A. Malik, *Synthesis and biodistribution of 99mTc-Vancomycin in a model of bacterial infection.* Radiochimica Acta, 2005. **93**: p. 415-18.
179. Roohi, S., et al., *Synthesis , quality control and biodistribution of 99m Tc-Kanamycin.* Journal of Radioanalytical and Nuclear Chemistry, 2006. **267**: p. 561-566.
180. Motaleb, M.A., *Preparation of 99mTc-cefoperazone complex, a novel agent for detecting sites of infection.* Journal of Radioanalytical and Nuclear Chemistry, 2007. **272**: p. 167-171.
181. Yurt Lambrecht, F., K. Durkan, and P. Unak, *Preparation, quality control and stability of 99mTc-cefuroxime axetil.* Journal of Radioanalytical and Nuclear Chemistry, 2007. **275**: p. 161-164.
182. Yurt Lambrecht, F., et al., *Evaluation of 99mTc-Cefuroxime axetil for imaging of inflammation.* Journal of Radioanalytical and Nuclear Chemistry, 2008. **277**: p. 491-494.
183. Shah, S.Q., M.R. Khan, and A.U. Khan, *99m Tc-Novobiocin: a~novel radiotracer for infection imaging.* Radiochimica Acta, 2011. **99**: p. 53-58.
184. Martin-Comin, J., et al., *Clinical usefulness of 111In-oxine-labeled autologous lymphocytes in kidney-graft rejection.* European Journal of Nuclear Medicine, 1985. **10**: p. 308-12.
185. Saverymuttu, S.H., et al., *111Indium autologous granulocytes in the detection of inflammatory bowel disease.* Gut, 1985. **26**: p. 955-960.
186. Bhattacharya, A., et al., *PET/CT with 18F-FDG-Labeled Autologous Leukocytes for the Diagnosis of Infected Fluid Collections in Acute Pancreatitis.* Journal of nuclear medicine, 2014. **55**: p. 1267-1272.
187. Blocklet, D., et al., *In-111-oxine and Tc-99m-HMPAO labelling of antigen-loaded dendritic cells: in vivo imaging and influence on motility and actin content.* European Journal of Nuclear Medicine and Molecular Imaging, 2003. **30**: p. 440-447.

188. Wang, G., *Positron Emission Tomography Plays a More Important Role in Health Care.* Journal of Integrative Oncology, 2014. **4**: p. 134-135.
189. Weinstein, E.A., et al., *Imaging Enterobacteriaceae infection in vivo with 18F-fluorodeoxysorbitol positron emission tomography.* Science Translational Medicine, 2015. **6**: p. 1-20.
190. Gowrishankar, G., et al., *Investigation of 6-[18F]-Fluoromaltose as a Novel PET Tracer for Imaging Bacterial Infection.* PLoS ONE, 2014. **9**: p. e107951.
191. Ning, X., et al., *PET Imaging of Bacterial Infections with Fluorine-18-Labeled Maltohexaose.* Angewandte Chemie International Edition, 2014. **53**: p. 14096-14101.
192. Li, Z.-B., et al., *The Synthesis of 18F-FDS and Its Potential Application in Molecular Imaging.* Molecular Imaging and Biology, 2008. **10**: p. 92-98.
193. Wang, X. and N. Murthy, *Bacterial Imaging Comes of Age.* Science Translational Medicine, 2014. **6**: p. 259fs43-259fs43.
194. Peters, A.M., *Antibodies in nuclear medicine.* Methods in Molecular Medicine, 2000. **40**: p. 179-192.
195. Young, H., *Applications of monoclonal antibodies in diagnostic nuclear medicine.* Radiography Today, 1989. **55**(631): p. 20-21.
196. Keenan, A.M., J.C. Harbert, and S.M. Larson, *Monoclonal antibodies in nuclear medicine.* Journal of Nuclear Medicine, 1985. **26**(5): p. 531-537.
197. Dams, E., et al., *Technetium-99m Labeled to Human Immunoglobulin G Through the Nicotinyl Hydrazine Derivative : A Clinical Study.* Journal of Nuclear Medicine, 1998. **39**: p. 119-124.
198. Krejcarek, G.E. and K.L. Tucker, *Covalent attachment of chelating groups to macromolecules.* Biochemical and Biophysical Research Communications, 1977. **77**: p. 581-585.
199. Khaw, B.A., et al., *Acute Myocardial Infarct Imaging with Indium-111-Labeled Monoclonal Antimyosin Fab.* Journal of Nuclear Medicine, 1987. **28**: p. 1671-1678.
200. Fischman, A., et al., *Detection of acute inflammation with 111In-labeled nonspecific polyclonal IgG.* Seminars in Nuclear Medicine., 1988. **18**: p. 335-344.
201. Abrams, M.J., et al., *Technetium-99m-Human Polyclonal IgG Radiolabeled via the Hydrazino Nicotinamide Derivative for Imaging Focal Sites of Infection in Rats.* Journal of Nuclear Medicine, 1990. **31**: p. 2022-2029.
202. Singh, T., et al., Bhatnagar A, *A new method for radiolabeling of human immunoglobulin-G and its biological evaluation.* Journal of Pharmacy and Bioallied Sciences., 2012. **4**: p. 286-290.
203. Callahan, R.J., et al., *Biodistribution and Dosimetry of Technetium- 99m-Hydrazino Nicotinamide IgG : Comparison Biodistribution and Dosimetry of Technetium-99m-Hydrazino Nicotinamide IgG : Comparison with Indium- 111-DTPA-IgG.* Journal of Nuclear Medicine, 1996. **37**: p. 843-846.
204. Cao, W., X. Lu and Z. Chang, *The Advancement of Human Serum Albumin-Based Molecular Probes for Molecular Imaging.* Current Pharmaceutical Design., 2015. **21**: p. 1908-1915.
205. Fu, Z., C. Zhang and R. Wang, *99mTc-HSA is a valuable tracer in monitoring acute lung injury induced by lipopolysaccharide in rats.* Journal of Nuclear Medicine, 2015. **56**: p. 2506.
206. Malviya, G., et al., *Radiolabelled Peptides and Monoclonal Antibodies for Therapy Decision Making in Inflammatory Diseases.* Current Pharmaceutical Design, 2008. **14**: p. 2401-2414.
207. Annovazzi, A., et al., *Radiolabelling of a monoclonal anti-TNF-α antibody with 99mTc: in vitro studies.* The Quarterly Journal of Nuclear Medicine and Molecular Imaging, 2002. **46**: p. 27.
208. Conti, F., et al., *Successful treatment with intraarticular infliximab for resistant knee monarthritis in a patient with spondylarthropathy: A role for scintigraphy with99mTc-infliximab.* Arthritis & Rheumatism, 2005. **52**: p. 1224-1226.
209. Bleeker-Rovers, C.P., et al., *99mTc-labeled interleukin 8 for the scintigraphic detection of infection and inflammation: first clinical evaluation.* Journal of Nuclear Medicine, 2007. **48**: p. 337-343.

210. Rennen, H.J.J.M., et al., *Specific and rapid scintigraphic detection of infection with 99mTc-labeled interleukin-8.* Journal of Nuclear Medicine, 2001. **42**: p. 117-123.
211. Dams, E.T., et al., *99mTc-PEG liposomes for the scintigraphic detection of infection and inflammation: clinical evaluation.* Journal of Nuclear Medicine, 2000. **41**: p. 622-630.
212. Phillips, W.T., *Delivery of gamma-imaging agents by liposomes.* Advanced Drug Delivery Reviews, 1999. **37**: p. 13-32.
213. Konteatis, Z.D., et al., *Development of C5a receptor antagonists. Differential loss of functional responses.* Journal of Immunology, 1994. **153**: p. 4200-4205.
214. Rennen, H.J., et al., *Tc-99m-labeled C5a and C5a des Arg74 for infection imaging.* Nuclear medicine and biology, 2003. **30**: p. 267-272.
215. Rubin, R.H., et al., *Specific and nonspecific imaging of localized Fisher immunotype 1 Pseudomonas aeruginosa infection with radiolabeled monoclonal antibody.* Journal of Nuclear Medicine, 1988. **29**(5): p. 651-656.
216. Blauenstein, P., et al., *Experience with the iodine-123 and technetium-99m labelled anti-granulocyte antibody MAb47: a comparison of labelling methods.* European Journal of Nuclear Medicine, 1995. **22**(7): p. 690-698.
217. Machulla, H.J. and E.J. Knust, *Recent developments in the field of 123I-radiopharmaceuticals.* Nuklearmedizin, 1984. **23**(3): p. 111-118.
218. Bourguignon, M.H., et al., *Iodine-123 labelled radiopharmaceuticals and single-photon emission tomography: a natural liaison.* European Journal of Nuclear Medicine, 1997. **24**(3): p. 331-344.
219. Signore, A., et al., *The Developing Role of Cytokines for Imaging Inflammation and Infection.* Cytokine, 2000. **12**: p. 1445-1454.
220. van der Laken, C.J., et al., *Specific targeting of infectious foci with radioiodinated human recombinant interleukin-1 in an experimental model.* European Journal of Nuclear Medicine, 1995. **22**: p. 1249-1255.
221. van der Laken, C.J., et al., *Imaging of infection in rabbits with radioiodinated interleukin-1 (alpha and beta), its receptor antagonist and a chemotactic peptide: A comparative study.* European Journal of Nuclear Medicine, 1998. **25**: p. 347-352.
222. Brock, J.H., T. Mainou-Fowler, and S.J. McGregor, *Transferrins and defence against infection.* Annali dell'Istituto Superiore di Sanita, 1987. **23**(4): p. 935-941.
223. Yeaman, M.R. and N.Y. Yount, *Mechanisms of Antimicrobial Peptide Action and Resistance.* Pharmacological Reviews, 2003. **55**: p. 27-55.
224. Ebenhan, T., et al., *Antimicrobial Peptides : Their Role as Infection-Selective Tracers for Molecular Imaging.* European Cells and Materials, 2014. **2014**.
225. Welling, M.M., et al., *Technetium-99m labeled antimicrobial peptides discriminate between bacterial infections and sterile inflammations.* European Journal of Nuclear Medicine, 2000. **27**: p. 292-301.
226. Guérin, B., et al., *Total Solid-Phase Synthesis of NOTA-Functionalized Peptides for PET Imaging.* Organic Letters, 2010. **12**: p. 280-283.
227. Ebenhan, T., et al., *Peptide synthesis, characterization and 68Ga-radiolabeling of NOTA-conjugated ubiquicidin fragments for prospective infection imaging with PET/CT.* Nuclear Medicine and Biology, 2014. **41**: p. 390-400.
228. Ebenhan, T., et al., *Preclinical Evaluation of 68Ga-Labeled 1,4,7-Triazacyclononane-1,4,7-Triacetic Acid-Ubiquicidin as a Radioligand for PET Infection Imaging.* Journal of Nuclear Medicine, 2014. **55**: p. 308-314.
229. Peschel, A., et al., *Inactivation of the dlt operon in Staphylococcus aureus confers sensitivity to defensins, protegrins, and other antimicrobial peptides.* Journal of Biological Chemistry, 1999. **274**: p. 8405-8410.
230. Welling, M.M., et al., *Imaging of bacterial infections with 99mTc-labeled human neutrophil peptide-1.* Journal of Nuclear Medicine, 1999. **40**: p. 2073-2080.
231. Pauwels, E.K., et al., *The labeling of proteins and LDL with 99mTc: a new direct method employing KBH4 and stannous chloride.* Nuclear Medicine and Biology, 1993. **20**: p. 825-833.

232. Liberatore, M., et al., *Microbial targeting of 99mTc-labeled recombinant human beta-defensin-3 in an animal model of infection: a feasibility pilot study.* Journal of Nuclear Medicine, 2009. **50**: p. 823-826.
233. Locke, L.W., et al., *A novel neutrophil-specific PET imaging agent: cFLFLFK-PEG-64Cu.* Journal of Nuclear Medicine, 2009. **50**(5): p. 790-797.
234. Silvola, J., et al., *Preliminary evaluation of novel 68 Ga-DOTAVAP-PEG-P2 peptide targeting vascular adhesion protein-1.* Clinical Physiology and Functional Imaging, 2010. **30**: p. 75-78.
235. Ujula, T., et al., *Synthesis, 68Ga labeling and preliminary evaluation of DOTA peptide binding vascular adhesion protein-1: a potential PET imaging agent for diagnosing osteomyelitis.* Nuclear Medicine and Biology, 2009. **36**: p. 631-641.
236. Ahtinen, H., et al., *^{68}Ga-DOTA-Siglec-9 PET/CT imaging of peri-implant tissue responses and staphylococcal infections.* European Journal of Nuclear Medicine and Molecular Imaging Research, 2014. **4**: p. 45.
237. Haubner, R. and H.-J. Wester, *Radiolabeled Tracers for Imaging of Tumor Angiogenesis and Evaluation of Anti-Angiogenic Therapies.* Current Pharmaceutical Design, 2004. **10**: p. 1439-1455.
238. Dijkgraaf, I., et al., *PET imaging of $\alpha v\beta_3$ integrin expression in tumours with ^{68}Ga-labelled mono-, di- and tetrameric RGD peptides.* European Journal of Nuclear Medicine and Molecular Imaging, 2011. **38**: p. 128-137.
239. Audi, S., et al., *Understanding the in vivo uptake kinetics of a phosphatidylethanolamine-binding agent 99mTc-Duramycin.* Nuclear Medicine and Biology, 2012. **39**: p. 821-825.
240. Thompson, C., *Apoptosis in the pathogenesis and treatment of disease.* Science, 1995. **267**: p. 1456-1462.
241. Carter, V., et al., *Killer Bee Molecules: Antimicrobial Peptides as Effector Molecules to Target Sporogonic Stages of Plasmodium.* PLoS Pathogens, 2013. **9**: p. e1003790.
242. Zhao, M., Z. Li, and S. Bugenhagen, *99mTc-Labeled Duramycin as a Novel Phosphatidylethanolamine-Binding Molecular Probe.* Journal of Nuclear Medicine, 2008. **49**: p. 1345-1352.
243. Zhao, M. and Z. Li, *A single-step kit formulation for the 99mTc-labeling of HYNIC-Duramycin.* Nuclear Medicine and Biology, 2012. **39**: p. 1006-1011.
244. Yao, S., et al., *Positron emission tomography imaging of cell death with [18F]FPDuramycin.* Apoptosis, 2014. **19**: p. 841-850.
245. Mokaleng, B.B., et al., *Synthesis, 68Ga-radiolabeling, and preliminary in vivo assessment of a depsipeptide-derived compound as a potential PET/CT infection imaging agent.* Biomed Res Int, 2015. **2015**.
246. Lazzeri, E., et al., *Scintigraphic Imaging of Vertebral Osteomyelitis With 111In-Biotin.* Spine, 2008. **33**: p. E198-E204.
247. Virzi, F., et al., *New indium-111 labeled biotin derivatives for improved immunotargeting.* International Journal of Radiation Applications and Instrumentation. Part B. Nuclear Medicine and Biology, 1991. **18**: p. 719-726.
248. Shoup, T.M., et al., *Synthesis of Fluorine-18-Labeled Biotin Derivatives: Biodistribution and Infection Localization.* Journal of Nuclear Medicine, 1994. **35**: p. 1685-90.
249. Wójtowicz-Rajchel, H., M. Migas, and H. Koroniak, *Simple Synthesis of Some Pentafluoropropenyl Derivatives of Pyrimidine and Purine Based on Addition−Elimination Reaction.* The Journal of Organic Chemistry, 2006. **71**: p. 8842-8846.
250. Peñuelas, I., et al., *A Fully Automated One Pot Synthesis of 9-(4-[18F]Fluoro-3-Hydroxymethylbutyl) Guanine for Gene Therapy Studies.* Molecular Imaging and Biology, 2002. **4**: p. 415 -424.
251. Tjuvajev, J.G., et al., *Comparison of radiolabeled nucleoside probes (FIAU, FHBG, and FHPG) for PET imaging of HSV1-tk gene expression.* Journal of Nuclear Medicine, 2002. **43**: p. 1072-83.

252. Vaidyanathan, G. and M.R. Zalutsky, *Preparation of 5-[131I]iodo- and 5-[211At]astato-1-(2-deoxy-2-fluoro-beta-D-arabinofuranosyl) uracil by a halodestannylation reaction.* Nuclear medicine and biology, 1998. **25**: p. 487-96.
253. Alauddin, M.M., et al., *Synthesis and evaluation of 2′-deoxy-2′-18F-fluoro-5-fluoro-1-beta-D-arabinofuranosyluracil as a potential PET imaging agent for suicide gene expression.* Journal of Nuclear Medicine, 2004. **45**: p. 2063-2069.
254. Lamare, F., et al., *Detection and Quantification of Large-Vessel Inflammation with 11C-(R)-PK11195 PET/CT.* Journal of Nuclear Medicine, 2011. **52**: p. 33-39.
255. Rojas, S., et al., *Imaging brain inflammation with [11C]PK11195 by PET and induction of the peripheral-type benzodiazepine receptor after transient focal ischemia in rats.* Journal of Cerebral Blood Flow & Metabolism, 2007. **27**: p. 1975-1986.
256. Cagnin, A., A. Gerhard, and R. Banati, *Neuroinflammation — From Bench to Bedside.* PET Neuroinflammation — From Bench to Bedside, 2002: p. 179-191.
257. Chauveau, F., et al., *Comparative evaluation of the translocator protein radioligands 11C-DPA-713, 18F-DPA-714, and 11C-PK11195 in a rat model of acute neuroinflammation.* Journal of Nuclear Medicine, 2009. **50**(3): p. 468-476.
258. Hacht, B., *Gallium (III) ion hydrolysis under physiological conditions.* Bulletin - Korean Chemical Society, 2008. **29**: p. 372-376.

Chapter 5
Imaging the Host Response

Catherine A. Foss, Nada M.S. Hammouda, Chentian Shen, Jun Li, and H. Charles Manning

5.1 Introduction

Inflammation is a host response to either a sterile physical or biochemical irritant or to the presence of a microbial pathogen such as bacteria, viruses, fungi, or parasites. Thus, inflammation and the detection thereof may report on either sterile or infectious processes. Celsus described almost 2000 years ago the concept of color (heat), dolor (pain), rubor (redness), and tumor (swelling) as the hallmark signs of inflammation [1]. Today, more tools are available to begin selectively labeling a given cellular lineage or labeling a specific biologic process such as fibrosis or assessing blood flow in three dimensions. Nuclear and fluorescent imaging combined with computed tomography (CT) and magnetic resonance imaging (MRI) provides biologic targeting with anatomic co-registration for context.

C.A. Foss (✉)
Russel H. Morgan Department of Radiology and Radiological Sciences,
Johns Hopkins University School of Medicine, Baltimore, MD, USA
e-mail: cfoss1@jhmi.edu

N.M.S. Hammouda
Icahn School of Medicine at Mount Sinai, New York, NY, USA

C. Shen
U.S. National Institutes of Health, Bethesda, MD, USA

J. Li
Vanderbilt Center for Molecular Probes and Molecular Imaging Research, Vanderbilt University, Nashville, TN, USA

H.C. Manning
Department of Radiology, Vanderbilt Center for Molecular Probes and Molecular Imaging Research, Vanderbilt University, Nashville, TN, USA

S.K. Jain (ed.), *Imaging Infections*, DOI 10.1007/978-3-319-54592-9_5

Before the advent of modern imaging, estimating the site and extent of an infection was mostly derived from external physiologic observations. Current plasma or serum analysis from patient blood for suspected infections includes measurement of the erythrocyte sedimentation rate (ESR) and C-reactive protein (CRP) concentration, both of which are markers of inflammation and not specifically of infection [2]. Blood and tissue samples can be cultured for the presence of living bacteria, fungi, protozoa, and viruses, while many bacteria and parasites may be viewed in histological samples depending on life cycle stage [3]. Host response imaging can do for the treating physician what conventional biochemistry and radiology cannot—imaging can localize the site(s) of infection, and noninvasive serial can also provide therapeutic monitoring and therapeutic endpoints for treatments.

5.2 Leukocyte Tracking

Leukocytes such as neutrophils, basophils, eosinophils, mast cells, and monocytes with their daughter lineages (dendritic cells, microglia, macrophages) are derived from their own lineage of multipotent hematopoietic stem cells [4]. Each cell type has its own function and molecular characteristics that can be exploited to report on the host response to various microbial exposures. Currently, novel immune cell tracers (largely tracking B and T cells) and infection-specific tracers are being tested in clinical trials for future use [5, 6]. Details of some of these tracers are already provided in Chapters 2 and 4. Here, we will outline some of the labeling strategies employed to track selected cell types with examples from the literature.

5.2.1 [^{111}In]Oxyquinoline and [^{99m}Tc]HMPAO

Pan-leukocyte labeling using [^{111}In]oxyquinoline and [^{99m}Tc]HMPAO (hexamethylpropyleneamineoxime) is an ex vivo labeling method utilizing nonspecific hydrophilic trapping of radiotracer to label all mononuclear cells isolated from fresh patient blood using the Ficoll-Hypaque technique [7, 8]. The washed, labeled granulocytes are then reinjected into the patient and allowed to circulate with the goal to image blood flow at early time points and accumulation of labeled granulocytes at sites of inflammation and infection at later time points. Drawbacks to this technique include the relatively nonspecific readout on inflammation regardless of the cause and high uptake in bone marrow in addition to the radiotracer preparation and incubation with patient cells. Nevertheless, these radiotracers and technique have been used to image diabetic foot [9], musculoskeletal infections including infected prostheses [10–15], and cardiac infections [16, 17], among others.

5.2.2 ^{18}F-2-Fluoro-Deoxy-D-Glucose (^{18}F-FDG) Ex Vivo Labeling of Leukocytes

The increased glycolytic activity of inflammatory cells causes higher ^{18}F-FDG uptake at the site of inflammation and infection. However, as a nonspecific tracer incapable of distinguishing bacterial uptake from inflammatory cell uptake, ^{18}F-FDG positron-emission tomography (PET) demonstrates a poor specificity. Based on this, ex vivo labeling of leukocytes with ^{18}F-FDG has been employed to specifically label leukocytes for reinjection into the patient following labeling. This approach combines cell-bound radionuclide trafficking from the blood-pool compartment to the lesion with the high spatial resolution of PET imaging [18]. When compared to ^{111}In-labeled leukocytes, ^{18}F-FDG PET imaging demonstrated a similar sensitivity with a much lower specificity due to false-positive uptake in aseptic inflammation as well as oncological diseases [19]. Yilmaz et al. compared ^{18}F-FDG and ^{18}F-FDG-labeled leukocytes PET/CT in the diagnosis of infection using different SUV and visual thresholds for interpretation in 49 consecutive patients, and they found ^{18}F-FDG-labeled leukocytes PET/CT was more valuable than ^{18}F-FDG PET/CT in the imaging of infection [20]. However, in clinical practice, ^{18}F-FDG is much easier to approach making it one of the most important agents for imaging infection diseases.

5.2.3 Iron Oxide Nanoparticle Labeling and T2-Weighted MRI

The physicochemical surface properties of iron oxide nanoparticles allow their efficient internalization into phagocytic cells like macrophages, and the presence of intracellular superparamagnetic iron oxide nanoparticles can be typically indicated by signal hypointensities in T2-weighted MRI [21]. These properties make them appropriate for use as a contrast agent of MRI for inflammation and infection. Macrophages can be either pre-labeled with iron oxide nanoparticles ex vivo, or free iron oxide nanoparticles are intravenously injected and taken up by macrophages in vivo [22].

5.2.4 ^{19}F-Labeled Perfluorocarbons and MRI

Emulsified perfluorocarbons can be efficiently and selectively enriched in the monocyte/macrophage system. ^{19}F can be detected by using magnetic resonance spectroscopic imaging (MRSI), and because of the lack of any ^{19}F background in the body, observed signals originating from ^{19}F-labeled agents result in high specificity. Therefore, this technology could be promising for imaging inflammatory diseases;

^{19}F-labeled perfluorocarbons targeting leukocytes have been evaluated in inflammatory disease states like cardiac and cerebral ischemia and pulmonary infection in animal models [23, 24].

5.2.5 Chemokine Receptor

CC chemokine receptor 2 (CCR2) is an important chemokine receptor in the recruitment and migration of monocytes and macrophages [25]. Probes targeting to CCR2 like a 7-amino acid CCR2 binding peptide (extracellular loop 1 inverso [ECL1i])-conjugated tetraazacyclododecane tetraacetic acid (DOTA) labeled with ^{64}Cu (^{64}Cu-DOTA-ECL1i) and 7-amino acid CCR2 binding peptide-conjugated gold nanoclusters doped with ^{64}Cu (^{64}CuAuNCs-ECL1i) have recently been developed and evaluated in animal models. ^{64}Cu-DOTA-ECL1i and ^{64}CuAuNCs-ECL 1i are potential tools for PET-based theranostics of CCR2-directed inflammation [26, 27].

5.2.6 Folate Receptor-β

Folate receptor-β (FR-β) is overexpressed on activated macrophages [28]. By now, multiple selectively targeting FR-β imaging agents have been designed and synthesized. Folate was conjugated to a variety of dyes or radionuclides, such as FITC, Texas Red, Alexa Fluor, Oregon Green, ^{99m}Tc, ^{67}Ga, ^{111}In, and ^{18}F, to generate different probes [28, 29]. Further, FR-β imaging might discriminate between M1-like and M2-like macrophage phenotype. Jager et al. found that higher numbers of M2-like macrophages were present in areas of high ^{99m}Tc-folate accumulation than areas with low accumulation in carotid endarterectomy specimens of 20 patients [30].

5.2.7 Translocator Protein (TSPO)

Previously termed as peripheral benzodiazepine receptor (PBR), TSPO is an 18 kDa protein typically localized to the outer mitochondrial membrane whose primary role is to facilitate cholesterol metabolism. TSPO expression and function is shown to be linked with steroid biosynthesis, cellular proliferation, and apoptosis [31, 32]. Given the important role of TSPO in imaging, several TSPO PET ligands have been synthesized based upon a diversity of core scaffolds, including benzodiazepines, isoquinoline carboxamides, phenoxypheylacetamide, indolacetamides, *N,N*-dialkyl-2-phenylindol-3-ylglyoxyamides, and pyrazolopyrimides (Figure 5.1) [33–36]. Some of the most widely imaged TSPO probes include PK 11195, DAA 1097, DAA 1106, and Ro 5-4864 [34, 35, 37–41]. Alpidem (Figure 5.2) was among the first TSPO ligands that exhibit nanomolar binding affinity to TSPO (Ki = 0.5–7 nM)

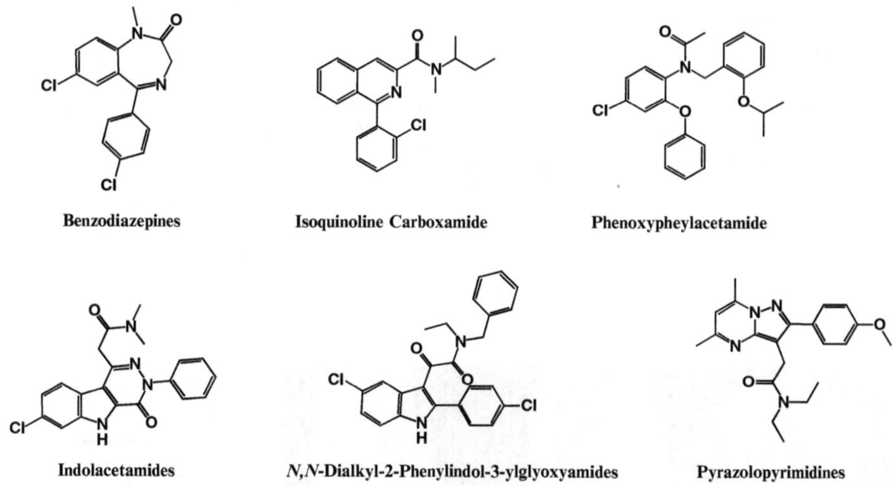

Figure 5.1 Common chemical scaffolds of translocator protein (TSPO) ligands

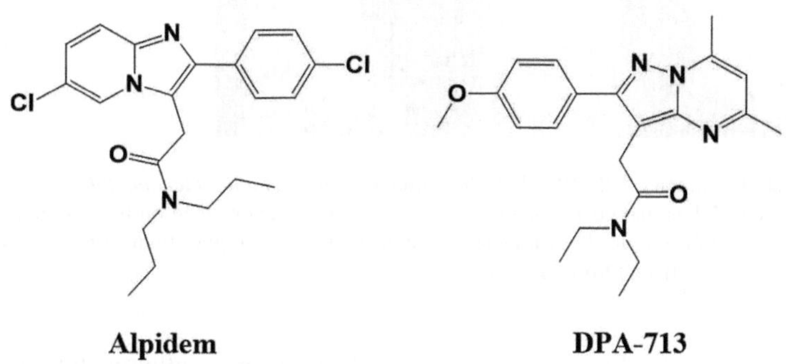

Figure 5.2 Structure of alpidem and DPA-713

[42–44]. However, further research illustrated that it also exhibited high binding affinity to central benzodiazepine receptor (CBR, $Ki = 1\text{–}28$ nM) [44]. Starting from this highly potent but nonselective ligand, Selleri et al. reported a novel ligand which can selectively bind to TSPO and maintain nanomolar affinity ($Ki = 4.7$ nM) through structural optimization [44, 45]. This ligand was later named DPA-713 (Figure 5.2) [35]. The 5, 6, and 7 positions of the pyrazolopyrimidine scaffold of DPA-713 were further optimized and developed as a novel PET tracer with improved affinity and pharmacokinetic properties (Figure 5.3) [46, 47]. TSPO is upregulated in active macrophages and microglia, and a variety of TSPO-specific radioligands have been synthesized and used to detect different disease-related inflammation both in patients and animal models. Gershen et al. successfully measured neuroinflammation in patients with temporal lobe epilepsy by using TSPO radioligand, ^{11}C PBR28, and ^{11}C DPA-713 [48]. In mice, ^{125}I-iodo-DPA-713 was found to

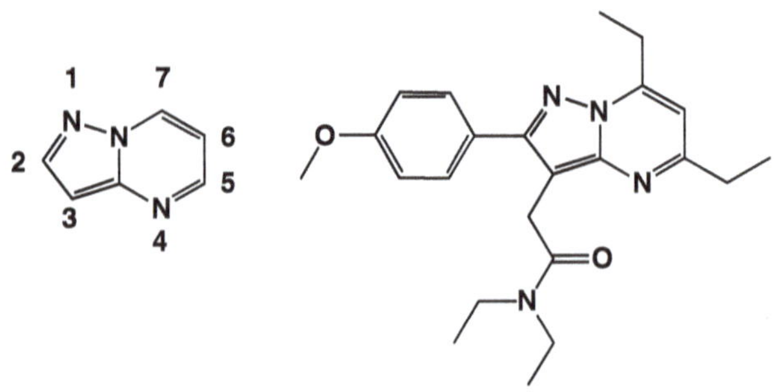

Figure 5.3 Pyrazolo-pyrimidine ring numbering and 2-(5,7-diethyl-2-(4-methoxyphenyl) pyrazolo[1,5-*a*]pyrimidin-3-yl)-*N,N*-diethylacetam ide

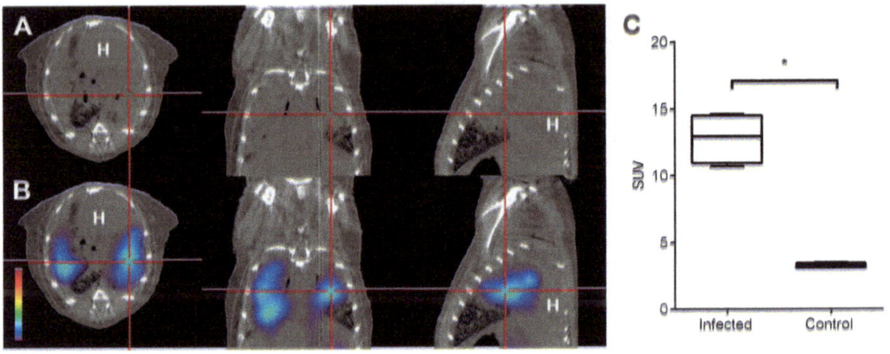

Figure 5.4 Pulmonary ^{124}I-DPA-713 PET imaging of a *Mycobacterium tuberculosis*-infected mouse. (**a**, **b**) PET signal co-localizes with the pulmonary lesion seen on the CT image. (**c**) The PET signal from *M. tuberculosis*-infected mice is significantly higher than from uninfected (control) mice. Adapted from Ordonez et al. [50]

accumulate specifically in tuberculosis (TB)-associated inflammatory lesions by selective retention within macrophages and phagocytic cells [49]. Pulmonary ^{125}I-DPA-713 single photon emission computed tomography (SPECT), but not ^{18}F-FDG PET, was able to correctly identify the bactericidal activities of the two TB treatments as early as 4 weeks after the start of treatment [50]. Furthermore, ^{124}I-DPA-713 PET was able to localize TB lesions with high-signal-to-noise ratios (Figure 5.4).

5.2.8 *CD206 Mannose Receptor*

Macrophage mannose receptor (MMR; CD206) is a 175-kDa C-type lectin predominantly expressed by mature macrophages and specific endothelial and dendritic cells. MMR targeting agents are mostly designed for imaging tumor-associated macrophages as well as some other inflammatory diseases like rheumatoid arthritis [51–53]. Put et al. investigated ^{99m}Tc-labeled nanobodies targeting to MMR with SPECT/CT imaging in a mouse model of rheumatoid arthritis, and they found that

MMR was expressed on macrophages in vitro and in vivo in synovial fluid of inflamed paws and the use of nanobodies against MMR with SPECT/CT could track inflammatory cells in vivo in arthritic joints [53].

5.2.9 MoAb Granulocyte Tracking

Anti-granulocyte scintigraphy using ^{99m}Tc-labeled monoclonal antibodies (MoAb) or fragments is introduced with the advantage of in vivo labeling of leukocytes. ^{99m}Tc-besilesomab which has been used since 1992 can recognize the nonspecific cross-reacting antigen 95 (NCA-95, also referred to as CD66b and CEACAM8) in the cytoplasm and on the cell membranes of granulocytes and granulocyte precursor cells during in vivo labeling [54].

5.2.10 CX3CR1

CX3CR1 is a seven-transmembrane G-protein-coupled receptor that plays a role in leukocyte migration and adhesion [55]. Peripheral blood monocytes, subsets of natural killer cells (NK) and dendritic cells, and also microglia naturally express CX3CR1 [56]. As CX3CR1 plays an important role in the regulation of neuroinflammation by microglia and the phagocytosis function of phagocytes, it can be a promising target to imaging inflammations and infections by using its radionuclide-labeled MoAbs and/or analogs.

5.2.11 Lymphocyte Tracking

Lymphocytes are a distinct lineage of leukocytes that comprise B cells, T cells and, natural killer cells. They constitute the effector arm of adaptive immunity and mediate responses to bacteria, viruses, fungi, and autoimmune-related reactions including cancer.

5.2.11.1 B Cells

Because in vitro immune cell studies do not accurately reflect how immune cells behave inside the body, it is important to study them in vivo. Thus the concept of in vivo cell labeling, where antibodies against immune cell markers are conjugated to radioactive, spin, or fluorescent labels (either before or after the antibodies are injected) [was developed] to study their behavior in the context of their biological environment. In vivo lymphocyte tracking has been of interest since the 1980s [57], although primarily for oncologic applications [58–61]. One of the first radiotracers to be employed successfully in the clinic—and later developed into radiologic and immune therapeutic treatments—is anti-CD20 antibody to target B cells [62–67]. In the case of oncology, the disease target is B-cell lymphomas. B-cell migration to sites of infection is an important host response and can also be followed using labeled antigen-specific antibodies including anti-CD19 antibody [68], and this target has been exploited in chimeric antigen receptor-modified T cell (CART) therapies [69–72] against B-cell lymphomas. While imaging of cell populations homing to sites of infection may help to identify foci of infection and extent of immune response, B-cell populations may also decrease in the presence of microbial superantigens [73]. B-lymphocyte behavior has been studied using two-photon and intravital microscopy techniques in the context of murine models of Friend Murine Leukemia Virus infection [74] in which the authors observed prolonged contact between fluorescent-infected and uninfected lymphocytes, resulting in viral spread. In the context of radionuclide imaging, in a 2011 study by Walther et al., DBA/1 mouse B cells were labeled ex vivo with anti-B-cell antibodies labeled with ^{89}Zr as the imaging marker [75]. PET imaging showed successful binding of the antibodies to B cells. Since then the technique has been used experimentally in oncology and rheumatology patients [76–78]; applying this technique toward tracking host-infection interactions is a logical extension of this technology. Whereas direct B-cell labeling has been attempted in vivo much less frequently, T-cell tracking is more common. Since T cells are among the class of effector cells, tracking their movement is perceived to be a better measure of active immune involvement in the context of infection and can potentially be distinguished between helper and effector T cells.

5.2.11.2 T Cells

T-cell imaging techniques are summarized in Table 5.1. Tavare et al. successfully produced PET-based CD8-antibody imaging agents to be used in preclinical as well as clinical studies, especially immune therapy protocols [79]. They achieved this by conjugating anti-CD8 minibody (Mb) fragments to a ^{64}Cu-radiotracer. Mice injected with the final product displayed high-contrast PET images with clear uptake in the spleen and lymph nodes. Thus, monitoring the live biology and kinetics of CD-8 T cells in vivo became feasible. Several examples of tracking T-cell migration and behavior using intravital or two-photon microscopy in the context of experimental *Toxoplasma gondii* infection in mice are present. One example includes investigation of the interaction of antigen-specific T cells with dendritic cells shortly after *Toxoplasma* infection [80] in which the authors discovered that both antigen-specific and naïve T cells reduce velocity and interactions with dendritic cells were not restricted to the T zone of draining lymph nodes. Another study using intravital microscopy to follow fluorescent T-cell movement in the brains of mice infected with fluorescent *T. gondii* [81] showed the interactions of CD8+ T cells with chronically infected brain tissue as well as interactions with fluorescent APCs. This imaging-based study allowed the researchers to discover that CD8+ T cells are

Table 5.1 T-cell imaging techniques

Labeling methods	Benefits	Drawbacks	Side effects on T-cell function	Clinical uses
Optical				
Direct (fluorescent dyes)	Simple preparation Cheap Easy administration	False signals (dead cells) Probe dilution Toxicity Limited tissue penetration	Rare	None
Indirect (fluorescent proteins/bioluminescent agents)	Highly specific Suitable for studying mechanisms	Altered T-cell function Difficult technique Limited tissue penetration	Genetic alterations	None
MRI				
Direct (gadolinium complexes, SPIO, CEST, and 19F-containing probes)	Simple preparation Efficient labeling No background noise	False signals (dead cells) Probe dilution Toxicity	T-cell toxicity	Stem cell and tumor cell tracking
Indirect (MRI reporter genes)	Endogenous or exogenous substrates can be used [38]	Altered T-cell function Difficult technique Low sensitivity	Genetic alterations	None
PET/SPECT				
Direct (e.g., 99mTc-HMPAO, 18F-FDG, 64Cu2 + gold nanoparticles, etc.)	Simple preparation	False signals (dead cells, probe leak) Longitudinal studies difficult due to short half-life	T-cell viability	Common in preclinical studies
Indirect (e.g., PET reporter genes such as HSV1-tk)	Allows tracking over time	Very complex technique Expensive	Genetic alterations	T-cells tracking in glioblastoma multiforme [5]

Adapted from Liu et al. [97]

arrested before making prolonged contacts with infected cells and never contacted infected astrocytes or neurons. A similar study involving similar methods showed that *T. gondii* gained entry to the brain via infection of vessel endothelial cells and, furthermore, did not utilize a Trojan horse method of entry via infected monocytes as had been hypothesized [82]. In the case of *Shigella flexneri*, T cells are actively targeted and invaded by the bacterium. One study tracked the movement of T cells to infected spleen compartments where the T cells became infected once their movement became arrested [83]. This group utilized ex vivo fluorescently labeled purified T cells adoptively transferred into mice subsequently infected with bacteria for two-photon microscopy measurement of cell movements and velocities. Another example involves host response against *Listeria monocytogenes* (LM). Using intravital microscopy with fluorescent protein-engineered mouse models, Waite et al. were able to directly visualize immune cell dynamics in response to LM foci within the subcapsular red pulp region of the spleen [84]. They found that subcapsular dendritic cells (scDCs) sequestrated LM from the blood directly, while neutrophils were attracted to cells infected with the bacteria. CD8+ T cells were later demonstrated to clear the infection by terminating both LM cells and infected DCs. Intravital fluorescence microscopy was used to follow individual T cells within living tissues at high resolution. This technique can be applied to any cell type or biomolecule of interest so long as a specific antibody or other ligand exists for labeling.

5.2.12 Glycoprotein IIb/IIIa in Platelets

Glycoprotein IIb/IIIa (GPIIb/IIIa) is a platelet receptor for fibrinogen and other clotting factors. It is a membrane glycoprotein integrin complex which aids platelet adhesion and aggregation [85]. While platelet involvement in infectious diseases is uncommon, it is directly involved in cases of infective endocarditis and inflammatory thrombosis. Early detection of activated platelets is critical to avoid major complications such as myocardial infarction. One of the earlier techniques of platelet imaging involved radiolabeling with ^{111}In, performed by Al and colleagues. ^{111}In-labeled platelets proved better indicators of infective endocarditis than leukocyte imaging as platelet uptake was evident in thrombotic, vegetative areas rather than broader areas of inflammation [86]. In another study, ^{99m}Tc was used to label glycoprotein IIb/IIIa receptors on platelets to study acute deep vein thrombosis although the accuracy of the scintigraphy technique proved operator dependent [87]. Kam Leung, PhD, combined microbubble-ultrasound technology with abciximab (abciximab microbubbles) to image acute arterial thrombotic arterial occlusion [88]. Abciximab is a glycoprotein IIb/IIIa antibody with high affinity to platelets and is successfully incorporated into ultrasound microbubbles. Hagisawa et al. used perfluorocarbon gas-containing bubble liposomes (BL) instead of MPIOs and followed the same protocol [89]. They were both able to detect acute thrombotic arterial occlusion noninvasively using ultrasound-based platelet imaging. Alternatively, Muhlen et al. employed microparticles of iron oxide (MPIOs) to label GP IIb/IIIa receptor antibodies bound to platelets [90]. Functional MR imaging showed binding of MPIO particles to atherosclerotic plaques under both venous and arterial flow chamber settings and at clinically detectable levels. Thus, this technique proved to be of high clinical value in detecting atherothrombotic clots. As mentioned previously, imaging of indications other than the context of infection predominates in the literature. Cancer imaging is by far the most common application for inflammation imaging with the exception of platelet/thrombus imaging in which noninfectious vascular pathologies have taken the lead. Nevertheless, the techniques described above can easily be applied to study processes in the context of infection such as in *E. coli* infections [91], certain strains of *Streptococcus* infections, and other thrombogenic infections [92].

5.2.13 Others

Host responses such as collagen deposition (fibrosis) [93], the local environment such as hypoxia [94–96], and soluble factors such as the release of cytokines and chemokines have not been discussed here but have also been targets of investigation.

5.3 Summary

Radiotracer and spin-labeled magnetic resonance technique development has greatly advanced in the last two decades providing myriad new targeted ligands and biologics for targeting a multitude of receptors, enzymes, saccharides, metabolites, and cellular processes. The majority of these new ligands have been validated in cancer models, reflecting the distribution of funding from federal and other sources. However, infections remain a prevalent scourge in developing nations and are re-emerging as a serious threat in developed nations in the form of antibiotic-resistant infections. The need to confirm and locate infections, especially in inaccessible anatomic locations, should be high priority both to understand the biological processes involved and as an aid to clinicians. Imaging the host response, in particular, can help scientists understand how effector and innate immune cells respond and understand the impact of antimicrobial treatments.

References

1. Serhan, C.N., P.A. Ward, and D.W. Gilroy, *Fundamentals of inflammation*. 2010, Cambridge; New York: Cambridge University Press. xiv, 473 p.
2. Harrison, M., *Erythrocyte sedimentation rate and C-reactive protein*. Aust Prescr, 2015. **38**(3): p. 93-4.
3. Eroschenko, V.P., *Atlas of histology with functional correlations*. 13th edition. ed. 2017, Philadelphia: Wolters Kluwer. p.
4. Till, J.E., et al., *Regulation of blood cell differentiation*. Fed Proc, 1975. **34**(13): p. 2279-84.
5. Nahrendorf, M., et al., *Imaging systemic inflammatory networks in ischemic heart disease*. J Am Coll Cardiol, 2015. **65**(15): p. 1583-91.
6. Mills, B., et al., *[(18)F]FDG-6-P as a novel in vivo tool for imaging staphylococcal infections*. EJNMMI Res, 2015. **5**: p. 13.

7. de Vries, E.F., et al., *Guidelines for the labelling of leucocytes with (99m)Tc-HMPAO. Inflammation/Infection Taskgroup of the European Association of Nuclear Medicine.* Eur J Nucl Med Mol Imaging, 2010. **37**(4): p. 842-8.
8. Axelsson, B., et al., *Comparison of In-111 granulocytes and Tc-99m albumin colloid for bone marrow scintigraphy by the use of quantitative SPECT imaging.* Clin Nucl Med, 1990. **15**(7): p. 473-9.
9. Filippi, L., et al., *Diabetic foot infection: usefulness of SPECT/CT for 99mTc-HMPAO-labeled leukocyte imaging.* J Nucl Med, 2009. **50**(7): p. 1042-6.
10. Filippi, L. and O. Schillaci, *Usefulness of hybrid SPECT/CT in 99mTc-HMPAO-labeled leukocyte scintigraphy for bone and joint infections.* J Nucl Med, 2006. **47**(12): p. 1908-13.
11. Bruni, C., et al., *Usefulness of hybrid SPECT/CT for the 99mTc-HMPAO-labeled leukocyte scintigraphy in a case of cranial osteomyelitis.* Braz J Infect Dis, 2008. **12**(6): p. 558-60.
12. Glaudemans, A.W., et al., *A large retrospective single-centre study to define the best image acquisition protocols and interpretation criteria for white blood cell scintigraphy with (9)(9) mTc-HMPAO-labelled leucocytes in musculoskeletal infections.* Eur J Nucl Med Mol Imaging, 2013. **40**(11): p. 1760-9.
13. Erba, P.A., et al., *Radiolabeled WBC scintigraphy in the diagnostic workup of patients with suspected device-related infections.* JACC Cardiovasc Imaging, 2013. **6**(10): p. 1075-86.
14. Erba, P.A., et al., *Radiolabelled leucocyte scintigraphy versus conventional radiological imaging for the management of late, low-grade vascular prosthesis infections.* Eur J Nucl Med Mol Imaging, 2014. **41**(2): p. 357-68.
15. Kim, H.O., et al., *Usefulness of adding SPECT/CT to 99mTc-hexamethylpropylene amine oxime (HMPAO)-labeled leukocyte imaging for diagnosing prosthetic joint infections.* J Comput Assist Tomogr, 2014. **38**(2): p. 313-9.
16. Erba, P.A., et al., *Added value of 99mTc-HMPAO-labeled leukocyte SPECT/CT in the characterization and management of patients with infectious endocarditis.* J Nucl Med, 2012. **53**(8): p. 1235-43.
17. Loke, K.S., et al., *Pseudoaneurysm and coronary abscess secondary to coronary stent fracture identified with Tc-99m hexamethylpropyleneamine oxime-labeled white blood cell SPECT/CT scintigraphy.* Clin Nucl Med, 2011. **36**(5): p. 397-9.
18. Dumarey, N., et al., *Imaging infection with 18F-FDG-labeled leukocyte PET/CT: initial experience in 21 patients.* J Nucl Med, 2006. **47**(4): p. 625-32.
19. Kjaer, A., et al., *Fever of unknown origin: prospective comparison of diagnostic value of 18F-FDG PET and 111In-granulocyte scintigraphy.* Eur J Nucl Med Mol Imaging, 2004. **31**(5): p. 622-6.
20. Yilmaz, S., et al., *Comparison of FDG and FDG-labeled leukocytes PET/CT in diagnosis of infection.* Nuklearmedizin, 2015. **54**(6): p. 262-71.
21. Corot, C., et al., *Macrophage imaging in central nervous system and in carotid atherosclerotic plaque using ultrasmall superparamagnetic iron oxide in magnetic resonance imaging.* Invest Radiol, 2004. **39**(10): p. 619-25.
22. Oweida, A.J., et al., *Iron-oxide labeling of hematogenous macrophages in a model of experimental autoimmune encephalomyelitis and the contribution to signal loss in fast imaging employing steady state acquisition (FIESTA) images.* J Magn Reson Imaging, 2007. **26**(1): p. 144-51.
23. Flogel, U., et al., *In vivo monitoring of inflammation after cardiac and cerebral ischemia by fluorine magnetic resonance imaging.* Circulation, 2008. **118**(2): p. 140-8.
24. Temme, S., et al., *19F magnetic resonance imaging of endogenous macrophages in inflammation.* Wiley Interdiscip Rev Nanomed Nanobiotechnol, 2012. **4**(3): p. 329-43.
25. Geissmann, F., S. Jung, and D.R. Littman, *Blood monocytes consist of two principal subsets with distinct migratory properties.* Immunity, 2003. **19**(1): p. 71-82.
26. Mojumdar, K., et al., *Inflammatory monocytes promote progression of Duchenne muscular dystrophy and can be therapeutically targeted via CCR2.* EMBO Mol Med, 2014. **6**(11): p. 1476-92.

27. Liu, Y., et al., *PET-based Imaging of Chemokine Receptor 2 in Experimental and Disease-related Lung Inflammation.* Radiology, 2017: p. 161409.
28. Yi, Y.S., *Folate Receptor-Targeted Diagnostics and Therapeutics for Inflammatory Diseases.* Immune Netw, 2016. **16**(6): p. 337-343.
29. Gent, Y.Y., et al., *Evaluation of the novel folate receptor ligand [18F]fluoro-PEG-folate for macrophage targeting in a rat model of arthritis.* Arthritis Res Ther, 2013. **15**(2): p. R37.
30. Jager, N.A., et al., *Folate receptor-beta imaging using 99mTc-folate to explore distribution of polarized macrophage populations in human atherosclerotic plaque.* J Nucl Med, 2014. **55**(12): p. 1945-51.
31. Papadopoulos, V., et al., *Translocator protein (18kDa): new nomenclature for the peripheral-type benzodiazepine receptor based on its structure and molecular function.* Trends in pharmacological sciences, 2006. **27**(8): p. 402-409.
32. Papadopoulos, V. and L. Lecanu, *Translocator protein (18 kDa) TSPO: an emerging therapeutic target in neurotrauma.* Experimental neurology, 2009. **219**(1): p. 53-57.
33. Le Fur, G., et al., *Peripheral benzodiazepine binding sites: effect of PK 11195, 1-(2-chlorophenyl)-N-methyl-N-(1-methylpropyl)-3-isoquinolinecarboxamide: I. In vitro studies.* Life sciences, 1983. **32**(16): p. 1839-1847.
34. Marangos, P.J., et al., *Characterization of peripheral-type benzodiazepine binding sites in brain using [3H] Ro 5-4864.* Molecular pharmacology, 1982. **22**(1): p. 26-32.
35. James, M.L., et al., *Synthesis and in vivo evaluation of a novel peripheral benzodiazepine receptor PET radioligand.* Bioorganic & medicinal chemistry, 2005. **13**(22): p. 6188-6194.
36. Denora, N., et al., *2-Phenyl-imidazo [1, 2-a] pyridine compounds containing hydrophilic groups as potent and selective ligands for peripheral benzodiazepine receptors: synthesis, binding affinity and electrophysiological studies.* Journal of medicinal chemistry, 2008. **51**(21): p. 6876-6888.
37. Müller, N., et al., *Anti-inflammatory treatment in schizophrenia.* Progress in Neuro-Psychopharmacology and Biological Psychiatry, 2013. **42**: p. 146-153.
38. Taliani, S., et al., *Translocator protein ligands as promising therapeutic tools for anxiety disorders.* Current medicinal chemistry, 2009. **16**(26): p. 3359-3380.
39. Chaki, S., et al., *Binding characteristics of [3H] DAA1106, a novel and selective ligand for peripheral benzodiazepine receptors.* European journal of pharmacology, 1999. **371**(2): p. 197-204.
40. Briard, E., et al., *Single-step high-yield radiosynthesis and evaluation of a sensitive 18F-labeled ligand for imaging brain peripheral benzodiazepine receptors with PET.* Journal of medicinal chemistry, 2009. **52**(3): p. 688-699.
41. Delavoie, F., et al., *In Vivo and in Vitro Peripheral-Type Benzodiazepine Receptor Polymerization: Functional Significance in Drug Ligand and Cholesterol Binding†.* Biochemistry, 2003. **42**(15): p. 4506-4519.
42. Gaillard, Y., J.-P. Gay-Montchamp, and M. Ollagnier, *Simultaneous screening and quantitation of alpidem, zolpidem, buspirone and benzodiazepines by dual-channel gas chromatography using electron-capture and nitrogen—phosphorus detection after solid-phase extraction.* Journal of Chromatography B: Biomedical Sciences and Applications, 1993. **622**(2): p. 197-208.
43. Byrnes, J.J., D.J. Greenblatt, and L.G. Miller, *Benzodiazepine receptor binding of nonbenzodiazepines in vivo: alpidem, zolpidem and zopiclone.* Brain research bulletin, 1992. **29**(6): p. 905-908.
44. Selleri, S., et al., *2-Arylpyrazolo [1, 5-a] pyrimidin-3-yl acetamides. New potent and selective peripheral benzodiazepine receptor ligands.* Bioorganic & medicinal chemistry, 2001. **9**(10): p. 2661-2671.
45. Selleri, S., et al., *Insight into 2-phenylpyrazolo [1, 5-a] pyrimidin-3-yl acetamides as peripheral benzodiazepine receptor ligands: synthesis, biological evaluation and 3D-QSAR investigation.* Bioorganic & medicinal chemistry, 2005. **13**(16): p. 4821-4834.
46. Tang, D., et al., *Synthesis and Structure–Activity Relationships of 5, 6, 7-Substituted Pyrazolopyrimidines: Discovery of a Novel TSPO PET Ligand for Cancer Imaging.* Journal of medicinal chemistry, 2013. **56**(8): p. 3429-3433.

47. Tang, D., et al., *Preclinical Imaging Evaluation of Novel TSPO-PET Ligand 2-(5, 7-Diethyl-2-(4-(2-[18F] fluoroethoxy) phenyl) pyrazolo [1, 5-a] pyrimidin-3-yl)-N, N-diethylacetamide ([18F] VUIIS1008) in Glioma.* Molecular Imaging and Biology, 2014. **16**(6): p. 813-820.
48. Gershen, L.D., et al., *Neuroinflammation in Temporal Lobe Epilepsy Measured Using Positron Emission Tomographic Imaging of Translocator Protein.* JAMA Neurol, 2015. **72**(8): p. 882-8.
49. Foss, C.A., et al., *Noninvasive molecular imaging of tuberculosis-associated inflammation with radioiodinated DPA-713.* J Infect Dis, 2013. **208**(12): p. 2067-74.
50. Ordonez, A.A., et al., *Radioiodinated DPA-713 imaging correlates with bactericidal activity of tuberculosis treatments in mice.* Antimicrob Agents Chemother, 2015. **59**(1): p. 642-9.
51. Movahedi, K., et al., *Nanobody-based targeting of the macrophage mannose receptor for effective in vivo imaging of tumor-associated macrophages.* Cancer Res, 2012. **72**(16): p. 4165-77.
52. Blykers, A., et al., *PET Imaging of Macrophage Mannose Receptor-Expressing Macrophages in Tumor Stroma Using 18F-Radiolabeled Camelid Single-Domain Antibody Fragments.* J Nucl Med, 2015. **56**(8): p. 1265-71.
53. Put, S., et al., *SPECT imaging of joint inflammation with Nanobodies targeting the macrophage mannose receptor in a mouse model for rheumatoid arthritis.* J Nucl Med, 2013. **54**(5): p. 807-14.
54. Richter, W.S., et al., *99mTc-besilesomab (Scintimun) in peripheral osteomyelitis: comparison with 99mTc-labelled white blood cells.* Eur J Nucl Med Mol Imaging, 2011. **38**(5): p. 899-910.
55. Imai, T., et al., *Identification and molecular characterization of fractalkine receptor CX3CR1, which mediates both leukocyte migration and adhesion.* Cell, 1997. **91**(4): p. 521-30.
56. Jung, S., et al., *Analysis of fractalkine receptor CX(3)CR1 function by targeted deletion and green fluorescent protein reporter gene insertion.* Mol Cell Biol, 2000. **20**(11): p. 4106-14.
57. Pozzilli, P., et al., *Tracking of indium-111-oxine labelled lymphocytes in autoimmune thyroid disease.* Clin Endocrinol (Oxf), 1983. **19**(1): p. 111-6.
58. Deane, M. and J.D. Norton, *Immunoglobulin gene 'fingerprinting': an approach to analysis of B lymphoid clonality in lymphoproliferative disorders.* Br J Haematol, 1991. **77**(3): p. 274-81.
59. Wallace, P.K., et al., *Mechanisms of adoptive immunotherapy: improved methods for in vivo tracking of tumor-infiltrating lymphocytes and lymphokine-activated killer cells.* Cancer Res, 1993. **53**(10 Suppl): p. 2358-67.
60. Rylova, S.N., et al., *Immuno-PET Imaging of CD30-Positive Lymphoma Using 89Zr-Desferrioxamine-Labeled CD30-Specific AC-10 Antibody.* J Nucl Med, 2016. **57**(1): p. 96-102.
61. Tavare, R., et al., *Immuno-PET of Murine T Cell Reconstitution Postadoptive Stem Cell Transplantation Using Anti-CD4 and Anti-CD8 Cys-Diabodies.* J Nucl Med, 2015. **56**(8): p. 1258-64.
62. Dietlein, M., et al., *Imaging of central nervous system lymphomas with iodine-123 labeled rituximab.* Eur J Haematol, 2005. **74**(4): p. 348-52.
63. Boucek, J.A. and J.H. Turner, *Validation of prospective whole-body bone marrow dosimetry by SPECT/CT multimodality imaging in (131)I-anti-CD20 rituximab radioimmunotherapy of non-Hodgkin's lymphoma.* Eur J Nucl Med Mol Imaging, 2005. **32**(4): p. 458-69.
64. Gmeiner Stopar, T., et al., *99mTc-labelled rituximab, a new non-Hodgkin's lymphoma imaging agent: first clinical experience.* Nucl Med Commun, 2008. **29**(12): p. 1059-65.
65. Esmaeli, B., et al., *Prospective trial of targeted radioimmunotherapy with Y-90 ibritumomab tiuxetan (Zevalin) for front-line treatment of early-stage extranodal indolent ocular adnexal lymphoma.* Ann Oncol, 2009. **20**(4): p. 709-14.
66. Natarajan, A., et al., *Validation of 64Cu-DOTA-rituximab injection preparation under good manufacturing practices: a PET tracer for imaging of B-cell non-Hodgkin lymphoma.* Mol Imaging, 2015. **14**.

67. Muylle, K., et al., *Tumour targeting and radiation dose of radioimmunotherapy with (90) Y-rituximab in CD20+ B-cell lymphoma as predicted by (89)Zr-rituximab immuno-PET: impact of preloading with unlabelled rituximab.* Eur J Nucl Med Mol Imaging, 2015. **42**(8): p. 1304-14.
68. Najjar, A.M., et al., *Imaging of Sleeping Beauty-Modified CD19-Specific T Cells Expressing HSV1-Thymidine Kinase by Positron Emission Tomography.* Mol Imaging Biol, 2016. **18**(6): p. 838-848.
69. Velasquez, M.P., et al., *T cells expressing CD19-specific Engager Molecules for the Immunotherapy of CD19-positive Malignancies.* Sci Rep, 2016. **6**: p. 27130.
70. Bai, Y., et al., *Enhancement of the in vivo persistence and antitumor efficacy of CD19 chimeric antigen receptor T cells through the delivery of modified TERT mRNA.* Cell Discov, 2015. **1**: p. 15040.
71. Long, A.H., et al., *4-1BB costimulation ameliorates T cell exhaustion induced by tonic signaling of chimeric antigen receptors.* Nat Med, 2015. **21**(6): p. 581-90.
72. Tasian, S.K. and R.A. Gardner, *CD19-redirected chimeric antigen receptor-modified T cells: a promising immunotherapy for children and adults with B-cell acute lymphoblastic leukemia (ALL).* Ther Adv Hematol, 2015. **6**(5): p. 228-41.
73. Silverman, G.J. and C.S. Goodyear, *Confounding B-cell defences: lessons from a staphylococcal superantigen.* Nat Rev Immunol, 2006. **6**(6): p. 465-75.
74. Sewald, X., et al., *In vivo imaging of virological synapses.* Nat Commun, 2012. **3**: p. 1320.
75. Walther, M., et al., *Implementation of 89Zr production and in vivo imaging of B-cells in mice with 89Zr-labeled anti-B-cell antibodies by small animal PET/CT.* Appl Radiat Isot, 2011. **69**(6): p. 852-7.
76. Zeman, M.N. and P.J. Scott, *Current imaging strategies in rheumatoid arthritis.* Am J Nucl Med Mol Imaging, 2012. **2**(2): p. 174-220.
77. Bruijnen, S., et al., *B-cell imaging with zirconium-89 labelled rituximab PET-CT at baseline is associated with therapeutic response 24 weeks after initiation of rituximab treatment in rheumatoid arthritis patients.* Arthritis Res Ther, 2016. **18**(1): p. 266.
78. Barrington, S.F., et al., *Role of imaging in the staging and response assessment of lymphoma: consensus of the International Conference on Malignant Lymphomas Imaging Working Group.* J Clin Oncol, 2014. **32**(27): p. 3048-58.
79. Tavare, R., et al., *Engineered antibody fragments for immuno-PET imaging of endogenous CD8+ T cells in vivo.* Proc Natl Acad Sci U S A, 2014. **111**(3): p. 1108-13.
80. John, B., et al., *Dynamic Imaging of CD8(+) T cells and dendritic cells during infection with Toxoplasma gondii.* PLoS Pathog, 2009. **5**(7): p. e1000505.
81. Schaeffer, M., et al., *Dynamic imaging of T cell-parasite interactions in the brains of mice chronically infected with Toxoplasma gondii.* J Immunol, 2009. **182**(10): p. 6379-93.
82. Konradt, C., et al., *Endothelial cells are a replicative niche for entry of Toxoplasma gondii to the central nervous system.* Nat Microbiol, 2016. **1**: p. 16001.
83. Salgado-Pabon, W., et al., *Shigella impairs T lymphocyte dynamics in vivo.* Proc Natl Acad Sci U S A, 2013. **110**(12): p. 4458-63.
84. Waite, J.C., et al., *Dynamic imaging of the effector immune response to listeria infection in vivo.* PLoS Pathog, 2011. **7**(3): p. e1001326.
85. Fullard, J.F., *The role of the platelet glycoprotein IIb/IIIa in thrombosis and haemostasis.* Curr Pharm Des, 2004. **10**(14): p. 1567-76.
86. Riba, A.L., et al., *Imaging experimental infective endocarditis with indium-111-labeled blood cellular components.* Circulation, 1979. **59**(2): p. 336-43.
87. Bates, S.M., et al., *Imaging characteristics of a novel technetium Tc 99m-labeled platelet glycoprotein IIb/IIIa receptor antagonist in patients With acute deep vein thrombosis or a history of deep vein thrombosis.* Arch Intern Med, 2003. **163**(4): p. 452-6.
88. Leung, K., *Abciximab microbubbles*, in *Molecular Imaging and Contrast Agent Database (MICAD).* 2004: Bethesda (MD).

89. Hagisawa, K., et al., *Enhancement of ultrasonic thrombus imaging using novel liposomal bubbles targeting activated platelet glycoprotein IIb/IIIa complex--in vitro and in vivo study.* Int J Cardiol, 2011. **152**(2): p. 202-6.
90. von Zur Muhlen, C., et al., *Functionalized magnetic resonance contrast agent selectively binds to glycoprotein IIb/IIIa on activated human platelets under flow conditions and is detectable at clinically relevant field strengths.* Mol Imaging, 2008. **7**(2): p. 59-67.
91. Sprouse, J.T., et al., *Thrombogenic alleles, Escherichia coli O157:H7 infections, and hemolytic uremic syndrome.* Blood Coagul Fibrinolysis, 2001. **12**(4): p. 283-8.
92. Stevens, D.L. and E.L. Kaplan, *Streptococcal infections: clinical aspects, microbiology, and molecular pathogenesis*. 2000, New York: Oxford University Press. xv, 449 p.
93. Rossleigh, M.A., *Scintigraphic imaging in renal infections.* Q J Nucl Med Mol Imaging, 2009. **53**(1): p. 72-7.
94. Liu, R.S., et al., *Detection of anaerobic odontogenic infections by fluorine-18 fluoromisonidazole.* Eur J Nucl Med, 1996. **23**(10): p. 1384-7.
95. Haralampieva, D., et al., *Noninvasive PET Imaging and Tracking of Engineered Human Muscle Precursor Cells for Skeletal Muscle Tissue Engineering.* J Nucl Med, 2016. **57**(9): p. 1467-73.
96. Belton, M., et al., *Hypoxia and tissue destruction in pulmonary TB.* Thorax, 2016.
97. Liu, Z. and Z. Li, *Molecular imaging in tracking tumor-specific cytotoxic T lymphocytes (CTLs).* Theranostics, 2014. **4**(10): p. 990-1001.

Chapter 6
Bacterial Imaging

Alvaro A. Ordonez, Lauren E. Bambarger, Niren Murthy, David M. Wilson, and Sanjay K. Jain

6.1 Introduction

Despite significant advances in health care, bacterial infections remain a major cause of mortality and morbidity worldwide, as well as in the USA. Moreover, the increasing use of invasive techniques and implants, immunosuppressive and cancer therapies, and the alarming rise of multidrug-resistant bacteria are a major threat to humanity [1–6], costing billions of dollars to the US economy alone [7]. Multidrug-resistant (MDR) bacteria are increasingly challenging to treat [5], cause life-threatening diseases [4], and often require the use of increasingly toxic antibiotics [8]. Finally, several bacteria are also recognized as biothreat pathogens by the US Centers for Disease Control and Prevention (CDC) [9]. Early diagnosis and targeted pharmaceutical intervention may significantly reduce morbidity and mortality caused by bacterial infections worldwide.

A.A. Ordonez • L.E. Bambarger
Department of Pediatrics, Johns Hopkins University School of Medicine, Baltimore, MD, USA

Center for Infection and Inflammation Imaging Research, Johns Hopkins University School of Medicine, Baltimore, MD, USA

N. Murthy
Department of Bioengineering, University of California at Berkeley, Berkley, CA, USA

D.M. Wilson
Department of Radiology, University of California, San Francisco, San Francisco, CA, USA

S.K. Jain (✉)
Department of Pediatrics, Johns Hopkins University School of Medicine, Baltimore, MD, USA

Center for Infection and Inflammation Imaging Research, Johns Hopkins University School of Medicine, Baltimore, MD, USA

Department of International Health, Johns Hopkins Bloomberg School of Public Health, Baltimore, MD, USA
e-mail: sjain5@jhmi.edu

S.K. Jain (ed.), *Imaging Infections*, DOI 10.1007/978-3-319-54592-9_6

The gold standard in diagnosing bacterial infections remains microbiologic culture or molecular techniques, which require a clinical sample for the assays. While easily obtained samples (blood, urine) can often be useful, in cases of a deep-seated infection, a biopsy is often required, which is invasive, costly, sometimes dangerous, and prone to sampling errors. Also commonly employed are conventional radiological techniques such as computerized tomography (CT), magnetic resonance imaging (MRI), X-ray, and ultrasound. However, these techniques rely on the presence of structural abnormalities and are unable to reliably differentiate infection from inflammation or oncologic processes. With increasing rates of MDR bacteria, there exists a need for rapid and accurate diagnosing and monitoring of deep-seated bacterial infections.

6.2 Imaging Techniques

Optical imaging techniques, including fluorescence and bioluminescence imaging, have been used extensively to detect bacteria in vivo in various small animal models as discussed in Chapter 3. These studies have helped significantly in understanding disease pathogenesis and in developing therapeutics for infections. Despite their widespread use in research laboratories, optical imaging probes have not been extensively evaluated in the clinical setting for bacterial infection, as they are limited by tissue penetration, i.e., signals from deep inside the body cannot be visualized well. However, recent advances in fluorophore design and imaging equipment, combined with the ongoing efforts toward the development of bacteria-specific compounds, could lead to interesting applications of optical imaging in the clinic [10]. Nuclear imaging techniques are usually not limited by tissue penetration and are therefore widely available for clinical use. The detection of infection with radionuclides that rely on physiological and biochemical changes at the site of disease is discussed in Chapter 4.

Both routine and advanced MRI methods have been used to diagnose acute pyogenic infection, taking advantage of the improved soft-tissue contrast of this modality. In particular, MRI is essential for workup of suspected central nervous system (CNS) and musculoskeletal infections. Pyogenic infection can have a variety of appearances depending on the organs involved, but typical findings include hyperintensity on T_2-weighted imaging, enhancement on post-gadolinium T_1-weighted imaging, and the presence of fluid signal reflecting abscess formation. Unfortunately, there is significant overlap between the appearance of pyogenic infection and other disorders on MRI. For example, active spine infection (discitis-osteomyelitis) may look similar to age-related degeneration, while cerebral abscesses can have a similar appearance to intracranial tumors, especially glioblastoma multiforme (GBM) and metastases. Therefore, biopsy is often required for definitive diagnosis, which can be difficult depending on location and subject patients to significant risk. Avoiding these unnecessary biopsies is an important goal of imaging techniques with improved diagnostic accuracy. Several advanced MRI methods have been applied to pyogenic infection, both in patients and preclinical models. In patients, diffusion-weighted imaging (DWI) is essential in the workup of pyogenic infection involving

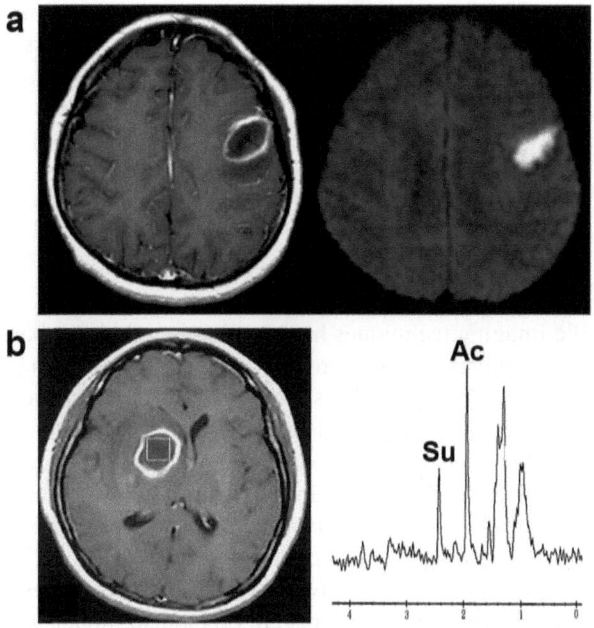

Figure 6.1 (**a**) MRI in a 44-year-old patient with suspected intracranial infection. The images show a left frontal rim-enhancing collection on post-gadolinium T_1-weighted imaging, with the diagnosis of pyogenic infection essentially confirmed by the bright signal on diffusion-weighted imaging. (**b**) MRS in a 43-year-old patient with surgically confirmed anaerobic pyogenic infection. T_1-weighted imaging shows the position of the volume element (voxel) from which a ^{1}H spectrum is generated. This spectrum (*right*) shows large acetate (Ac) and succinate (Su) resonances that are not typically observed in the normal human brain or other intracranial lesions. Adapted from Lai et al. [11]

the CNS. This technique used the variable movement of water molecules to generate contrast in MR images, with reduced diffusion characteristic of pyogenic infection. The reduced diffusion seen in pyogenic cerebral abscesses distinguishes them from tumors, an essential distinction in the neurosurgical approach to these lesions. Figure 6.1a shows the MRI of a 44-year-old patient with acute onset aphasia, with a DWI-positive brain lesion. Proton magnetic resonance spectroscopy (^{1}H-MRS) can also provide helpful information in suspected cerebral abscesses. This technique uses the variable ^{1}H chemical shifts of brain metabolites to identify their relative steady-state concentrations, in health and disease. In cerebral abscesses, several metabolites not found in the normal brain can be detected this way. Figure 6.1b shows an example of a patient with an enhancing cerebral lesion, whose workup included ^{1}H-MRS demonstrating both succinate and acetate resonances [11]. While ^{1}H-MRS can demonstrate differences in steady-state metabolite concentration, a recently developed technique hyperpolarized ^{13}C-MRS allows real-time analysis of in vivo metabolism. Since metabolic pathways used by mammals and prokaryotic cells are fundamentally different, this technology could also be leveraged to differentiate "them" from "us" using bacteria-specific metabolic signatures.

Hyperpolarized ^{13}C-MRS has been used in humans to show real-time metabolism of ^{13}C-enriched pyruvate in prostate cancer patients and is a promising new tool to diagnose acute pyogenic infections. MRI techniques such as chemical exchange saturation transfer (CEST) have also been utilized to image specifically bacteria in a mouse model [12].

6.3 Bacteria-Specific Imaging

Pathogen-specific imaging techniques have predominantly been based upon radiolabeling existing antibiotics or antimicrobial peptides (reviewed in [13, 14]). While antibiotics and antimicrobial peptides should in principle bind specifically to bacterial targets, they are designed to kill or disable bacteria at the lowest possible concentration and may not accumulate sufficiently for sensitive detection of living microorganisms. For example, ^{99m}Tc-ciprofloxacin was evaluated in patients for diagnosing infections [15], but subsequent detailed studies demonstrated nonspecific binding and an inability to differentiate infection from sterile inflammation [16, 17], presumably due to the relative few target binding sites per bacterium. Radiolabeled peptides have shown promise in preclinical models [18, 19], but lack specific binding or uptake mechanisms [20]. Immuno-PET imaging has also been evaluated [21], and although reported results are promising, antibodies have several pharmacokinetic challenges including slow clearance from nontarget sites. The metabolism-directed probes discussed here address some of these important limitations. Some of the promising imaging approaches are discussed below.

6.3.1 Metabolism-Based Tracers

There have been significant efforts to develop novel imaging tracers that will specifically target bacteria and aid in diagnosing bacterial infections and monitoring the efficacy of antibiotic treatments. Clinical microbiology has provided the means to differentiate microbes by selective metabolism [22], and a selection strategy based on this selective metabolism of small molecules by bacteria could be exploited to discover and develop novel bacteria-specific imaging tracers. By utilizing metabolic pathways selectively expressed by different classes of bacteria, and not by mammalian cells, novel imaging tracers could be developed not only to detect the presence of bacterial infection but also to identify the class of bacteria causing the infections [23]. This technology would allow for immediate and appropriate pathogen-directed antibacterial therapy. Easy penetration into diseased tissues and rapid clearance of small molecules, such as radiofluorinated sugars and sugar alcohols, combined with favorable radiation dosimetry due to short half-life isotopes (e.g., ^{18}F), are some of the favorable characteristics of this approach. Finally, clinically apparent (acute) infections have high pathogen burdens, e.g., 8.3 $\log_{10}$ CFU/ml of bacteria [24], with volumes of tens to hundreds of milliliters [25, 26]. Therefore, pathogen-specific imaging agents in development could indeed prove to be sensitive enough for the early detection of infection in patients.

6.3.1.1 Sugars

^{18}F-Fluorodeoxyglucose (^{18}F-FDG) is a fluorinated analog of glucose. Since its development in 1976, ^{18}F-FDG is the most widely available PET imaging tracer and is heavily employed in clinical oncology. Along with identifying rapidly growing malignant tumors, ^{18}F-FDG is presently the most used PET tracer for imaging bacterial infections by identifying infection-associated inflammatory responses. Immune cells increase the use of glucose as an energy source during metabolic bursts associated with inflammatory responses due to infection [27]. Even during chronic inflammation, increased cell glycolysis persists [28]. It is therefore not surprising that ^{18}F-FDG has potential to image infections with high sensitivity [27]. Currently, the Society of Nuclear Medicine and Molecular Imaging (SNMMI) and the European Association of Nuclear Medicine (EANM) guidelines recommend ^{18}F-FDG PET imaging in clinical cases of peripheral bone osteomyelitis, suspected spinal infection, and fever of unknown origin (FUO) [29] and suggest it can be used in other infection settings. ^{18}F-FDG PET has also been used to monitor tuberculosis (TB) patients [30], help distinguish between septic and aseptic loosening in joint prosthesis infection [31], and diagnose diabetic foot infections [32]. More information on the clinical applications of ^{18}F-FDG PET can be found in Chapter 2. However, since ^{18}F-FDG is metabolized by the same pathways as glucose, and given the widespread expression of glucose surface transporters in eukaryotic cells, ^{18}F-FDG is not specific enough to differentiate true infection from sterile inflammation. In an effort to facilitate specific uptake of ^{18}F-FDG by bacterial hexose phosphate transporters, Mills et al. developed the phosphate analog ^{18}F-FDG-6-P [33]. However, in vivo PET imaging with ^{18}F-FDG-6-P in a foreign body *Staphylococcus aureus* infection mouse model demonstrated that the biodistribution was similar to ^{18}F-FDG.

Sorbitol, a sugar alcohol, is a metabolic substrate for Enterobacteriaceae (*K. pneumoniae*, *E. coli*, *Yersinia* spp., *Enterobacter* spp., etc.) which represent the largest group of Gram-negative bacterial pathogens in humans. Similar to glucose, sorbitol is taken up by bacteria via surface transporters, phosphorylated and further metabolized by bacteria [34] (Figure 6.2). Mammalian cells do not have transporters for this sugar [35]. The radiolabeled sorbitol analog, ^{18}F-fluorodeoxysorbitol (^{18}F-FDS), was first synthesized from commercial ^{18}F-FDG by Li et al., using a 30-min reduction reaction [36]. In 2014, Weinstein and Ordonez et al. demonstrated that ^{18}F-FDS was rapidly taken up by Enterobacteriaceae [37]. In vitro uptake assays indicated that ^{18}F-FDS accumulated selectively in Enterobacteriaceae (~1000-fold higher than mammalian cells), but not in Gram-positive bacteria or mammalian/cancer cells. There was also significant uptake in drug-resistant clinical strains. Moreover, addition of excess unlabeled sorbitol blocked accumulation of

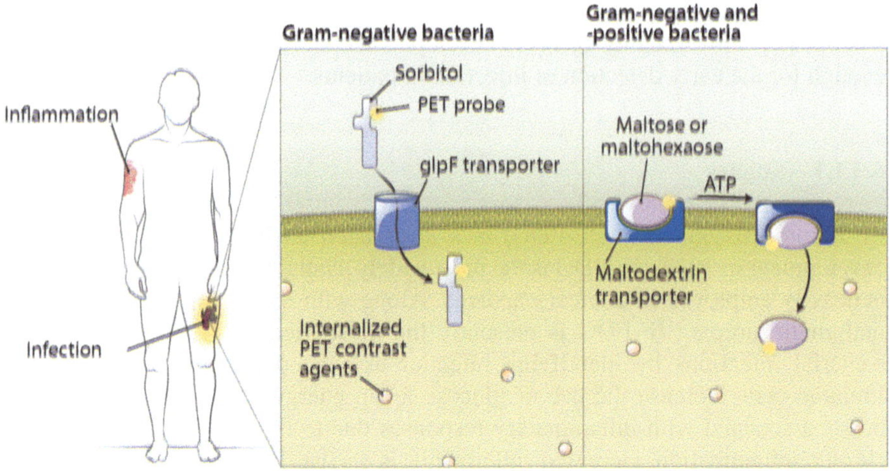

Figure 6.2 Metabolism-based tracers for bacterial infection imaging. ^{18}FFDS internalization through glpF. Other transporters may contribute to the uptake of sorbitol by bacteria as well. Mammalian cells do not take up sorbitol. Maltodextrin transporter–mediated uptake of ^{18}F-maltose and ^{18}F-maltohexaose. Neither glpF nor maltodextrin transporter is expressed by mammalian cells, thus the specificity in distinguishing bacterial infections from general inflammation. Adapted from Wang et al. [150]

bacteria-associated activity. In a murine myositis model, ^{18}F-FDS PET rapidly differentiated infection from sterile inflammation with a limit of detection of 6.2 ± 0.2 $\log_{10}$ colony forming units (CFU) for *Escherichia coli* (Figure 6.3). This is a promising threshold, since clinically relevant infections have much higher burdens of approximately 8 $\log_{10}$ CFU bacteria per mL [24]. These findings were extended to models of mixed Gram-positive and Gram-negative thigh coinfections, brain infection, *Klebsiella* spp. pneumonia, and mice undergoing immunosuppressive chemotherapy. Last, ^{18}F-FDS PET monitored the efficacy of antimicrobial treatment, demonstrating a signal proportional to the bacterial burden. Therapeutic failures associated with drug-resistant ESBL-producing *E. coli* infections were detected in real time (Figure 6.4). These data demonstrate that ^{18}F-FDS could be a candidate imaging tool to clinically detect infections due to Enterobacteriaceae. Recently, ^{18}F-FDS was determined to be safe and well tolerated after a single intravenous dose injected into healthy human volunteers to assess biodistribution and radiation dosimetry [38].

Maltose and maltodextrin are polysaccharides consisting of two or multiple glucose units, respectively. In *E. coli*, these sugars are incorporated with high specificity using the maltose-maltodextrin transport system [39]. Similar transporter systems are present in multiple Gram-negative and Gram-positive bacterial species, but not in mammalian cells (Figure 6.2). In 2011, Ning et al. reported maltodextrin-based optical imaging probes that could specifically detect *E. coli* myositis in mice with high specificity [40]. Subsequent work led to the development of ^{18}F-labeled

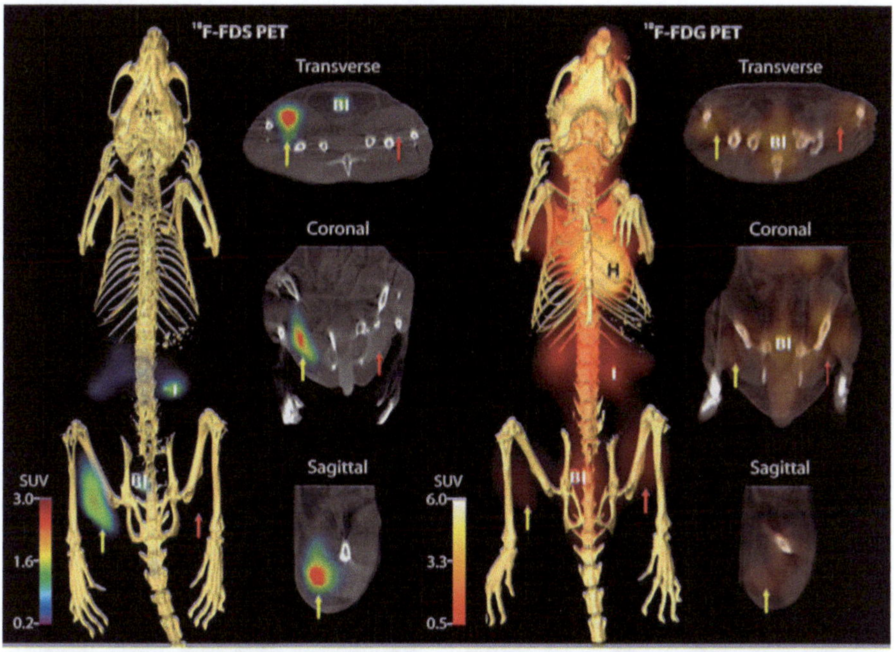

Figure 6.3 ^{18}F-FDS PET/CT imaging of *E. coli* myositis in immunocompetent mice. ^{18}F-FDS signal is noted in the infected (*yellow arrow*) but not in the inflamed (control) sterile thigh (*red arrow*). ^{18}F-FDG signal was noted in both infected and inflamed thighs. *H* heart, *I* intestine, *Bl* bladder. Adapted from Weinstein and Ordonez et al. [37]

maltohexaose (MH^{18}F) [41]. Using ^{19}F NMR spectroscopy, MH^{19}F was found to have high specificity for bacteria over mammalian cells, accumulating two times more in *E. coli* compared to hepatocytes. Using a rat *E. coli* myositis model, MH^{18}F PET was able to localize the infected tissue as early as 10-min postinjection, and 60 min later the signal in infected muscle was 8.5-fold higher compared to uninfected control muscle. Unlike ^{18}F-FDG, MH^{18}F was able to differentiate between live (infection) and dead (inflammation) bacteria in muscle (Figure 6.5). MH^{18}F was also used to effectively measure drug resistance and monitor the therapeutic effect of antibiotics in vivo. Therefore, MH^{18}F could be a useful PET imaging agent for a broad spectrum of Gram-positive and Gram-negative infections. A similar approach was adopted by Gowrishankar et al. in the development of 6-^{18}F-fluoromaltose [42]. 6-^{18}F-Fluoromaltose accumulated in in vitro cultures of *E. coli*, *P. aeruginosa*, and *L. monocytogenes* but not in mammalian cells. PET imaging with this compound was able to differentiate infected from inflamed muscle: however, there was high background signal, with slow elimination from the liver, kidneys, and brain, which the authors attribute to possible lack of complete trapping and increased efflux from bacteria.

Due to a key role in cell wall biosynthesis, trehalose is essential for mycobacterial growth and virulence [43]. Therefore, in an effort to develop mycobacteria-

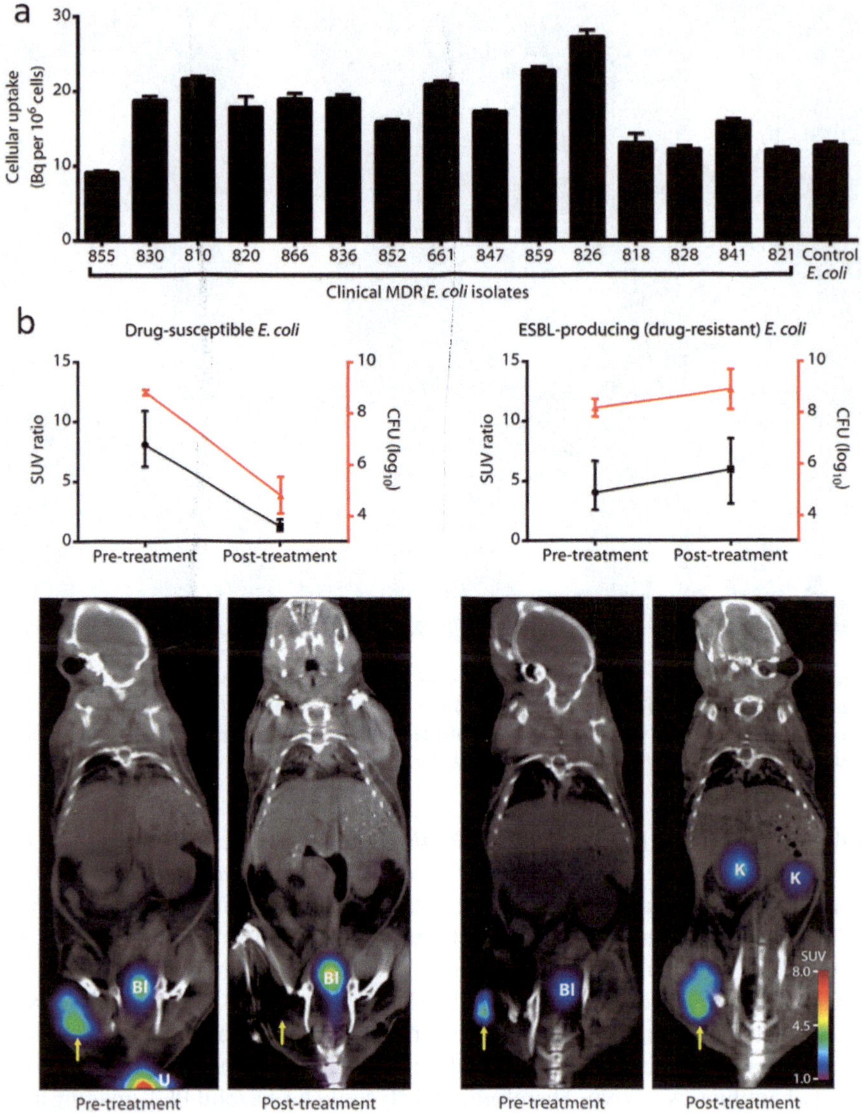

Figure 6.4 Monitoring the efficacy of antimicrobial treatment using ^{18}F-FDS PET. (**a**) ^{18}F-FDS demonstrates substantial uptake in 15 random extended-spectrum beta-lactamase (ESBL)-producing clinical strains of *E. coli*. (**b**) Mice were inoculated with drug-susceptible or drug-resistant (ESBL-producing) *E. coli* into the right thigh and a tenfold higher burden of the corresponding heat-killed *E. coli* strain into the left thigh. Imaging was performed before and after the administration of ceftriaxone, a commonly used antimicrobial effective against drug-susceptible *E. coli* but ineffective against ESBL-producers. Corresponding to the bacterial burden, ^{18}F-FDS PET signal disappears with treatment in mice infected with drug-susceptible *E. coli*, but not in mice infected with the drug-resistant *E. coli*. Thus, therapeutic failures associated with multidrug-resistant infections can be detected in real-time. *K* kidney, *Bl* bladder, *U* extravasated urine. Adapted from Weinstein and Ordonez et al. [37]

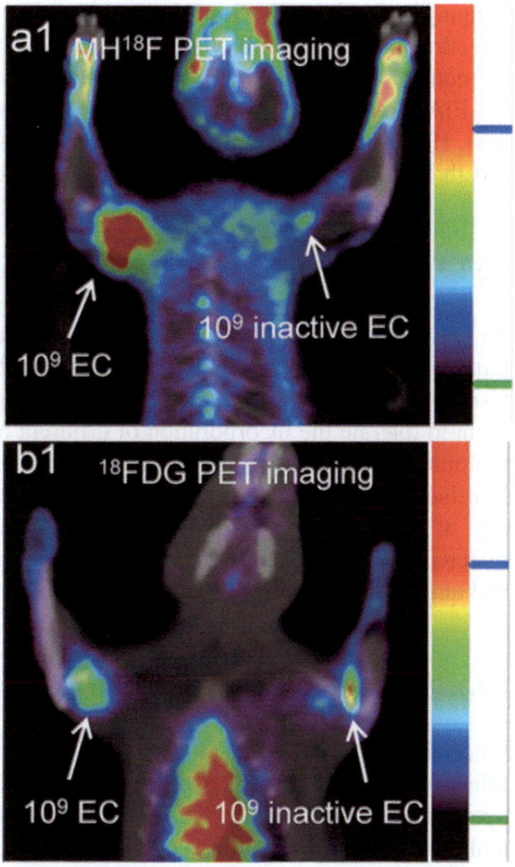

Figure 6.5 MH^{18}F PET/CT imaging of *E. coli* myositis. MH^{18}F can distinguish between live versus dead bacteria and can discriminate infections from inflammation. (**a**) MH^{18}F can distinguish between live versus dead bacteria in vivo. Rats were infected with 10^9 live and dead *E. coli* and imaged with MH^{18}F using a microPET/CT. The image of the rat is a representative result of four experiments and demonstrates that MH^{18}F does not accumulate in dead bacteria. (**b**) ^{18}F-FDG accumulates in tissues infected with both live and dead bacteria. Adapted from Ning et al. [41]

specific radiotracers, initial studies have shown uptake of trehalose analogs by *Mycobacterium tuberculosis* [44]. More recently, Rundell et al. reported that fluorinated trehalose analogs (^{19}F-FDTre) accumulate in *M. smegmatis* and also presented a viable synthesis of a ^{18}F-radiolabeled version [45].

6.3.1.2 Nucleoside Analogs

Some of the initial efforts to develop bacteria-specific agents were focused on imaging tumor-targeting bacteria to aid in the development of novel cancer treatments. These efforts led to the development of the thymidine analogue FIAU (1-(2′-deoxy-2′-fluoro-β-D-arabinofuranosyl)-5-iodouracil), which was found to be a substrate for the native thymidine kinases (TK) of herpes viruses and a wide variety of bacterial species. Once inside the bacterial cell, FIAU gets phosphorylated by TK and subsequently trapped. In 2004, Bettegowda et al. reported successful in vivo imaging of bacterial infections in a mouse model using ^{125}I-FIAU [46]. Using a lung infection murine model, Pullambhatla et al. also showed that the tracer can be used to monitor the efficacy of antimicrobial therapy [47]. Subsequent studies with ^{124}I-FIAU reported promising results in patients with musculoskeletal infections [48]. However, one recent study found that FIAU lacks specificity in patients with prosthetic joint infections, presumably due to host mitochondrial metabolism [49].

6.3.1.3 Amino Sugars

To build the cell wall, Gram-positive and Gram-negative bacteria incorporate a number of amino sugars into the peptidoglycan layer. By labeling the peptidoglycan "building blocks," bacteria can be directly imaged, and given that diverse bacteria seem to tolerate the incorporation of different nonnatural D-amino acids, there are multiple potential targets that could be radiolabeled [50]. Exploring this pathway, Martinez et al. reported the synthesis, preliminary characterization, and PET imaging of 2-deoxy-2-^{18}F-fluoroacetamido-D-glucopyranose (^{18}F-FAG) in *E. coli*-infected mice and rats [51]. ^{18}F-FAG PET was able to differentiate between infection and turpentine oil-induced inflammation.

6.3.1.4 Iron Metabolism

Since the early 1970s, ^{67}Ga-citrate SPECT has been extensively used to detect infection/inflammation [52]. Multiple pathways have been proposed for ^{67}Ga-citrate uptake in inflamed/infected tissues: increased vascular permeability [53], uptake by leukocytes [54], direct uptake by bacteria [55], and binding to plasma transferrin, lactoferrin, and/or bacterial siderophores [56, 57]. Despite the lack of specificity for bacterial infection, ^{67}Ga-citrate is still widely used around the world to identify sites of infection in patients with fever of unknown origin (FUO) [58]. ^{68}Ga-citrate was developed to improve the long waiting time required for imaging after a ^{67}Ga-citrate injection (usually 48–72 h). ^{68}Ga-citrate has been evaluated in animal models of osteomyelitis and myositis [59, 60], as well as in patients with tuberculosis, where ^{68}Ga-citrate accumulated in both pulmonary and extrapulmonary tuberculous lesions [61]. More information on clinical imaging with $^{67/68}$Ga-citrate can be found in Chapters 2 and 4. Based on the same principle of iron accumulation in infected tissues, Kumar et al. developed a ^{68}Ga-radiolabeled apo-transferrin complex (^{68}Ga-TF), which provided a 7.5 times higher signal in the PET images of *S. aureus* muscle infection in rats, compared to uninfected uninflamed muscle [62]. No signal from the infected sites was evident within the first 2-h postinjection in additional unconjugated ^{68}Ga-Cl_3 PET scans, suggesting some specificity of the transferrin-bound compound. However, these mechanisms are nonspecific and do not detect bacteria specifically, and there has been interest in the use of pathogen-specific radiolabeled siderophores [63], which could also be applied to specifically imaging bacteria.

6.3.1.5 Activity-Based Probes

Bacterial specificity and subsequent amplification of the signal have also been achieved by targeting key bacterial enzymes. For example, Kong et al. developed a near-infrared (NIR) fluorogenic substrates for β-lactamase, an enzyme expressed by tubercle bacilli, but not by their eukaryotic hosts. This allowed real-time imaging of pulmonary infections and rapid quantification of bacteria in living animals [64]. Similarly, Lentz et al. optimized reporter substrates and activity-based probes for *M. tuberculosis* Hip1 serine protease. Hip1 is a cell-envelope-associated enzyme with minimal homology to host proteases and therefore an excellent target for probe development [65]. However, both these probes are based on optical imaging and therefore not yet clinically translatable.

6.3.2 *Antibiotics*

Antibiotics are natural or synthetic compounds designed to kill (bactericidal) or impair the growth (bacteriostatic) of bacterial pathogens. Radiolabeled antibiotics can localize specifically to the site of an infection and exhibit dual potential in infectious disease: antibiotics offer a targeted imaging approach to diagnose infection in the clinic as well as noninvasive techniques for studying pharmacokinetics and pharmacodynamics in vivo (see Chapters 9 and 10). ^{99m}Tc is the predominant radionuclide used to label antibiotics as the tracer preparation is easily accomplished using a cold kit format within 30 min [66] (also see Chapter 4). Ideally, the radiolabeled antibiotic will bind to their bacterial targets with high specificity. However, excess unlabeled antibiotic may compete with the radiolabeled antibiotic or kill the pathogen, both of which will impair the imaging efficacy of the tracer. Table 6.1 provides a list of radiolabeled antibiotics evaluated in animal models.

6.3.2.1 Fluoroquinolones

The broad-spectrum bactericidal fluoroquinolone ciprofloxacin was initially labeled with ^{99m}Tc and evaluated in preclinical infection models with promising results [67]. Commercially known as Infecton, ^{99m}Tc-ciprofloxacin imaging was used in large clinical trials that reported high sensitivity and specificity in the diagnosis of bacterial infections [68, 69]. Subsequent preclinical and clinical trials with ^{99m}Tc-ciprofloxacin or ^{18}F-ciprofloxacin demonstrated variable specificity and an inability to reliably differentiate infection from sterile inflammatory processes [16, 70–72]. Development of this tracer proved controversial due to low specificity attributed to nonspecific binding to dead bacteria [73], as well as nonspecific binding of host neutrophil DNA [20]. After an unsuccessful phase II trial in which ^{99m}Tc-ciprofloxacin failed to differentiate sterile inflammation from infection [74], commercial development was suspended. Nevertheless, ^{99m}Tc-ciprofloxacin has

Table 6.1 Evaluation of radiolabeled antibiotics in animal models

Radiopharmaceutical	Animal model	Max target/nontarget ratio					Reference
		Bacterial strain	Background (nontarget)	Target/nontarget	Control experiment	Target/nontarget (control)	
^{99m}Tc-Clinafloxacin	Mouse	MRSA	Muscle	6.0	Turpentine oil	4.3	[106]
^{99m}Tc-Difloxacin	Rat	*S. aureus*	Muscle	5.5	Turpentine oil/ heat-killed bacteria	5/5.2	[107]
^{99m}Tc-Enrofloxacin	Rat	*S. aureus*	Muscle	4.8	Turpentine oil/ heat-killed bacteria	3.85/3.8	[108]
	Rabbit	*S. typhi*	Muscle	4.8	Normal	n.a.	[109]
^{99m}Tc-Gatifloxacin	Rat	*E. coli*	Muscle	4.5	Turpentine oil/ heat-killed bacteria	4.1/4.4	[110]
^{99m}Tc-Gemifloxacin	Rabbit	*S. typhi*, *P. aeruginosa*, *K. pneumoniae*	Muscle	8/8.8/16	Normal	n.a.	[111]
	Rat	*S. pneumoniae*	Muscle	4.88	Heat-killed bacteria	1.4	[112]
^{99m}Tc-Levofloxacin	Rabbit	*E.coli*, *P. aeruginosa*	Muscle	1.3/8.09	Normal	n.a.	[113]
^{99m}Tc-Lomefloxacin	Rat	*S. aureus*	Muscle	6.5	n.a.	n.a.	[114]
^{99m}Tc-Moxifloxacin	Rat, rabbit	*E. coli*	Muscle	1.62	n.a.	n.a.	[115]
^{99m}Tc-*N*-Norfloxacin dithiocarbamate	Mouse	*S. aureus*	Muscle	3.46	Turpentine oil	1.23	[116]
^{99m}Tc-Norfloxacin	Rat	*S. aureus*	Muscle	6.9	Turpentine oil/ heat-killed bacteria	4.5/6	[117]
	Rat	*S. aureus*	Muscle	2.87	Turpentine oil	1	[118]
^{99m}Tc-Ofloxacin	Mouse	*S. aureus*	Muscle	2.02	n.a.	n.a.	[119]
	Rat	*S. aureus*	Muscle	4.3	n.a.	n.a.	[114]

^{99m}Tc-Pefloxacin	Mouse	*E. coli*	Muscle	5.6	Turpentine oil	0.75	[120]
	Rat	*S. aureus*	Muscle	5	Turpentine oil/ heat-killed bacteria	5.2/2.6	[107]
^{99m}Tc-Rufloxacin	Mouse	*E. coli*	Muscle	8.5	Turpentine oil/ heat-killed bacteria	3/4.5	[121]
^{99m}Tc-Sarafloxacin	Mouse	*S. aureus*	Muscle	4.2	Turpentine oil/ heat-killed bacteria	3.4/3.3	[122]
^{99m}Tc-Sitafloxacin	Rat	*S. aureus*	Muscle	23.13	Turpentine oil	1.13	[123]
^{99m}Tc-*N*-Sitafloxacin dithiocarbamate	Rat	*S. aureus*	Muscle	7.6	Heat-killed bacteria	1	[124]
^{99m}Tc-Sparafloxacin	Rat	*S. aureus*	Muscle	5.9	None	n.a.	[125]
^{99m}Tc-Cefazolin	Mouse	*S. aureus*	Muscle	8.57	Turpentine oil	1.4	[126]
^{99m}Tc-Cefepime	Rat	*E. coli*	Muscle	8.4	Turpentine oil/ heat-killed bacteria	3.31/4.13	[127]
^{99m}Tc-Cefoperazone	Rat	*S. aureus*	Muscle	4.66	n.a.	n.a.	[128]
^{99m}Tc-Cefotaxime	Mouse	*S. aureus*	Muscle	2.89	Normal	n.a.	[129]
^{99m}Tc-Cefotaxime sodium	Rat	*E. coli*	Muscle	3.77	Turpentine oil	3.3	[130]
^{99m}Tc-Ceftazimide	Mouse	*S. aureus*	Muscle	1.4	n.a.	n.a.	[131]
^{99m}Tc-Ceftizoxime	Rat	*E. coli*	Muscle	3.24	Zymosan	1.65	[132]
	Rat	n.a.	n.a.	n.a.	Bone wax	n.a.	[133]
	Rat	*S. aureus*	n.a.	n.a.	Sterile implant	n.a.	[134]
^{99m}Tc-Ceftriaxone	Mouse	*E. coli*	Muscle	5.6	Turpentine oil/ heat-killed bacteria	1.49	[77]
	Rabbit	*S. aureus*	Right forearm	4.5	Turpentine oil	1.4	[80]
	Mouse	*S. aureus*	Muscle	3.39	Turpentine oil/ heat-killed bacteria	3.12/2.48	[78]
	Rat	*E. coli, S. aureus*	Muscle	12.6/2.36	Turpentine oil	1.4	[79]

(continued)

Table 6.1 (continued)

Radiopharmaceutical	Animal model	Max target/nontarget ratio					Reference
		Bacterial strain	Background (nontarget)	Target/nontarget	Control experiment	Target/nontarget (control)	
^{99m}Tc-Cefuroxime	Rat	*E. coli*	Muscle	1.8	Normal	n.a.	[135]
^{99m}Tc-Cefuroxime acetil	Rat	*S. aureus*	Muscle	2.5	Turpentine oil	1.2	[136]
^{99m}Tc-Nitrofurantoin	Rat	*E. coli*	Muscle	4.83	Turpentine oil/ normal	1	[137]
^{99m}Tc-Rifampicin	Rat	MRSA	Muscle	7.34	Turpentine oil	1.2	[138]
^{99m}Tc-*N*-Sulfanilamide	Mouse	*E. coli*	Muscle	2.9	Heat-killed bacteria	1.4	[139]
^{99m}Tc-Alafosfalin	Rat	*S. aureus*	Muscle	4.32	99mTc-DTPA/99mTc-WBC	1.93/20.09	[140]
^{99m}Tc-Amoxicillin	Rabbit	*S. pneumoniae*	Muscle	4.6	n.a.	–	[141]
^{99m}Tc-Vancomycin	Rat	*S. aureus*	Muscle	5.1	Turpentine oil	1.2	[142]
^{99m}Tc-Azithromycin	Mouse	*S. aureus*	Muscle	6.2	Turpentine oil/ heat-killed bacteria	2.60/3.13	[143]
^{99m}Tc-Clarithromycin	Mouse	*S. aureus*	Muscle	7.33	Turpentine oil/ heat-killed bacteria	3.1/3.26	[144]
^{99m}Tc-Clindamycin	Rat	*S. aureus*	Muscle	3.1	Turpentine oil/ heat-killed bacteria	2.47/1.6	[145]
^{99m}Tc-Doxycycline hyclate	Rat	*E. coli*	Muscle	2.24	n.a.	n.a.	[146]
^{99m}Tc-Erythromycin	Mouse	*S. aureus*	Muscle	5	Turpentine oil	4.8	[147]
^{99m}Tc-Kanamycin	Rat	*S. aureus*	Muscle	2.5	n.a.	–	[148]
^{99m}Tc-Vibramycin	Rat	*S. aureus*	Muscle	2.64	Turpentine oil/ heat-killed bacteria	1.80/2.15	[149]

Adapted from Auletta et al. [82]
n.a., data was not available
MRSA, methicillin-resistant *S. aureus*

continued to be used by some investigators for the diagnosis of infections [75, 76]. Multiple additional fluoroquinolones have been radiolabeled and preliminary studies have demonstrated inconsistent results (Table 6.1). Although some might seem promising for bacteria-specific imaging, in order to avoid past mistakes, extensive preclinical evaluation for the uptake mechanisms should be performed before further development.

6.3.2.2 Cephalosporins

Initial experiments with ^{99m}Tc-ceftriaxone in animal models (mice, rats, and rabbits) suggested higher accumulation in infected versus inflamed tissues [77–79]. In 2012, Kaul et al. reported SPECT imaging with ^{99m}Tc-ceftriaxone in 36 patients with clinical and radiological suspicion of an orthopedic infection. They reported a sensitivity and specificity of 85.2% and 77.8%, respectively, for the diagnosis of infection [80]. The high protein binding of ^{99m}Tc-ceftriaxone (>90%) led to delayed elimination and a high background.

6.3.2.3 Glycopeptides

Fluorescently labeled vancomycin (vanco-800CW) has been used to specifically target and detect infections caused by Gram-positive bacteria. Vanco-800CW could discriminate bacterial infections from sterile inflammation in a murine myositis model and detect biomaterial-associated infections in ex vivo analyses of human cadaver tissues [81]. However, this probe is based on optical imaging and therefore not yet clinically translatable.

Several other radiolabeled antibiotics with different mechanisms of action have been evaluated, but using different models and end points, making comparison among them difficult. The variability between animal models (mice, rats, or rabbits), injected activities, and image acquisition times are significant, and, most importantly, the number of bacteria used for inducing the infection ranges from 5 to 10 $\log_{10}$ colony forming units (CFU) [82]. Moreover, given the rapid growth of bacteria in tissues (generation time ~20 min for most pyogenic bacteria), information on the bacterial burden at the time of imaging/radioactivity quantification rather than at the time of injection will be the critical determinant of sensitivity.

6.3.3 Antibodies

Multiple radiolabeled antibodies (e.g., ^{99m}Tc-besilesomab, ^{111}In-IgG) and antibody fragments (e.g., ^{99m}Tc-sulesomab) have been developed and evaluated with promising results [66, 83]. While most of these compounds target the inflammation associated with infection, antibodies specifically targeting bacteria have also been reported. Due to the difficulties in diagnosis and high risk of mortality, bacterial endocarditis was one of the initial targets in the development of bacteria-specific antibody imaging [84]. Early research with a ^{99m}Tc-labeled anti-*S. aureus* antibody showed encouraging results in the rabbit endocarditis model [85]. In 2014, Pinkston et al. reported a monoclonal antibody (MAb 69) against the major component of *Enterococcus faecalis* pili, EbpC [86]. After radiolabeling, ^{64}Cu-DOTA-MAb 69 PET imaging successfully identified enterococcal infection in a rat endocarditis model. Targeting a different pathogen, Rubin et al. reported a ^{125}I-labeled anti-*Pseudomonas aeruginosa*-specific monoclonal antibody that was able to discriminate between *P. aeruginosa* and *S. aureus* infection sites in a rat model [87]. Recently, Wiehr et al. developed a ^{64}Cu-labeled polyclonal antibody targeting YadA, an outer membrane protein, essential for in vivo virulence of *Yersinia enterocolitica* [88]. PET imaging with ^{64}Cu-NODAGA-YadA allowed the detection of bacteria in the spleen. A clear identification of the pathogen in the liver tissue was not possible due to the nonspecific uptake of the radiolabeled antibody and free-copper accumulation. A similar approach has been used to detect *M. tuberculosis*. Given the similarities between *M. tuberculosis* and *Mycobacterium bovis* (Bacillus Calmette–Guérin, BCG), Malpani et al. developed a ^{131}I-labeled anti-BCG antibody. Localization of ^{131}I-anti BCG was observed at the site of TB lesions in a rabbit model, but significant concentration of ^{131}I-anti BCG also noted in background and major organs like the heart, liver, spleen, and kidneys [89]. Subsequently, Lee et al. reported the use of a ^{131}I-labeled antibody against BCG [90]. They demonstrated that the BCG-specific antibody $F(ab')_2$ accumulated in TB lesions of rabbits (induced with by the inoculation of heat-killed, sonicated *M. tuberculosis* in muscle) while washing away from syphilitic lesions. However, there are suggestions that the results could be attributed to nonspecific iodine uptake in the inflammation site [91].

6.3.4 Other Agents

Antimicrobial peptides have been evaluated extensively and reviewed in [13, 14]. Additional information can also found in Chapters 2 and 4. Unlike healthy mammalian cells, bacterial membranes contain negatively charged phospholipids which can bind to bis(zinc(II)-dipicolylamine) (Zn-DPA). This property has been extensively used to develop bacteria-specific imaging agents. Initial experiments with fluorescent Zn-DPA showed that it only accumulated in vitro in Gram-positive and Gram-negative bacteria, and optical imaging was used to monitor in vivo imaging of infection mouse models [92, 93]. Subsequently, Liu et al. developed ^{111}In-DOTA-biotin and Zn-DPA-biotin, non-covalently linked by streptavidin (SA) to form the complex ^{111}In-DOTA-biotin-SA-Zn-DPA-biotin [94]. Using mice infected intramuscularly with *S. pyogenes* (infection) or LPS (inflammation control), SPECT imaging of the ^{111}In-labeled Zn-DPA complex was 2.8-fold higher in the infected animals compared to inflamed controls. Using a different chelator, Rice et al. used

^{111}In-DTPA-Zn-DPA SPECT to successfully identify the *S. pyogenes* infection in a mouse model [95]. The structure of the membrane of mammalian cells is a bilayer composed of different lipids and proteins. The neutral electrostatic charge of the exterior surface is maintained by an ATP-dependent translocase that catalyzes the transport of phospholipids to the internal membrane surface. However, during the process of programmed cell death or apoptosis in mammalian cells, the translocase activity is attenuated leading to increased negative charge on the cell exterior [96]. Therefore, despite the promising results for bacterial imaging, Zn-DPA was found to also bind to necrotic and apoptotic tissues reducing its specificity for bacteria. ^{99m}Tc and ^{18}F-labeled analogs of Zn-DPA have been reported to successfully evaluate death and cardiomyocyte apoptosis following acute myocardial infarction [97–99].

Biotin, also known as vitamin B7, is a precursor of acetyl CoA carboxylase in bacteria and eukaryotic cells [100]. ^{111}In-labeled biotin, alone or combined with streptavidin, has been reported for bacterial SPECT imaging in patients and animal models [101–103], with promising results in the diagnosis of vertebral osteomyelitis. Biotin analogs have also been radiolabeled with ^{18}F and successfully evaluated in *E. coli*-infected rats [104]. Recently, Baldoni et al. reported an analog of cyanocobalamin (vitamin B12) labeled with ^{99m}Tc, ^{99m}Tc-PAMA(4)-Cbl [105]. This tracer had a time-dependent accumulation in vitro in *S. aureus* and *E. coli*, and ex vivo tissue biodistribution showed higher concentration of tracer in the infected implants.

6.4 Summary

Bacterial infections are a major threat to human health in the USA and globally. The modern patient is increasingly susceptible to severe infections due to the use of invasive implants, cancer therapies, and the rapid emergence of multidrug-resistant bacteria. Overuse and misuse of antimicrobials are costing billions of dollars to the US health system with similar patterns in other developed and developing countries. Molecular imaging is a promising tool for the early diagnosis, and targeted pharmaceutical intervention of bacterial infection, which could significantly improve patient care and reduce costs worldwide.

References

1. Keen, E.F., III, et al., *Changes in the incidences of multidrug-resistant and extensively drug-resistant organisms isolated in a military medical center.* Infect.Control Hosp.Epidemiol., 2010. **31**(7): p. 728-732.
2. McKenna, M., *Antibiotic resistance: the last resort.* Nature, 2013. **499**(7459): p. 394-6.
3. Nordmann, P., L. Dortet, and L. Poirel, *Carbapenem resistance in Enterobacteriaceae: here is the storm!* Trends Mol Med, 2012. **18**(5): p. 263-72.

4. Melzer, M. and I. Petersen, *Mortality following bacteraemic infection caused by extended spectrum beta-lactamase (ESBL) producing E. coli compared to non-ESBL producing E. coli.* J Infect, 2007. **55**(3): p. 254-9.
5. Salazar-Austin, N., et al., *Extensively drug-resistant tuberculosis in a young child after travel to India.* Lancet Infect Dis, 2015. **15**(12): p. 1485-91.
6. Velayati, A.A., et al., *Emergence of new forms of totally drug-resistant tuberculosis bacilli: super extensively drug-resistant tuberculosis or totally drug-resistant strains in Iran.* Chest, 2009. **136**(2): p. 420-5.
7. McCaughey, B. *Unnecessary Deaths: The Human and Financial Costs of Hospital Infections.* 2nd Edition November 13, 2016]; Available from: http://emerald.tufts.edu/med/apua/consumers/faqs_2_4154863510.pdf.
8. Falagas, M.E., et al., *Antibiotic treatment of infections due to carbapenem-resistant Enterobacteriaceae: systematic evaluation of the available evidence.* Antimicrob Agents Chemother, 2014. **58**(2): p. 654-63.
9. Donnenberg, M.S., *Enterobacteriaceae*, in *Mandell, Douglas, and Bennett's principles and practice of infectious diseases.*, J.E.B. Gerald L. Mandell, and Raphael Dolin, Editor. 2010, Elsevier Inc: Philadelphia, PA. p. 2815-2833.
10. Zackrisson, S., S.M. van de Ven, and S.S. Gambhir, *Light in and sound out: emerging translational strategies for photoacoustic imaging.* Cancer Res, 2014. **74**(4): p. 979-1004.
11. Lai, P.H., et al., *Pyogenic brain abscess: findings from in vivo 1.5-T and 11.7-T in vitro proton MR spectroscopy.* AJNR Am J Neuroradiol, 2005. **26**(2): p. 279-88.
12. Liu, G., et al., *Noninvasive imaging of infection after treatment with tumor-homing bacteria using Chemical Exchange Saturation Transfer (CEST) MRI.* Magn Reson Med, 2013. **70**(6): p. 1690-8.
13. Gemmel, F., N. Dumarey, and M. Welling, *Future diagnostic agents.* Semin Nucl Med, 2009. **39**(1): p. 11-26.
14. van Oosten, M., et al., *Targeted imaging of bacterial infections: advances, hurdles and hopes.* FEMS Microbiol Rev, 2015. **39**(6): p. 892-916.
15. Vinjamuri, S., et al., *Comparison of 99mTc infecton imaging with radiolabelled white-cell imaging in the evaluation of bacterial infection.* Lancet, 1996. **347**(8996): p. 233-5.
16. Sarda, L., et al., *Inability of 99mTc-ciprofloxacin scintigraphy to discriminate between septic and sterile osteoarticular diseases.* J Nucl Med, 2003. **44**(6): p. 920-6.
17. Palestro, C., et al., *Phase II study of 99mTc-ciprofloxacin uptake in patients with high suspicion of osteomyelitis.* J Nucl Med, 2006. **47**(suppl 1): p. 152P.
18. Ebenhan, T., et al., *Preclinical evaluation of 68Ga-labeled 1,4,7-triazacyclononane-1,4,7-triacetic acid-ubiquicidin as a radioligand for PET infection imaging.* J Nucl Med, 2014. **55**(2): p. 308-14.
19. Vilche, M., et al., *68Ga-NOTA-UBI-29-41 as a PET Tracer for Detection of Bacterial Infection.* J Nucl Med, 2016. **57**(4): p. 622-7.
20. Welling, M., et al., *The many roads to infection imaging.* Eur J Nucl Med Mol Imaging, 2008. **35**(4): p. 848-9.
21. Wiehr, S., et al., *New pathogen-specific immunoPET/MR tracer for molecular imaging of a systemic bacterial infection.* Oncotarget, 2016. **7**(10): p. 10990-1001.
22. Mac Faddin, J.F., *Biochemical tests for identification of medical bacteria.* 1976, Baltimore, MD: The Williams & Wilkins Company. 312.
23. Ordonez, A.A., et al., *A Systematic Approach for Developing Bacteria-Specific Imaging Tracers.* J Nucl Med, 2017. **58**(1): p. 144-150.
24. Konig, C., H.P. Simmen, and J. Blaser, *Bacterial concentrations in pus and infected peritoneal fluid--implications for bactericidal activity of antibiotics.* J Antimicrob Chemother, 1998. **42**(2): p. 227-32.
25. Jang, K., et al., *Treatment of prostatic abscess: case collection and comparison of treatment methods.* Korean J Urol, 2012. **53**(12): p. 860-4.

26. Yamamoto, M., et al., *Treatment of bacterial brain abscess by repeated aspiration--follow up by serial computed tomography.* Neurol Med Chir (Tokyo), 2000. **40**(2): p. 98-104.; discussion 104-5.
27. Vaidyanathan, S., et al., *FDG PET/CT in infection and inflammation--current and emerging clinical applications.* Clin Radiol, 2015. **70**(7): p. 787-800.
28. Marjanovic, S., et al., *Expression of glycolytic isoenzymes in activated human peripheral lymphocytes: cell cycle analysis using flow cytometry.* Exp Cell Res, 1991. **193**(2): p. 425-31.
29. Jamar, F., et al., *EANM/SNMMI guideline for 18F-FDG use in inflammation and infection.* J Nucl Med, 2013. **54**(4): p. 647-58.
30. Chen, R.Y., et al., *PET/CT imaging correlates with treatment outcome in patients with multidrug-resistant tuberculosis.* Sci Transl Med, 2014. **6**(265): p. 265ra166.
31. Love, C., S.E. Marwin, and C.J. Palestro, *Nuclear medicine and the infected joint replacement.* Semin Nucl Med, 2009. **39**(1): p. 66-78.
32. Treglia, G., et al., *Diagnostic performance of Fluorine-18-Fluorodeoxyglucose positron emission tomography for the diagnosis of osteomyelitis related to diabetic foot: a systematic review and a meta-analysis.* The Foot, 2013. **23**(4): p. 140-148.
33. Mills, B., et al., *[(18)F]FDG-6-P as a novel in vivo tool for imaging staphylococcal infections.* EJNMMI Res, 2015. **5**: p. 13.
34. Lengeler, J., *Nature and properties of hexitol transport systems in Escherichia coli.* J Bacteriol, 1975. **124**(1): p. 39-47.
35. Scott, M.E. and R.E. Viola, *The use of fluoro-and deoxy-substrate analogs to examine binding specificity and catalysis in the enzymes of the sorbitol pathway.* Carbohydrate research, 1998. **313**(3): p. 247-253.
36. Li, Z.-B., et al., *The Synthesis of 18F-FDS and Its Potential Application in Molecular Imaging.* Molecular Imaging and Biology, 2008. **10**: p. 92-98.
37. Weinstein, E.A., et al., *Imaging Enterobacteriaceae infection in vivo with 18F-fluorodeoxysorbitol positron emission tomography.* Science translational medicine, 2014. **6**(259): p. 259ra146-259ra146.
38. Zhu, W., et al., *Biodistribution and Radiation Dosimetry of the Enterobacteriaceae-Specific Imaging Probe [18F]Fluorodeoxysorbitol Determined by PET/CT in Healthy Human Volunteers.* Molecular Imaging and Biology, 2016. **18**(5): p. 782-787.
39. Shuman, H.A. and N.A. Treptow, *The Maltose-Maltodextrin-Transport System of Escherichia coli K-12*, in *The Enzymes of Biological Membranes*, A. Martonosi, Editor. 2012, Springer Science & Business Media. p. 561-572.
40. Ning, X., et al., *Maltodextrin-based imaging probes detect bacteria in vivo with high sensitivity and specificity.* Nat Mater, 2011. **10**(8): p. 602-607.
41. Ning, X., et al., *PET Imaging of Bacterial Infections with Fluorine-18-Labeled Maltohexaose.* Angewandte Chemie International Edition, 2014. **53**(51): p. 14096-14101.
42. Gowrishankar, G., et al., *Investigation of 6-[18F]-Fluoromaltose as a Novel PET Tracer for Imaging Bacterial Infection.* PLOS ONE, 2014. **9**(9): p. e107951.
43. Tournu, H., A. Fiori, and P. Van Dijck, *Relevance of Trehalose in Pathogenicity: Some General Rules, Yet Many Exceptions.* PLOS Pathogens, 2013. **9**(8): p. e1003447.
44. Backus, K.M., et al., *Uptake of unnatural trehalose analogs as a reporter for Mycobacterium tuberculosis.* Nat Chem Biol, 2011. **7**(4): p. 228-35.
45. Rundell, S.R., et al., *Deoxyfluoro-d-trehalose (FDTre) analogues as potential PET probes for imaging mycobacterial infection.* Org Biomol Chem, 2016. **14**(36): p. 8598-609.
46. Bettegowda, C., et al., *Imaging bacterial infections with radiolabeled 1-(2'-deoxy-2'-fluoro-beta-D-arabinofuranosyl)-5-iodouracil.* Proc Natl Acad Sci U S A, 2005. **102**(4): p. 1145-50.
47. Pullambhatla, M., et al., *[(125)I]FIAU imaging in a preclinical model of lung infection: quantification of bacterial load.* Am J Nucl Med Mol Imaging, 2012. **2**(3): p. 260-70.

48. Diaz, L.A., Jr., et al., *Imaging of musculoskeletal bacterial infections by [124I]FIAU-PET/CT.* PLoS One, 2007. **2**(10): p. e1007.
49. Zhang, X.M., et al., *[124I]FIAU: Human dosimetry and infection imaging in patients with suspected prosthetic joint infection.* Nuclear Medicine and Biology, 2016. **43**(5): p. 273-279.
50. Kuru, E., et al., *In Situ probing of newly synthesized peptidoglycan in live bacteria with fluorescent D-amino acids.* Angew Chem Int Ed Engl, 2012. **51**(50): p. 12519-23.
51. Martínez, M.E., et al., *New radiosynthesis of 2-deoxy-2-[18F]fluoroacetamido-d-glucopyranose and its evaluation as a bacterial infections imaging agent.* Nuclear Medicine and Biology, 2011. **38**(6): p. 807-817.
52. Littenberg, R.L., et al., *Gallium-67 for localization of septic lesions.* Ann Intern Med, 1973. **79**(3): p. 403-6.
53. Tzen, K.Y., et al., *Role of iron-binding proteins and enhanced capillary permeability on the accumulation of gallium-67.* J Nucl Med, 1980. **21**(1): p. 31-5.
54. Weiner, R., P.B. Hoffer, and M.L. Thakur, *Lactoferrin: its role as a Ga-67-binding protein in polymorphonuclear leukocytes.* J Nucl Med, 1981. **22**(1): p. 32-7.
55. Menon, S., H.N. Wagner, Jr., and M.F. Tsan, *Studies on gallium accumulation in inflammatory lesions: II. Uptake by Staphylococcus aureus: concise communication.* J Nucl Med, 1978. **19**(1): p. 44-7.
56. Kumar, V. and D.K. Boddeti, *68Ga-Radiopharmaceuticals for PET Imaging of Infection and Inflammation*, in *Theranostics, Gallium-68, and Other Radionuclides: A Pathway to Personalized Diagnosis and Treatment*, R.P. Baum and F. Rösch, Editors. 2013, Springer Berlin Heidelberg: Berlin, Heidelberg. p. 189-219.
57. Tsan, M.F., *Mechanism of gallium-67 accumulation in inflammatory lesions.* J Nucl Med, 1985. **26**(1): p. 88-92.
58. Palestro, C.J., *The current role of gallium imaging in infection.* Semin Nucl Med, 1994. **24**(2): p. 128-41.
59. Makinen, T.J., et al., *Comparison of 18F-FDG and 68Ga PET imaging in the assessment of experimental osteomyelitis due to Staphylococcus aureus.* Eur J Nucl Med Mol Imaging, 2005. **32**(11): p. 1259-68.
60. Kumar, V., et al., *(68)Ga-Citrate-PET for diagnostic imaging of infection in rats and for intra-abdominal infection in a patient.* Curr Radiopharm, 2012. **5**(1): p. 71-5.
61. Vorster, M., et al., *68Ga-citrate PET/CT in Tuberculosis: A pilot study.* The quarterly journal of nuclear medicine and molecular imaging: official publication of the Italian Association of Nuclear Medicine (AIMN)[and] the International Association of Radiopharmacology (IAR), [and] Section of the Society of 2014.
62. Kumar, V., et al., *Potential use of 68Ga-apo-transferrin as a PET imaging agent for detecting Staphylococcus aureus infection.* Nuclear Medicine and Biology, 2011. **38**(3): p. 393-398.
63. Petrik, M., et al., *68Ga-siderophores for PET imaging of invasive pulmonary aspergillosis: proof of principle.* J Nucl Med, 2010. **51**(4): p. 639-45.
64. Kong, Y., et al., *Imaging tuberculosis with endogenous beta-lactamase reporter enzyme fluorescence in live mice.* Proc Natl Acad Sci U S A, 2010. **107**(27): p. 12239-44.
65. Lentz, C.S., et al., *Design of Selective Substrates and Activity-Based Probes for Hydrolase Important for Pathogenesis 1 (HIP1) from Mycobacterium tuberculosis.* ACS Infect Dis, 2016. **2**(11): p. 807-815.
66. Tsopelas, C., *Radiotracers used for the scintigraphic detection of infection and inflammation.* ScientificWorldJournal, 2015. **2015**: p. 676719.
67. Solanki, K., et al., *Tc-99m Infecton: a new class of radiopharmaceutical for imaging infection.* Journal of Nuclear Medicine, 1993. **34**(5): p. P119-P119.
68. Britton, K.E., et al., *Clinical evaluation of technetium-99m infecton for the localisation of bacterial infection.* European Journal of Nuclear Medicine, 1997. **24**(5): p. 553-556.
69. Britton, K.E., et al., *Imaging bacterial infection with 99mTc-ciprofloxacin (Infecton).* Journal of Clinical Pathology, 2002. **55**(11): p. 817-823.

70. Sarda, L., et al., *Evaluation of (99m)Tc-ciprofloxacin scintigraphy in a rabbit model of Staphylococcus aureus prosthetic joint infection.* J Nucl Med, 2002. **43**(2): p. 239-45.
71. Dumarey, N. and A. Schoutens, *Renal abscess: filling in with Tc-99m ciprofloxacin of defects seen on Tc-99m DMSA SPECT.* Clin Nucl Med, 2003. **28**(1): p. 68-9.
72. Langer, O., et al., *In vitro and in vivo evaluation of [18F]ciprofloxacin for the imaging of bacterial infections with PET.* Eur J Nucl Med Mol Imaging, 2005. **32**(2): p. 143-50.
73. Alexander, K., et al., *Binding of ciprofloxacin labelled with technetium Tc 99m versus 99mTc-pertechnetate to a live and killed equine isolate of Escherichia coil.* Can J Vet Res, 2005. **69**(4): p. 272-7.
74. Palestro, C., et al., *Phase II study of 99mTc-ciprofloxacin uptake in patients with high suspicion of osteomyelitis.* J NUCL MED MEETING ABSTRACTS, 2006. **47**(suppl_1): p. 152P-.
75. Malamitsi, J., et al., *The value of successive Infecton scans in assessing the presence of chronic bone and joint infection and in predicting its evolution after treatment and after a prolonged follow-up.* Nucl Med Commun, 2011. **32**(11): p. 1060-9.
76. Bhardwaj, V., et al., *Evaluation of adequacy of short-course chemotherapy for extraspinal osteoarticular tuberculosis using 99mTc ciprofloxacin scan.* Int Orthop, 2011. **35**(12): p. 1869-74.
77. Mostafa, M., M. Motaleb, and T. Sakr, *Labeling of ceftriaxone for infective inflammation imaging using 99m Tc eluted from 99 Mo/99m Tc generator based on zirconium molybdate.* Applied Radiation and Isotopes, 2010. **68**(10): p. 1959-1963.
78. Fazli, A., M. Salouti, and M. Mazidi, *99mTc-ceftriaxone, as a targeting radiopharmaceutical for scintigraphic imaging of infectious foci due to Staphylococcus aureus in mouse model.* Journal of Radioanalytical and Nuclear Chemistry, 2013. **298**(2): p. 1227-1233.
79. Sohaib, M., Z. Khurshid, and S. Roohi, *Labelling of ceftriaxone with 99mTc and its bio-evaluation as an infection imaging agent.* Journal of Labelled Compounds and Radiopharmaceuticals, 2014. **57**(11): p. 652-657.
80. Kaul, A., et al., *Preliminary evaluation of technetium-99m-labeled ceftriaxone: infection imaging agent for the clinical diagnosis of orthopedic infection.* International Journal of Infectious Diseases, 2013. **17**(4): p. e263-e270.
81. van Oosten, M., et al., *Real-time in vivo imaging of invasive- and biomaterial-associated bacterial infections using fluorescently labelled vancomycin.* Nat Commun, 2013. **4**: p. 2584.
82. Auletta, S., et al., *Imaging bacteria with radiolabelled quinolones, cephalosporins and siderophores for imaging infection: a systematic review.* Clinical and Translational Imaging, 2016. **4**(4): p. 229-252.
83. Rubin, R.H., et al., *111In-labeled nonspecific immunoglobulin scanning in the detection of focal infection.* N Engl J Med, 1989. **321**(14): p. 935-40.
84. Panizzi, P., J.R. Stone, and M. Nahrendorf, *Endocarditis and molecular imaging.* Journal of Nuclear Cardiology, 2014. **21**(3): p. 486-495.
85. Wong, D.W., et al., *Imaging endocarditis with Tc-99m-labeled antibody--an experimental study: concise communication.* J Nucl Med, 1982. **23**(3): p. 229-34.
86. Pinkston, K.L., et al., *Targeting Pili in Enterococcal Pathogenesis.* Infection and Immunity, 2014. **82**(4): p. 1540-1547.
87. Rubin, R.H., et al., *Specific and nonspecific imaging of localized Fisher immunotype 1 Pseudomonas aeruginosa infection with radiolabeled monoclonal antibody.* J Nucl Med, 1988. **29**(5): p. 651-6.
88. Wiehr, S., et al., *New pathogen-specific immunoPET/MR tracer for molecular imaging of a systemic bacterial infection.* Oncotarget, 2016. **7**(10): p. 10990-11001.
89. Malpani, B.L., G.V. Kadival, and A.M. Samuel, *Radioimmunoscintigraphic approach for the in vivo detection of tuberculomas--a preliminary study in a rabbit model.* Int J Rad Appl Instrum B, 1992. **19**(1): p. 45-53.
90. Lee, J.D., et al., *Immunoscintigraphy in the detection of tuberculosis with radiolabelled antibody fragment against Mycobacterium bovis bacillus Calmette-Guérin: a preliminary study in a rabbit model.* European Journal of Nuclear Medicine and Molecular Imaging, 1992. **19**(12): p. 1011-1015.

91. Oyen, W.J.G., et al., *Specific antibody uptake in tuberculosis?* European Journal of Nuclear Medicine, 1993. **20**(6): p. 568-569.
92. Leevy, W.M., et al., *Optical imaging of bacterial infection in living mice using a fluorescent near-infrared molecular probe.* J Am Chem Soc, 2006. **128**(51): p. 16476-7.
93. Leevy, W.M., et al., *Noninvasive optical imaging of staphylococcus aureus bacterial infection in living mice using a Bis-dipicolylamine-Zinc(II) affinity group conjugated to a near-infrared fluorophore.* Bioconjug Chem, 2008. **19**(3): p. 686-92.
94. Liu, X., et al., *Radiolabeled Zn-DPA as a potential infection imaging agent.* Nucl Med Biol, 2012. **39**(5): p. 709-14.
95. Rice, D.R., et al., *Evaluation of [(1)(1)(1)In]-labeled zinc-dipicolylamine tracers for SPECT imaging of bacterial infection.* Mol Imaging Biol, 2015. **17**(2): p. 204-13.
96. Rice, D.R., K.J. Clear, and B.D. Smith, *Imaging and therapeutic applications of zinc (II)-dipicolylamine molecular probes for anionic biomembranes.* Chemical Communications, 2016. **52**(57): p. 8787-8801.
97. Wyffels, L., et al., *Synthesis and preliminary evaluation of radiolabeled bis(zinc(II)-dipicolylamine) coordination complexes as cell death imaging agents.* Bioorg Med Chem, 2011. **19**(11): p. 3425-33.
98. Wang, H., et al., *Noninvasive positron emission tomography imaging of cell death using a novel small-molecule probe, (18)F labeled bis(zinc(II)-dipicolylamine) complex.* Apoptosis, 2013. **18**(8): p. 1017-27.
99. Sun, T., et al., *Positron emission tomography imaging of cardiomyocyte apoptosis with a novel molecule probe [18F]FP-DPAZn2.* Oncotarget, 2015. **6**(31): p. 30579-91.
100. Kennedy, D.O., *B Vitamins and the Brain: Mechanisms, Dose and Efficacy--A Review.* Nutrients, 2016. **8**(2): p. 68.
101. Rusckowski, M., B. Fritz, and D.J. Hnatowich, *Localization of infection using streptavidin and biotin: an alternative to nonspecific polyclonal immunoglobulin.* J Nucl Med, 1992. **33**(10): p. 1810-5.
102. Lazzeri, E., et al., *Clinical impact of SPECT/CT with In-111 biotin on the management of patients with suspected spine infection.* Clin Nucl Med, 2010. **35**(1): p. 12-7.
103. Lazzeri, E., et al., *Scintigraphic imaging of vertebral osteomyelitis with 111in-biotin.* Spine (Phila Pa 1976), 2008. **33**(7): p. E198-204.
104. Shoup, T.M., et al., *Synthesis of fluorine-18-labeled biotin derivatives: biodistribution and infection localization.* J Nucl Med, 1994. **35**(10): p. 1685-90.
105. Baldoni, D., et al., *Evaluation of a Novel Tc-99m Labelled Vitamin B12 Derivative for Targeting Escherichia coli and Staphylococcus aureus In Vitro and in an Experimental Foreign-Body Infection Model.* Molecular Imaging and Biology, 2015. **17**(6): p. 829-837.
106. Shah, S.Q., M.R. Khan, and S.M. Ali, *Radiosynthesis of (99m)Tc(CO)3-Clinafloxacin Dithiocarbamate and Its Biological Evaluation as a Potential Staphylococcus aureus Infection Radiotracer.* Nucl Med Mol Imaging, 2011. **45**(4): p. 248-54.
107. Motaleb, M.A., *Radiochemical and biological characteristics of 99mTc-difloxacin and 99mTc-pefloxacin for detecting sites of infection.* Journal of Labelled Compounds and Radiopharmaceuticals, 2010. **53**(3): p. 104-109.
108. Siaens, R.H., et al., *Synthesis and comparison of 99mTc-enrofloxacin and 99mTc-ciprofloxacin.* Journal of Nuclear Medicine, 2004. **45**(12): p. 2088-2094.
109. Shahzad, S., et al., *A new method for synthesis of 99m Tc-enorfloxacin: an infection imaging agent.* Lat Am J Pharm, 2016. **35**: p. 259-264.
110. Motaleb, M.A., et al., *Study on the preparation and biological evaluation of 99mTc–gatifloxacin and 99mTc–cefepime complexes.* Journal of Radioanalytical and Nuclear Chemistry, 2011. **289**(1): p. 57-65.
111. Shahzad, S., et al., *Synthesis of 99m Tc-gemifloxacin freeze dried kits and their biodistribution in Salmonella typhi, Pseudomonas aeruginosa and Klebsiella pneumoniae.* Arabian Journal of Chemistry, 2015.

112. Shah, S.Q. and M.R. Khan, *Radiolabeling of gemifloxacin with technetium-99m and biological evaluation in artificially Streptococcus pneumoniae infected rats.* Journal of Radioanalytical and Nuclear Chemistry, 2011. **288**(1): p. 307-312.
113. Shahzad, S., et al., *In vivo studies 99m Tc-levofloxacin freeze dried kits in Salmonella typhi, Pseudoman aeruginosa, and Escherichia coli.* Lat Am J Pharm, 2015. **34**: p. 760-765.
114. Motaleb, M., *Preparation and biodistribution of 99mTc-lomefloxacin and 99mTc-ofloxacin complexes.* Journal of Radioanalytical and Nuclear Chemistry, 2007. **272**(1): p. 95-99.
115. Chattopadhyay, S., et al., *Synthesis and evaluation of 99m Tc-moxifloxacin, a potential infection specific imaging agent.* Applied Radiation and Isotopes, 2010. **68**(2): p. 314-316.
116. Zhang, S., et al., *Synthesis and biodistribution of a novel 99mTcN complex of norfloxacin dithiocarbamate as a potential agent for bacterial infection imaging.* Bioconjugate chemistry, 2011. **22**(3): p. 369-375.
117. Ibrahim, I., M. Motaleb, and K. Attalah, *Synthesis and biological distribution of 99mTc–norfloxacin complex, a novel agent for detecting sites of infection.* Journal of radioanalytical and nuclear chemistry, 2010. **285**(3): p. 431-436.
118. Sazonova, S.I., et al., *Synthesis and experimental study of norfloxacin labeled with technecium-99m as a potential agent for infection imaging.* Iranian Journal of Nuclear Medicine, 2015. **23**(2): p. 73-81.
119. Erfani, M., et al., *99mTc-tricabonyl labeling of ofloxacin and its biological evaluation in Staphylococcus aureus as an infection imaging agent.* Journal of Labelled Compounds and Radiopharmaceuticals, 2013. **56**(12): p. 627-631.
120. El-Ghany, E., et al., *Synthesis of 99mTc-pefloxacin: a new targeting agent for infectious foci.* Journal of Radioanalytical and Nuclear Chemistry, 2005. **266**(1): p. 131-139.
121. Motaleb, M. and S. Ayoub, *Preparation, quality control, and biodistribution of 99mTc-rufloxacin complex as a model for detecting sites of infection.* Radiochemistry, 2013. **55**(6): p. 610-614.
122. Moustapha, M., et al., *Synthesis and biological evaluation of technetium-sarafloxacin complex for infection imaging.* Journal of Radioanalytical and Nuclear Chemistry, 2016. **307**(1): p. 699-705.
123. Qaiser, S., A. Khan, and M. Khan, *Synthesis, biodistribution and evaluation of 99mTc-Sitafloxacin kit: a novel infection imaging agent.* Journal of radioanalytical and nuclear chemistry, 2010. **284**(1): p. 189-193.
124. Shah, S.Q., A.U. Khan, and M.R. Khan, *Radiosynthesis and biological evaluation of 99mTcN-sitafloxacin dithiocarbamate as a potential radiotracer for Staphylococcus aureus infection.* Journal of Radioanalytical and Nuclear Chemistry, 2011. **287**(3): p. 827-832.
125. Motaleb, M., *Preparation, quality control and stability of 99mTc-sparafloxacin complex, a novel agent for detecting sites of infection.* Journal of Labelled Compounds and Radiopharmaceuticals, 2009. **52**(10): p. 415-418.
126. El-Tawoosy, M., *Preparation and biological distribution of 99mTc-cefazolin complex, a novel agent for detecting sites of infection.* Journal of Radioanalytical and Nuclear Chemistry, 2013. **298**(2): p. 1215-1220.
127. Motaleb, M., et al., *Study on the preparation and biological evaluation of 99mTc–gatifloxacin and 99mTc–cefepime complexes.* Journal of Radioanalytical and Nuclear Chemistry, 2011. **289**(1): p. 57-65.
128. Motaleb, M., *Preparation of 99mTc-cefoperazone complex, a novel agent for detecting sites of infection.* Journal of Radioanalytical and Nuclear Chemistry, 2007. **272**(1): p. 167-171.
129. Mirshojaei, S., et al., *Radio labeling, quality control and biodistribution of 99mTc-cefotaxime as an infection imaging agent.* Journal of Radioanalytical and Nuclear Chemistry, 2011. **287**(1): p. 21-25.
130. Ilem-Ozdemir, D., et al., *Gamma scintigraphy and biodistribution of 99mTc-cefotaxime sodium in preclinical models of bacterial infection and sterile inflammation.* Journal of Labelled Compounds and Radiopharmaceuticals, 2016. **59**(3): p. 109-116.

131. Mirshojaei, S., M. Erfani, and M. Shafiei, *Evaluation of 99mTc-ceftazidime as bacterial infection imaging agent.* Journal of Radioanalytical and Nuclear Chemistry, 2013. **298**(1): p. 19-24.
132. Barreto, V.G., et al., *Gammagrafía con 99mTc-ceftizoxima en ratas normales y en ratas con absceso inducido.* Revista Española de Medicina Nuclear, 2005. **24**(5): p. 312-318.
133. Costa, P.H.N., et al., *Scintigraphic imaging with technetium-99M-labelled ceftizoxime is a reliable technique for the diagnosis of deep sternal wound infection in rats.* Acta Cirurgica Brasileira, 2015. **30**(9): p. 632-638.
134. Teixeira, L.E.M., et al., *Efficacy of 99mTc-labeled ceftizoxime in the diagnosis of subclinical infections associated with titanium implants in rats.* Surgical infections, 2015. **16**(3): p. 352-357.
135. Chattopadhyay, S., et al., *Preparation and evaluation of 99m Tc-cefuroxime, a potential infection specific imaging agent: A reliable thin layer chromatographic system to delineate impurities from the 99m Tc-antibiotic.* Applied Radiation and Isotopes, 2012. **70**(10): p. 2384-2387.
136. Yurt Lambrecht, F., et al., *Evaluation of 99mTc-Cefuroxime axetil for imaging of inflammation.* Journal of Radioanalytical and Nuclear Chemistry, 2008. **277**(2): p. 491-494.
137. Shah, S.Q., A.U. Khan, and M.R. Khan, *Radiosynthesis of 99mTc-nitrofurantoin a novel radiotracer for in vivo imaging of Escherichia coli infection.* Journal of Radioanalytical and Nuclear Chemistry, 2011. **287**(2): p. 417-422.
138. Shah, S.Q., A.U. Khan, and M.R. Khan, *Radiosynthesis and biodistribution of 99m Tc-rifampicin: a novel radiotracer for in-vivo infection imaging.* Applied Radiation and Isotopes, 2010. **68**(12): p. 2255-2260.
139. Essouissi, I., et al., *Synthesis and evaluation of 99mTc-N-sulfanilamide ferrocene carboxamide as bacterial infections detector.* Nuclear Medicine and Biology, 2010. **37**(7): p. 821-829.
140. Tsopelas, C., et al., *99m Tc-Alafosfalin: an antibiotic peptide infection imaging agent.* Nuclear medicine and biology, 2003. **30**(2): p. 169-175.
141. Shahzadi, S.K., et al., *99mTc-amoxicillin: A novel radiopharmaceutical for infection imaging.* Arabian Journal of Chemistry.
142. Roohi, S., A. Mushtaq, and S.A. Malik, *Synthesis and biodistribution of 99mTc-vancomycin in a model of bacterial infection.* Radiochimica Acta, 2005. **93**(7): p. 415-418.
143. Sanad, M., *Labeling and biological evaluation of 99mTc-azithromycin for infective inflammation diagnosis.* Radiochemistry, 2013. **55**(5): p. 539-544.
144. Borai, E., M. Sanad, and A. Fouzy, *Optimized chromatographic separation and biological evaluation of 99m Tc-clarithromycin for infective inflammation diagnosis.* Radiochemistry, 2016. **58**(1): p. 84-91.
145. Hina, S., et al., *Preparation, biodistribution, and scintigraphic evaluation of 99mTc-clindamycin: an infection imaging agent.* Applied biochemistry and biotechnology, 2014. **174**(4): p. 1420-1433.
146. İlem-Özdemir, D., et al., *99mTc-Doxycycline hyclate: a new radiolabeled antibiotic for bacterial infection imaging.* Journal of Labelled Compounds and Radiopharmaceuticals, 2014. **57**(1): p. 36-41.
147. Abdel-Ghaney, I. and M. Sanad, *Synthesis of 99mTc-erythromycin complex as a model for infection sites imaging.* Radiochemistry, 2013. **55**(4): p. 418-422.
148. Roohi, S., et al., *Synthesis, quality control and biodistribution of 99mTc-Kanamycin.* Journal of radioanalytical and nuclear chemistry, 2006. **267**(3): p. 561-566.
149. Hina, S., et al., *Labeling, quality control and biological evaluation of 99m Tc-vibramycin for infection sites imaging.* Bulg Chem Comm, 2015. **47**: p. 747-754.
150. Wang, X. and N. Murthy, *Bacterial imaging comes of age.* Sci Transl Med, 2014. **6**(259): p. 259fs43.

Chapter 7
Fungal Imaging

Greetje Vande Velde and Stefan Wiehr

7.1 Introduction

Fungal infections caused by yeasts (e.g., *Candida albicans*, *Cryptococcus neoformans*) and molds (e.g., *Aspergillus fumigatus*) have emerged over the past two decades to become more and more significant in clinical practice, due to an increase in the number of severely ill or immunocompromised [1–4]. The traditional, laboratory-based diagnostic modalities such as blood cultures, PCR, antigen tests, and microscopy often result in long turnaround times, making it more difficult when dealing with contaminants, thereby compelling clinicians to treat patients empirically with broad-spectrum medication until diagnostic results are available [5–7]. Molecular imaging could allow early and accurate detection of infections and monitoring of treatment efficacies, thereby limiting incorrect or unnecessary treatments and the intrinsic burdens of cost, drug resistance, and damage to the patient's health [6, 8]. An increasing number of innovative positron emission tomography (PET) radiopharmaceuticals, employing monoclonal antibodies or their fragments, peptides, and small molecules, have been developed and evaluated for infectious disease imaging [9], but compared to cancer research, tracer development for the specific detection of fungi and parasites is in its infancy. While no specific imaging modalities exist clinically, we will discuss some examples of imaging techniques that have been utilized in preclinical settings.

G. Vande Velde
Biomedical MRI Unit/MoSAIC, KU Leuven – University of Leuven, Leuven, Belgium

S. Wiehr (✉)
Department of Preclinical Imaging and Radiopharmacy, Werner Siemens Imaging Center, University Hospital Tuebingen, Tübingen, Germany
e-mail: Stefan.Wiehr@med.uni-tuebingen.de

S.K. Jain (ed.), *Imaging Infections*, DOI 10.1007/978-3-319-54592-9_7

7.2 Optical Imaging Techniques

Several transgenic fungi and parasites have already been engineered to express either a fluorescent or a bioluminescent reporter gene in order to facilitate their specific monitoring with whole body imaging or intravital microscopy and have been reviewed in Chapter 3. Host immune cells can also be labeled (e.g., with a different "color" fluorophore or luciferase), to monitor the host and the pathogen simultaneously. Intravital microscopy, using either two-photon laser scanning microscopy (TPLSM) or fibered confocal fluorescence microscopy (FCFM), can visualize cell-cell or cell-protein interactions. The limitations of intravital microscopy are its invasiveness and the small field of view. In spite of that, many efforts have already been made to get a better view on the parasite's or micro-pathogen's life inside its host [10]. Intravital microscopy has permitted the visualization in real time of *C. neoformans* cells trapped in superficial cortical mouse brain capillaries crossing the endothelial wall [11], shedding some light on how fungi manage to cross an apparently intact blood–brain barrier. Technological and methodological advances aim at minimizing invasiveness, thereby enabling repeated intravital microscopy at previously inaccessible, deeper located sites in order to investigate more physiological infection models. Intravital microscopy by FCFM is a technique used in both clinical and preclinical settings for microscopic probing inside the body [12, 13]. The use of a very small fiber optic probe connected to a laser unit for fluorescence imaging has very recently been developed for the noninvasive, repeated visualization of *Aspergillus* and *Cryptococcus* hyphae and cells in infected mouse lungs with cellular resolution (Figure 7.1a). The fiber optics approach lends itself for use in combination with MRI or CT, opening avenues for the global localization of lesions and simultaneous detailed microscopic examination with intravital microscopy at identified lesion sites (Figure 7.1b). In the clinic, the fiber optic probe can be introduced into the working channel of a bronchoscope, down to the distal lung areas to investigate, for example, airway microstructures in patients at risk for lung cancer or identified with suspicious findings on chest x-ray examinations [13–15]. The preclinical availability of such technology will be useful as a testing platform for the development of fungus-specific optical probes for direct labeling. Optimizing this technique for the visualization of fungi of parasites in a preclinical setting can result in a future clinical application for the differential diagnosis of such infections. Fluorescent dyes conjugated to a targeting moiety are already safely used in the clinic [16]. The development of an imaging approach combined with fluorescent probes specifically targeting different species of fungal cells or parasites would enable more efficient differential diagnosis and the immediate start of adequate specific antibiotic therapy. To unravel pathogenesis and host-pathogen interactions, the use of intravital microscopy in the zebrafish model has proven to be highly useful [17]. Similarly, whole body BLI has been used in mouse infection models [18–23]. Although BLI is a well-established technique, it can be particularly challenging for fungi [24, 25], due to difficulties in genetic engineering; existence of extra barriers such as a cell wall, capsule (*Cryptococcus* spp.), different morphological forms, and transitions (e.g., yeast and hyphal *Candida*, filamentous *Aspergillus*); and hypoxic

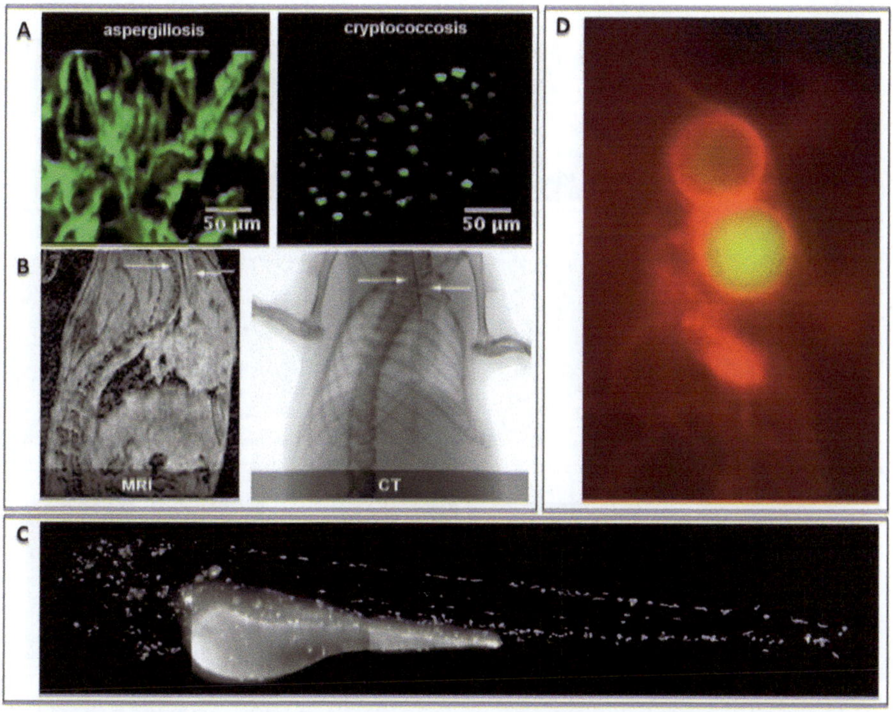

Figure 7.1 Intravital microscopy. (**a**) Intravital fibered confocal fluorescence microscopy (FCFM) in the lungs of mouse models of invasive pulmonary aspergillosis and pulmonary cryptococcosis, infected through inhalation of GFP-expressing *Aspergillus fumigatus* or *Crypotoccus gattii*, respectively. Note the clear visualization of the typical fungal morphology at cellular resolution: hyphae for *Aspergillus* and round yeastlike cells for *Cryptococcus*. (**b**) Simultaneous FCFM and MRI or CT, here shown for a mouse with pulmonary aspergillosis, allow for complementary visualization of lung lesions at macroscopic and microscopic level and localization of the FCFM probe at the exact lesion location. (**c**) Intravital microscopy in zebrafish allows monitoring of different cell populations, such as, in this example, by visualizing all the macrophages of a temporarily anesthetized animal or (**d**) by the simultaneous imaging of a host macrophage (*red*) containing a cryptococcal cell (*green*) (zebrafish IVM image courtesy of Dr. Simon Johnston, University of Sheffield; FCFM images courtesy of L. Vanherp, J. Poelmans and G. Vande Velde)

conditions in the infected environment that may hamper the light-producing reaction, obscuring the interpretation and quantification of the imaging results [26]. A *Gaussia* luciferase (*gLuc*) enzyme that is engineered to be located extracellularly sticking out of the cell wall has made BLI of hyphal cells possible, thereby showing substantial improvement in the use of BLI as a tool to monitor superficial *Candida albicans* infections and biofilm formation [27–29]. Noninvasive, dynamic imaging and quantification of *C. albicans* biofilm formation including morphogenesis from the yeast to hyphae state was feasible by using growth phase-dependent bioluminescent *C. albicans* strains in a subcutaneous catheter model in rodents (Figure 7.2) [27, 28]. Also for pulmonary and cutaneous *Aspergillus* infections in living animals, the use

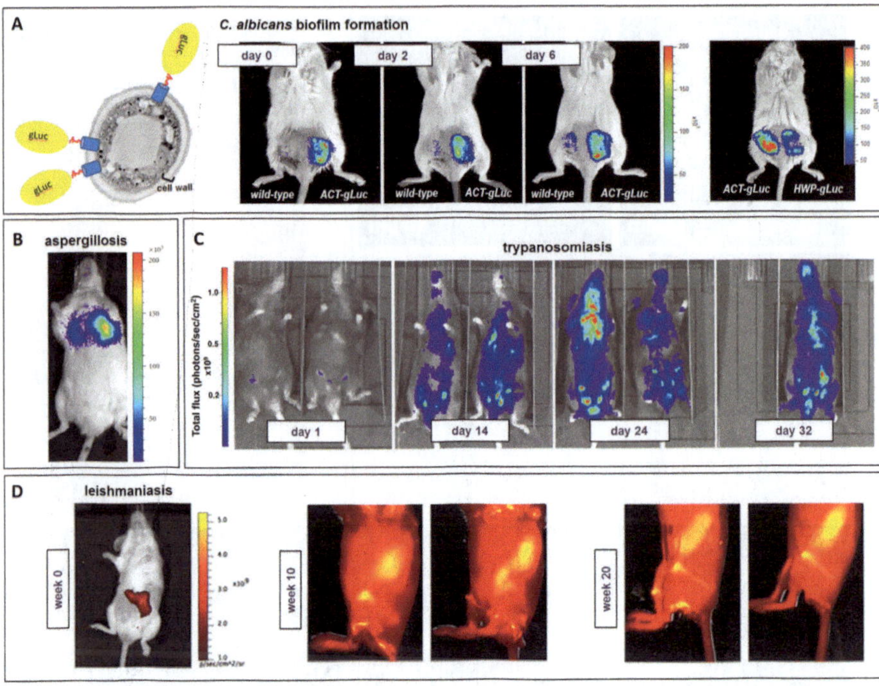

Figure 7.2 Bioluminescence and fluorescence imaging. (**a**) *Candida albicans* cells have been engineered to express *Gaussia* luciferase (*gLuc*) extracellularly, by targeting the luciferase through fusion with a GPI anchor protein coding sequence to the cell wall. (**b**) Using constitutively expressed (ACT-promoter) gLuc to genetically label *C. albicans* cells, longitudinal monitoring in the same mouse of biofilm formation on the inside of subcutaneously implanted catheters became possible. Using a promoter that is only active in the hyphal stage of *C. albicans* cell growth (HWP) to drive gLuc expression enabled BLI of the morphological switch from the yeast to the hyphal stage, an important step in pathogenesis. (**b**) Bioluminescence imaging of invasive aspergillosis. The depicted mouse was immunosuppressed with cortisone acetate and infected intranasally with the bioluminescent *A. fumigatus* strain C3. Bioluminescence was acquired 28 h after infection. Light emission is detected from both lung lobes indicating the establishment of bronchopulmonary aspergillosis (adapted with permission from [24]). (**c**) In vivo BLI (total flux) for monitoring the course of infection in mice inoculated *i.p.* with 3×10^4 *T. brucei* GVR35 expressing a red-shifted luciferase revealed the rapid growth and dissemination of parasites during the course of infection. Parasites can be detected in the heads of both mice by day 24 (adapted with permission from reference [35]). (**d**) Monitoring the course of in vivo visceral infection with NIR fluorescence imaging in mice infected with 10^7 metacyclic promastigotes of iRFP-expressing HSP70+ *L. infantum* after 10 and 20 weeks after infection (adapted with permission from [39])

of BLI has been explored and found to be useful for in vivo testing of antifungal strategies (Figure 7.2b) [21, 30–32]. Although the use of BLI for imaging of fungal infections is currently limited to *C. albicans* and *Aspergillus* spp. [24], it is likely that its use will expand to more different organisms because of its usefulness as an alternative readout for survival analyses. For example, the use of transgenic *Toxoplasma gondii* strains engineered to express luciferase enabled the visualization of parasites spreading to different organs, strain-related differences in virulence, and the noninvasive evaluation of antiparasitic treatment [22, 23, 33]. The use of reporter parasites in combination with reporter hosts has enabled the study of not only the parasite but also the immune response [34]. The construction of a *Trypanosoma brucei* and *T. cruzi* emitting red-shifted luciferase [35, 36] (Figure 7.2c) and the use of BLI have identified new sites of parasite persistence and have shed light on the presence of the parasite in the CNS and facilitated drug discovery also for this family of parasites [37, 38]. The oxygen and substrate dependence of the light-producing reaction is a drawback as it makes the imaging results dependent of the host response at the site of infection and limits quantification of the results. A first step to improve this has been taken by the construction of iRFP transgenic parasites for whole body fluorescence imaging utilizing the optimal tissue penetration capability of near-infrared light. *Leishmania infantum* strains were engineered to fluoresce in the near-infrared, enabling in vivo detection of visceral parasitic infection using whole body fluorescence imaging [39] (Figure 7.2d).

7.3 Clinical Translation

In spite of its proven usefulness in infectious disease research, the fundamental limitation and disadvantage of optical imaging are the depth dependence of the signal because of low tissue penetration of light and the lack of absolute quantification of the imaging results. Combinatory imaging techniques can provide more details and complement this technique. In a study by Mello et al., for example, BLI was used to track the homing of putative immunomodulatory therapeutic cells in a mouse model of *Trypanosoma cruzi* infection. Heart disease and therapeutic effects were evaluated in vivo by acquiring echocardiograms and cardiac MR images [40]. In another example, in addition to the fungal biomass quantification by BLI, CT or MRI can give information on the exact anatomical location of the implanted catheter and in the case of MRI provide information about scar tissue formation or bleeding that can help in interpreting the imaging results (Figure 7.3) [28]. In particular, for fungal lung infections, recent advances made in both MRI and micro-CT have been successfully applied to monitor onset and progression of pulmonary cryptococcosis and invasive aspergillosis in mouse inhalation infection models (Figure 7.4), providing several different biomarkers describing different aspects of lung infection progression [41–43]. High-resolution lung images can be safely obtained by micro-CT [44, 45], though MRI has several other advantages, including high spatial resolution, lack of radiation exposure, and use of different MR sequences that can provide additional information; however, specific diagnosis remains difficult [46]. MR spectroscopy on the other hand is able to identify specific metabolites that in theory could enable differentiation between brain glioma and bacterial and different fungal infections. For example, high levels of trehalose detectable by MR spectroscopy in cryptococcomas in experimentally infected animals could have significance for clinical translation [47, 48].

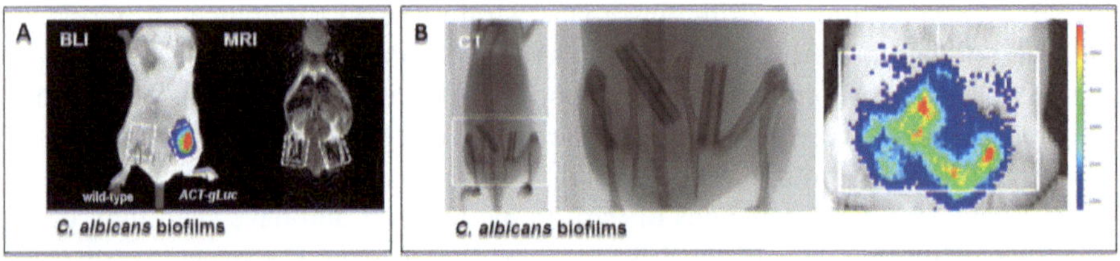

Figure 7.3 Multimodal imaging. (**a**) The use of MRI complementary to BLI for the longitudinal monitoring of in vivo biofilm formation on subcutaneously implanted medical devices by *C. albicans* provides additional information about the location of the catheters, potential edema, bleeding, or scar tissue formation, relevant for the interpretation and quantification of the BLI results. (**b**) Also micro-CT (here, a projection image is shown) provides anatomical information about the exact three-dimensional anatomical location of implanted medical devices. After reconstruction, the CT data can be coregistered with the BLI results for improved quantification of fungal load during biofilm formation, here illustrated for intraperitoneally implanted catheter pieces

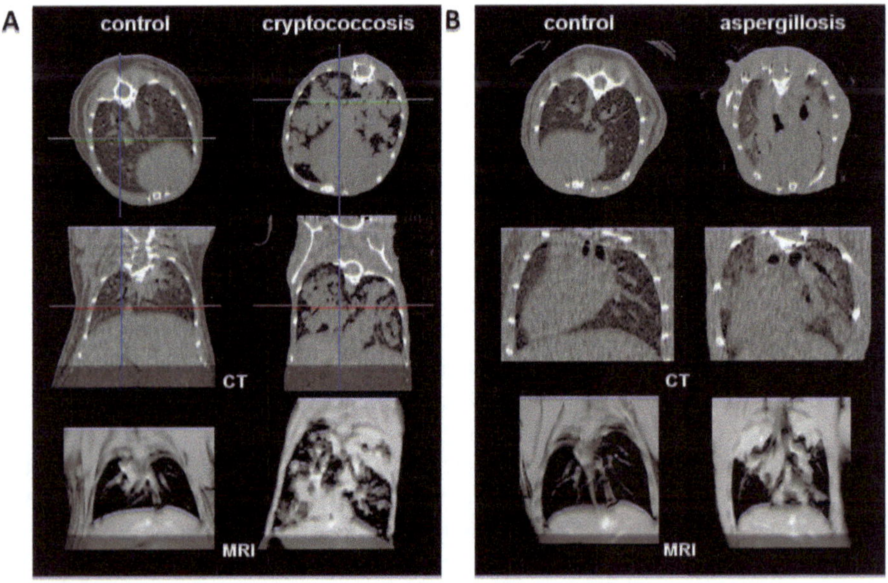

Figure 7.4 MRI and micro-CT of fungal lung infections. (**a**) Reconstructed micro-CT and self-gated MR images for a control mouse and a mouse infected with a pulmonary *Cryptococcus gattii* infection (4 weeks after infection), illustrating the noninvasive visualization of the progressed lung infection. Note the shape of the lung lesions, typical for cryptococcomas in the lung. (**b**) Micro-CT and self-gated MR images for immune suppressed control mice and mice infected with *Aspergillus fumigatus*, demonstrating that the progression of the lung pathology caused by this fungal infection can be noninvasively monitored by both MRI and micro-CT. Adapted from Poelmans et al. [42]

7.4 Invasive Pulmonary Aspergillosis

Humans with impaired immunity, e.g., those with hematological malignancies or bone marrow transplant recipients, are at a substantially elevated risk of severe, invasive *Aspergillus fumigatus* infection known as invasive aspergillosis (IA). Definitive diagnosis of IA is only obtained at autopsy or relies on invasive biopsy, which is not always possible. A convenient, fast, and specific diagnosis of IA is currently not available, forcing clinicians to implement empiric treatments with costly and toxic antifungal drugs. Consequently, there is the potential to increase the survival rates of aspergillosis patients, if a definitive diagnosis of IA could be obtained early and its response to treatment monitored and adjusted accordingly.

While it has been reported that ^{18}F-2-fluoro-deoxy-D-glucose (^{18}F-FDG) might serve as a useful imaging tool for initial diagnosis and therapy monitoring of IPA [49], our investigations have shown that increased ^{18}F-FDG uptake in *A. fumigatus*-infected lungs is indistinguishable from the uptake seen during inflammatory reactions due to sterile triggers or other pathogens. Recently, *A. fumigatus* detection based on single photon emission tomography (SPECT) with ^{99m}Tc-labeled morpholino-oligonucleotides (MORFs) specific for fungal 28S rRNA has been investigated [50]. Attempts have also been made to visualize *A. fumigatus*-infected animals with microPET/CT using ^{68}Ga radiolabeled siderophores [51, 52]. These small high-affinity chelating compounds are produced by fungi and bacteria to scavenge iron from the host and by gram-negative bacterial pathogens as virulence factors [53]. While rapid uptake of ^{68}Ga by the *A. fumigatus* siderophore TAFC has been shown to occur under conditions of iron depletion, TAFC-mediated ^{68}Ga uptake has also been demonstrated in *Fusarium solani* and *Rhizopus oryzae*, invasive fungal pathogens that cause fusariosis and mucormycosis in immunocompromised patients [54]. More recently, an immunoPET approach utilizing ^{64}Cu-DOTA-labeled anti-*A. fumigatus* mAb was developed for the detection of *A. fumigatus* [55]. Neutropenic mice were infected with *A. fumigatus*, the probe was delivered intravenously, and subsequent PET images were acquired. Figure 7.5 shows the localization of the tracer in the lungs of infected mice 48 h after the initial pulmonary infection. The advantages of simultaneous PET/MRI compared to PET/CT include the functional information of the MRI complementing the molecular information of the PET, outstanding localization of the PET signal in the soft tissue, and the absence of radiation from the MRI system [9]. The chance to image infectious diseases at an early stage of the disease and at a molecular and cellular level might allow early diagnosis and more accurate disease monitoring.

7.5 Summary

Imaging techniques provide huge potential to improve fundamental understanding of the host-pathogen interplay and to aid in the search for novel treatment targets. Not only will this be useful at the patients' bedside but help basic research.

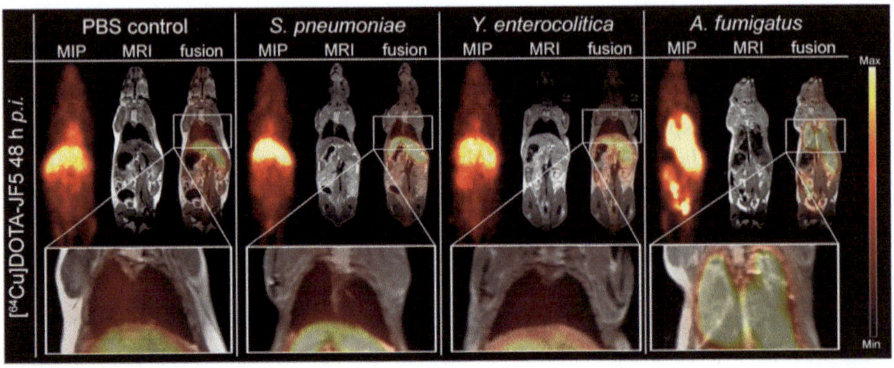

Figure 7.5 Coronal maximum intensity projections (MIP), magnetic resonance imaging (MRI), and fused positron emission tomography (PET)/MRI images of PBS-treated and *Streptococcus pneumoniae*-, *Yersinia enterocolitica*-, and *Aspergillus fumigatus*-infected mice injected with [^{64}Cu]DOTA-JF5 (48 h after infection). Tracer injection demonstrates highly specific accumulation in *A. fumigatus*-infected lung tissue compared to bacterial-infected or sham-treated animals. Lungs of the respective animals are detailed in the *lower panel*. Adapted from Rolle et al. [55]

Indeed, several fungal pathogens and parasites have the ability to disseminate widely in the body to organs such as the brain, often causing severe complications and life-threatening disease. Noninvasive in vivo imaging has the potential to provide dynamic data from live animals over a biologically relevant time scale, obviating the need to sacrifice animals at different time points during the course of disease, with significant clinical translation potential. Optical imaging methods with limited depth penetration, such as bioluminescence (BLI) or fluorescence imaging and intravital microscopy techniques, are extremely valuable in mouse experimental models as they allow monitoring of cell viability and proliferation at a relatively low cost. However, multimodality imaging can ultimately overcome limitations of individual techniques, provide complementary information on the macroscopic and microscopic level, and allow in vivo monitoring of different cell populations, not only fungal but also parasites and host immune cells.

References

1. Warnock, D.W., *Fungal diseases: an evolving public health challenge.* Med Mycol, 2006. **44**(8): p. 697-705.
2. Nucci, M. and K.A. Marr, *Emerging fungal diseases.* Clin Infect Dis, 2005. **41**(4): p. 521-6.
3. Chen, S.C., E.G. Playford, and T.C. Sorrell, *Antifungal therapy in invasive fungal infections.* Curr Opin Pharmacol, 2010. **10**(5): p. 522-30.
4. Eggimann, P., J. Garbino, and D. Pittet, *Epidemiology of Candida species infections in critically ill non-immunosuppressed patients.* Lancet Infect Dis, 2003. **3**(11): p. 685-702.
5. Bates, D.W., et al., *Predicting bacteremia in patients with sepsis syndrome. Academic Medical Center Consortium Sepsis Project Working Group.* J Infect Dis, 1997. **176**(6): p. 1538-51.

6. Weinstein, E.A., et al., *Imaging Enterobacteriaceae infection in vivo with 18F-fluorodeoxysorbitol positron emission tomography.* Sci Transl Med, 2014. **6**(259): p. 259ra146.
7. Nakamura, T., et al., *Clinical prediction rules for bacteremia and in-hospital death based on clinical data at the time of blood withdrawal for culture: An evaluation of their development and use.* J Eval Clin Pract, 2006. **12**(6): p. 692-703.
8. Stevens, V., et al., *Inpatient costs, mortality and 30-day re-admission in patients with central-line-associated bloodstream infections.* Clin Microbiol Infect, 2014. **20**(5): p. O318-24.
9. Glaudemans, A.W., A.M. Quintero, and A. Signore, *PET/MRI in infectious and inflammatory diseases: will it be a useful improvement?* Eur J Nucl Med Mol Imaging, 2012. **39**(5): p. 745-9.
10. Coombes, J.L. and E.A. Robey, *Dynamic imaging of host-pathogen interactions in vivo.* Nat Rev Immunol, 2010. **10**(5): p. 353-64.
11. Shi, M., et al., *Real-time imaging of trapping and urease-dependent transmigration of Cryptococcus neoformans in mouse brain.* J Clin Invest, 2010. **120**(5): p. 1683-93.
12. Morisse, H., et al., *In vivo and in situ imaging of experimental invasive pulmonary aspergillosis using fibered confocal fluorescence microscopy.* Med Mycol, 2012. **50**(4): p. 386-95.
13. Fuchs, F.S., et al., *Confocal laser endomicroscopy for diagnosing lung cancer in vivo.* Eur Respir J, 2013. **41**(6): p. 1401-8.
14. Thiberville, L., et al., *In vivo imaging of the bronchial wall microstructure using fibered confocal fluorescence microscopy.* Am J Respir Crit Care Med, 2007. **175**(1): p. 22-31.
15. Salaun, M., et al., *In vivo imaging of pulmonary alveolar proteinosis using confocal endomicroscopy.* Eur Respir J, 2010. **36**(2): p. 451-3.
16. van Dam, G.M., et al., *Intraoperative tumor-specific fluorescence imaging in ovarian cancer by folate receptor-alpha targeting: first in-human results.* Nat Med, 2011. **17**(10): p. 1315-9.
17. Gratacap, R.L. and R.T. Wheeler, *Utilization of zebrafish for intravital study of eukaryotic pathogen-host interactions.* Dev Comp Immunol, 2014. **46**(1): p. 108-15.
18. Hutchens, M. and G.D. Luker, *Applications of bioluminescence imaging to the study of infectious diseases.* Cell Microbiol, 2007. **9**(10): p. 2315-22.
19. Sjolinder, H. and A.B. Jonsson, *Imaging of disease dynamics during meningococcal sepsis.* PLoS One, 2007. **2**(2): p. e241.
20. Jacobsen, I.D., et al., *In vivo imaging of disseminated murine Candida albicans infection reveals unexpected host sites of fungal persistence during antifungal therapy.* J Antimicrob Chemother, 2014. **69**(10): p. 2785-96.
21. Slesiona, S., et al., *Murine Infection Models for Aspergillus terreus Pulmonary Aspergillosis Reveal Long-term Persistence of Conidia and Liver Degeneration.* Journal of Infectious Diseases, 2012. **205**(8): p. 1268-1277.
22. Saeij, J.P.J., et al., *Bioluminescence Imaging of Toxoplasma gondii Infection in Living Mice Reveals Dramatic Differences between Strains.* Infection and Immunity, 2005. **73**(2): p. 695-702.
23. Lambert, H., et al., *Induction of dendritic cell migration upon Toxoplasma gondii infection potentiates parasite dissemination.* Cell Microbiol, 2006. **8**(10): p. 1611-23.
24. Brock, M., *Application of bioluminescence imaging for in vivo monitoring of fungal infections.* Int J Microbiol, 2012. **2012**(2012): p. 956794.
25. d'Enfert, C., A. Vecchiarelli, and A.J.P. Brown, *Bioluminescent fungi for real-time monitoring of fungal infections.* Virulence, 2010. **1**(3): p. 174-176.
26. Ibrahim-Granet, O., et al., *In vivo bioluminescence imaging and histopathologic analysis reveal distinct roles for resident and recruited immune effector cells in defense against invasive aspergillosis.* BMC Microbiology, 2010. **10**: p. 105-105.
27. Enjalbert, B., et al., *A multifunctional, synthetic Gaussia princeps luciferase reporter for live imaging of Candida albicans infections.* Infect Immun, 2009. **77**(11): p. 4847-58.
28. Vande Velde, G., et al., *Towards non-invasive monitoring of pathogen-host interactions during Candida albicans biofilm formation using in vivo bioluminescence.* Cellular Microbiology, 2014. **16**(1): p. 115-130.

29. Vande Velde, G., et al., *Bioluminescence imaging of fungal biofilm development in live animals.* Methods Mol Biol, 2014. **1098**: p. 153-167.
30. Brock, M., et al., *Bioluminescent Aspergillus fumigatus, a new tool for drug efficiency testing and in vivo monitoring of invasive aspergillosis.* Appl Environ Microbiol, 2008. **74**(22): p. 7023-35.
31. Galiger, C., et al., *Assessment of efficacy of antifungals against Aspergillus fumigatus: value of real-time bioluminescence imaging.* Antimicrob Agents Chemother, 2013. **57**(7): p. 3046-59.
32. Donat, S., et al., *Surface display of Gaussia princeps luciferase allows sensitive fungal pathogen detection during cutaneous aspergillosis.* Virulence, 2012. **3**(1): p. 51-61.
33. Hitziger, N., et al., *Dissemination of Toxoplasma gondii to immunoprivileged organs and role of Toll/interleukin-1 receptor signalling for host resistance assessed by in vivo bioluminescence imaging.* Cell Microbiol, 2005. **7**(6): p. 837-48.
34. McGovern, K.E. and E.H. Wilson, *Dark side illuminated: imaging of Toxoplasma gondii through the decades.* Parasit Vectors, 2013. **6**(1): p. 334.
35. McLatchie, A.P., et al., *Highly Sensitive In Vivo Imaging of Trypanosoma brucei Expressing "Red-Shifted" Luciferase.* PLoS Negl Trop Dis, 2013. **7**(11): p. e2571.
36. Lewis, M.D., et al., *Bioluminescence imaging of chronic Trypanosoma cruzi infections reveals tissue-specific parasite dynamics and heart disease in the absence of locally persistent infection.* Cellular Microbiology, 2014. **16**(9): p. 1285-1300.
37. Goyard, S., et al., *In vivo imaging of trypanosomes for a better assessment of host–parasite relationships and drug efficacy.* Parasitology International, 2014. **63**(1): p. 260-268.
38. MacLean, L., et al., *Imaging African trypanosomes.* Parasite Immunology, 2013. **35**(9-10): p. 283-294.
39. Calvo-Álvarez, E., et al., *Infrared Fluorescent Imaging as a Potent Tool for In Vitro, Ex Vivo and In Vivo Models of Visceral Leishmaniasis.* PLoS Negl Trop Dis, 2015. **9**(3): p. e0003666.
40. Mello, D.B., et al., *Adipose Tissue-Derived Mesenchymal Stromal Cells Protect Mice Infected with <italic>Trypanosoma cruzi</italic> from Cardiac Damage through Modulation of Anti-parasite Immunity.* PLoS Negl Trop Dis, 2015. **9**(8): p. e0003945.
41. Vande Velde, G., et al., *The course of mouse pulmonary cryptococcosis visualized by multimodal imaging in live animals.* Mycoses 2014. **57**(S1): p. 12.
42. Poelmans, J., et al., *Longitudinal, in vivo assessment of invasive pulmonary aspergillosis in mice by computed tomography and magnetic resonance imaging.* Lab Invest, 2016. **96**(6): p. 692-704.
43. Vande Velde, G., et al., *Longitudinal micro-CT provides biomarkers of lung disease that can be used to assess the effect of therapy in preclinical mouse models, and reveal compensatory changes in lung volume.* Dis Model Mech, 2016. **9**(1): p. 91-98.
44. De Langhe, E., et al., *Quantification of lung fibrosis and emphysema in mice using automated micro-computed tomography.* PLoS One, 2012. **7**(8): p. e43123.
45. Vande Velde, G., et al., *Longitudinal in vivo microcomputed tomography of mouse lungs: No evidence for radiotoxicity.* Am J Physiol Lung Cell Mol Physiol, 2015. **309**(3): p. L271-9.
46. Starkey, J., T. Moritani, and P. Kirby, *MRI of CNS fungal infections: review of aspergillosis to histoplasmosis and everything in between.* Clin Neuroradiol, 2014. **24**(3): p. 217-30.
47. Himmelreich, U., et al., *Cryptococcomas Distinguished from Gliomas with MR Spectroscopy: An Experimental Rat and Cell Culture Study.* Radiology, 2001. **220**(1): p. 122-128.
48. Dzendrowskyj, T.E., et al., *Diagnosis of cerebral cryptococcoma using a computerized analysis of 1H NMR spectra in an animal model.* Diagn Microbiol Infect Dis, 2005. **52**(2): p. 101-5.
49. Hot, A., et al., *Diagnostic contribution of positron emission tomography with [18F]fluorodeoxyglucose for invasive fungal infections.* Clin Microbiol Infect, 2011. **17**(3): p. 409-17.
50. Wang, Y., et al., *Detection of Aspergillus fumigatus pulmonary fungal infections in mice with (99m)Tc-labeled MORF oligomers targeting ribosomal RNA.* Nucl Med Biol, 2013. **40**(1): p. 89-96.

51. Haas, H., M. Petrik, and C. Decristoforo, *An iron-mimicking, Trojan horse-entering fungi--has the time come for molecular imaging of fungal infections?* PLoS Pathog, 2015. **11**(1): p. e1004568.
52. Petrik, M., et al., *68Ga-siderophores for PET imaging of invasive pulmonary aspergillosis: proof of principle.* J Nucl Med, 2010. **51**(4): p. 639-45.
53. Holden, V.I. and M.A. Bachman, *Diverging roles of bacterial siderophores during infection.* Metallomics, 2015. **7**(6): p. 986-95.
54. Thornton, C.R. and O.E. Wills, *Immunodetection of fungal and oomycete pathogens: established and emerging threats to human health, animal welfare and global food security.* Crit Rev Microbiol, 2015. **41**(1): p. 27-51.
55. Rolle, A.M., et al., *ImmunoPET/MR imaging allows specific detection of Aspergillus fumigatus lung infection in vivo.* Proc Natl Acad Sci U S A, 2016. **113**(8): p. E1026-33.

Chapter 8
Neuroimaging

Dima A. Hammoud

8.1 Introduction

Since the advent of cross-sectional magnetic resonance (MR) and computed tomography (CT) imaging techniques, the diagnosis and characterization of various intracranial infectious processes has advanced significantly. Specific imaging characteristics for different pathogens were thoroughly described and now represent the first step in the management and follow-up of those patients. Structural cross-sectional techniques, however, reach their limits when questions of molecular nature are asked, such as differentiating active infection from sterile inflammation and/or immune response or from other etiologies such as primary or metastatic malignancies (Figure 8.1). Molecular imaging, on the other hand, has the potential of transcending the limitations of structural imaging, providing molecular and cellular level information. Multiple examples of preclinical central nervous system (CNS) imaging applications in the setting of viral, bacterial, parasitic, and fungal infections can be found in the literature. Clinical and human translational applications however remain limited in number and in scope.

Optical imaging and PET/SPECT imaging are the two most commonly used molecular imaging modalities in animal models of CNS infection. While only a few studies have attempted targeting the unmodified pathogen directly, tracking genetically modified pathogens in animal models, generally using optical imaging, remains the main approach. There are also multiple studies describing host responses

D.A. Hammoud (✉)
Center for Infectious Disease Imaging, Radiology and Imaging Sciences, Clinical Center, U.S. National Institutes of Health, Bethesda, MD, USA
e-mail: hammoudd@cc.nih.gov

S.K. Jain (ed.), *Imaging Infections*, DOI 10.1007/978-3-319-54592-9_8

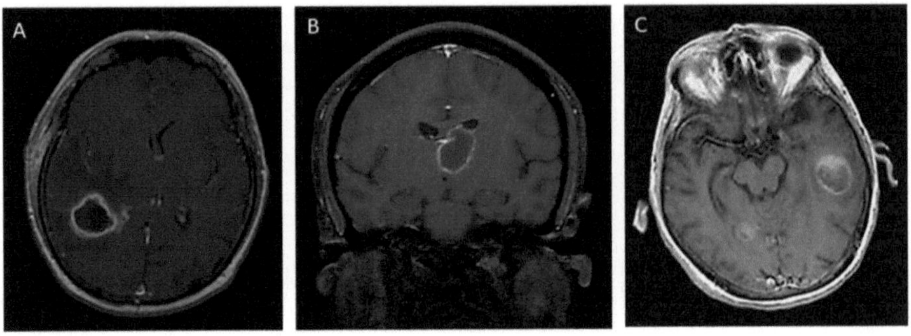

Figure 8.1 Conventional structural MR imaging showing nonspecific ring-enhancing lesions: (**a**) bacterial abscess; (**b**) toxoplasmosis in HIV-positive patient; and (**c**) metastatic disease from primary lung cancer

to infection such as activation of microglia or other components of the immune system. Among those approaches, direct targeting of the pathogen is probably of most clinical significance and would be most interesting to translate.

8.2 Targeting the Pathogen

Targeting the pathogen is limited by lack of pathogen-specific imaging ligands. Another limitation inherent to the CNS is the presence of the blood–brain barrier limiting brain access to few molecules with special characteristics (e.g., small size, appropriate lipophilicity). Even though the BBB can be disrupted in infectious processes, this is not always the case. In fact, with indolent less aggressive pathogens, the BBB can remain intact or minimally breached. In theory, directly imaging the infectious agent can be performed using ligands incorporated only by the pathogen but not by eukaryotic cells or through targeting of pathogen enzymes with labeled substrates. One example of the latter approach is imaging herpetic (HSV-1) encephalitis using ^{18}F-FHPG, a fluorinated derivative of ganciclovir, which is selectively phosphorylated by the HSV thymidine kinase (Tk) enzyme and subsequently trapped within infected cells [1]. Selective uptake of the ligand is then visualized using PET imaging of rats that received intranasal injection of HSV-1 compared to sham animals. This approach however is limited to pathogens that possess the Tk enzyme, but more importantly by the inability of Tk substrates such as FHPG, FHBG, and FIAU to cross an intact BBB. Even when the BBB is disrupted, the substrate can "leak" resulting in nonspecific accumulation. A well-designed experiment by Buursma et al. used a freezing injury model causing sterile disruption of the BBB; even though ^{18}F-FHPG accumulated initially, it washed out quickly suggesting that the FHPG uptake in actual infections is due to irreversible trapping of the ligand in phosphorylated form within the infected cells [1].

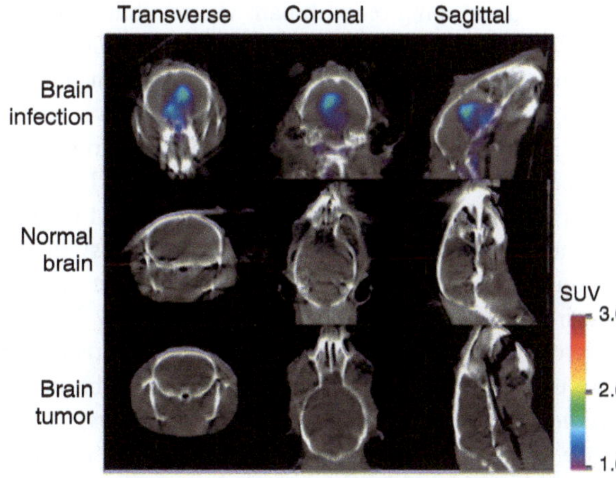

Figure 8.2 ^{18}F-FDS PET signal in an *E. coli*-infected brain (*top row*), normal brain (*middle row*), and brain tumor tissues (*lower row*). Uptake of the ligand is only noted in association with Gram-negative infection suggesting specific uptake by the pathogen. Adapted from Weinstein and Ordonez et al. [2]

Another recently described ligand, 2-[^{18}F]-fluorodeoxysorbitol (^{18}F-FDS), depends on its selective uptake by bacteria, in this case, the Enterobacteriaceae family of Gram-negative bacteria. Sorbitol is not taken by eukaryotic cells and was found to be readily incorporated in Gram-negative but not Gram-positive bacterial cells [2]. ^{18}F-FDS was previously synthesized through chemical reduction of the widely available ligand, ^{18}F-2-fluoro-deoxy-D-glucose (^{18}F-FDG) [3]. Even though originally designed to image brain tumors [3], a significantly higher uptake of ^{18}F-FDS was seen in the *E. coli*-infected brain versus brain tumor or normal brain, suggesting specific uptake and retention by the bacteria (Figure 8.2) [2]. This is rendered even more sensitive by the demonstrated lack of background uptake in the normal brain. Even though FDS can only detect infections due to the Enterobacteriaceae family, it can be greatly used in the right clinical setting, providing localization of the infection, differentiation of active infection from host inflammatory reaction, and evaluation of response to treatment. Development of pathogen-specific ligands with wider detection range and low background uptake is the ultimate goal.

8.3 Genetically Modified Pathogens and Reporter Mice

Much more commonly seen than direct pathogen detection in the brain is molecular imaging using genetically modified pathogens that are traceable through a reporter gene mechanism. A common approach is the use of recombinant viruses engineered to express a luciferase enzyme which allows performing longitudinal imaging, accurately determining the site(s) of infection, describing the temporal systemic dissemination of the virus, and eventually quantifying viral titers in various organs. A major limitation however is the inherent potential for attenuation of viral replication and/or loss of virulence of the pathogen [4–8]. Both latter factors thus need to be carefully evaluated prior to starting imaging experiments. Early examples included developing recombinant viruses that expressed various luciferase reporter proteins such as HSV-1 [6], vaccinia virus [9], and the mouse hepatitis virus (MHV), a member of the *Coronavirus* family [10]. An interesting finding in the paper by Raaben et al. is the detection of the protective role of type I interferon in MHV infection, with widespread viral dissemination, elucidated through bioluminescence, seen in mice lacking a functional type I interferon response and reversal of the process through the administration of type I interferons to the mice [10]. This is an example of molecular imaging providing insight into potential therapeutic applications. More recent examples include the use of recombinant murine gammaherpesvirus 68 (MHV-68) expressing the firefly luciferase (Fluc) to monitor virus progression after CNS infection [11] and of recombinant *Dengue virus*, for real-time evaluation of replication kinetics in the brain of infected mice [12]. *Western equine encephalitis virus* (WEEV; *Alphavirus*), a mosquito-borne virus that can cause severe encephalitis in humans, was also evaluated in a recombinant form (expressing Fluc) in intranasally infected mice [13].

The genetically engineered reporter gene approach however is not limited to viruses and has been used with other pathogens such as parasites. A genetically modified and fully virulent African IL1392 *Trypanosoma vivax* strain that stably expresses Fluc was monitored in vivo in the brain of infected immunocompetent mice. Light emitted by the brain increased slightly up till day 20 post-infection (<400-fold the background) then rose substantially by day 25, reaching up to 2000-fold the background, thus providing evidence of parenchymal infiltration [14]. Other examples of reporter gene use include imaging of *Toxoplasma gondii* encephalitis with spatiotemporal demonstration of recrudescence of the infection from the CNS of immunocompromised mice [15].

Virulent recombinant pathogens can also be used to assess responsiveness to treatment. For example, a *Streptococcus pneumoniae* strain modified by the integration of a luminescent lux operon was used to determine responsiveness of the infection to daptomycin, an alternative antibiotic, eventually found to be as effective as vancomycin [16]. Similarly, the use of luciferase-expressing *Trypanosoma brucei brucei* allowed the identification of pathogen entry into the brain (using multiphoton microscopy) in early stages and determination of their responsiveness to various drugs (bioluminescent parasites were permanently eliminated by treatment with melarsoprol and DB829 but not with diminazene). The interesting finding in this paper is that the investigators did not have to wait for the clinical development of the encephalitic stage of disease which could take as late as 180 days after the initial stage of the infection. Instead, by using serial noninvasive bioluminescence imaging, they reduced the time needed to assess drug efficacy by two-thirds [17].

An alternative model to reporter gene-expressing pathogens is to genetically modify the animal model, usually mice. For example, Luker et al. developed a transgenic reporter mouse that uses the promoter from HSV-1 thymidine kinase to control expression of Fluc [6]. Exposure to HSV-1 (three different strains tested) would then activate the expression of Fluc with bioluminescence increasing in proportion to increasing input titers of the virus. This study however did not detect brain involvement with HSV-1. More complex models such as the transgenic reporter mouse strain that expresses Fluc under the regulatory control of a concatenated Gal4 promoter [18] and the transgenic reporter mouse in which luciferase expression is driven by the nuclear factor B (NF-B)-dependent portion of the human immunodeficiency virus-1 long terminal repeat (HIV-1 LTR) [19] allowed the visualization of brain luciferase expression in response to adenovirus infection [18] and LPS intraperitoneal injection [19], respectively.

A particularly interesting example combines the two approaches (reporter gene and reporter mouse), using *Streptococcus pneumoniae* strain engineered for bioluminescence (lux) in a transgenic mouse model containing an inducible Fluc reporter gene under transcriptional control of the mouse glial fibrillary acidic protein (GFAP) promoter. The two reporters were then separated based on the different spectra of light emission and substrate requirements for lux and Fluc, using a highly sensitive in vivo imaging system. This approach allowed the monitoring of disease progression and response to treatment on one hand while documenting brain damage at the same time [20].

8.4 Imaging the Host

An indirect way of imaging the sequelae of intracranial infection is by imaging the host reaction. Perhaps the most commonly used approach in this setting is imaging infection-associated neuroinflammation. This can be achieved through targeting of the translocator protein (TSPO), an outer mitochondrial membrane receptor that gets upregulated in activated microglia, astrocytes, and blood- derived macrophages in response to CNS central nervous system injury. The classical ligand for TSPO has always been ^{11}C-PK11195; however a multitude of newer (second-generation) ligands designed to overcome the limitations of PK11195 have been developed over the last couple of decades [21]. Using two of the second-generation ligands, ^{11}C-DPA-713 and ^{18}F-DPA-714, along with the prototype ligand ^{11}C-PK11195 [22], neuroinflammation in the setting of HSV encephalitis could be imaged, with ^{11}C-DPA713 showing the lowest nonspecific uptake, suggesting it may be the most suitable for visualizing mild inflammation. Other pathogens in which neuroinflammation was visualized using TSPO ligands include simian immunodeficiency virus (SIV) in macaques [21] and *Taenia solium* (neurocysticercosis) in patients [23]. In the latter study, perilesional edema surrounding calcified lesions was visualized using ^{11}C-PBR28 suggesting resurgence of inflammation despite the chronicity of the infectious process.

Major limitations of TSPO imaging however exist. The main limitation is its inability to specifically visualize infection with ligand accumulation readily seen with sterile inflammation such as that induced by injection of quinolinic acid in the rat striatum [24] (Figure. 8.3). Another main limitation in human translation of TSPO imaging is a recently described polymorphism (rs6971) located in exon 4 of the TSPO gene which results in nonconservative amino acid substitution at position 147 from alanine to threonine (Ala147Thr) in the fifth transmembrane domain of

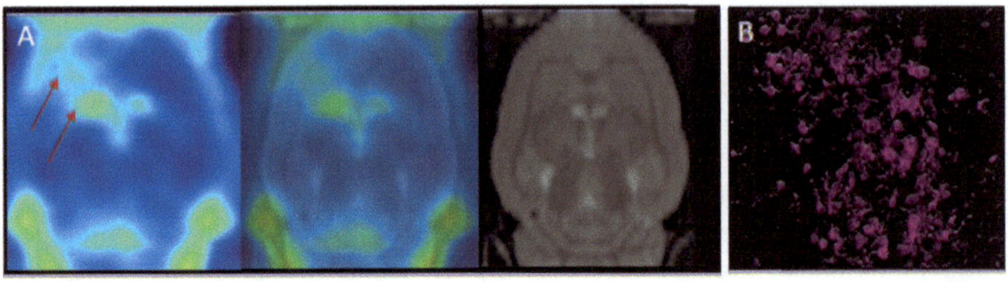

Figure 8.3 (**a**) ^{18}F-DPA-714 PET images (with MRI co-registration) showing increased uptake associated with microglial activation in an animal model of quinolinic acid injection (*red arrows*). (**b**) Increased Iba1staining on immunofluorescence corresponding to increased ^{18}F-DPA-714 uptake

the TSPO protein [25]. This polymorphism results in three binding levels: high, medium, and low binding. To account for the variability, in most cases, genotyping of subjects prior to quantitative assessments of TSPO upregulation using PET is necessary. Another problem with TSPO imaging in non-focal brain infections such as neuro-HIV is the lack of a reference region due to diffuse involvement of the brain. Analysis of the data in such cases requires labor-intensive arterial blood sampling and analysis of metabolites. Recent description of TSPO ligands that are not sensitive to polymorphism is encouraging [26]. Other currently evaluated neuroinflammation imaging targets include the cannabinoid receptors CB1 and CB2 which together constitute the endocannabinoid system [27]. Multiple ligands targeting CB2 are being developed [28–30] with encouraging animal applications [29]. Targeting leukocytes and platelets changes associated with different infectious processes has also been attempted. One example is the use of single-chain antibodies that recognize the ligand-induced binding sites (LIBS) of GPIIb/IIIa in activated platelets [31]. GPIIb/IIIa becomes exposed upon activation and therefore offers the opportunity to target activated platelets [32]. By conjugating the LIBS antibody to iron oxide nanoparticles, they used it in an animal model of cerebral malaria and were able to detect abnormal vascular platelet aggregation in vivo. This approach allowed imaging of the infection before pathology could be visualized by conventional in vivo MRI [31].

As an offshoot of optical imaging, two-photon microscopy has further opened the doors to better understanding of pathogen-host interaction in the brain. Up till now a handful of studies have used this technology in the evaluation of infectious processes; however the available literature points toward a big role for this technique in better understanding the role of specific immune cells such as CD+ lymphocytes and antigen-presenting cells (APCs) in the pathophysiology of CNS infection. The potential applications are limitless. For example, in the brains of mice chronically infected with *Toxoplasma gondii*, two-photon microscopy showed that antigen (Ag)-specific CD8 T cells were recruited and persisted in the presence of ongoing Ag recognition. The dynamics of the interactions between T cells and the parasite could then be visualized real time: while CD8 T cells made transient contacts with granuloma-like structures containing parasites and with individual

CD11b+ APCs, including some that did not contain parasites, they ignored intact Ag-bearing cysts, astrocytes, and neurons, including infected neurons [33]. In another example, two-photon imaging was used in mice infected with different strains of malaria, showing that CD8+ T cells tended to accumulate mainly in the perivascular spaces of experimental cerebral malaria (ECM) mice. This however was also seen with strains that did not cause ECM, indicating that the presence of perivascular T cells per se is insufficient to cause ECM [34]. What differentiated the strains however were dynamic time-lapse movies that showed distinct differences in T-cell motility rather than localization, with the arrest of T cells in the perivascular spaces correlating with the pathogenic potential [34]. This dynamic real-time demonstration of host–pathogen (immune system) interactions within living tissue will surely facilitate and improve our understanding of immune responses to persistent pathogens in the brain.

8.5 Summary

Imaging of infection in the CNS has been handled using cross-sectional imaging for more than two decades now resulting in a large array of descriptive diagnostic criteria, capable, in most circumstances of narrowing the differential diagnosis, detecting life-threatening complications and establishing baseline for assessment of treatment response. Limitations however exist, and in many circumstances, both cross-sectional imaging and nonspecific molecular imaging, such as ^{18}F-FDG, fail to establish a diagnosis. The availability of pathogen-specific imaging agents/ligands would have a great effect on the management of patients with CNS infection. Besides early diagnosis, avoidance of diagnostic brain biopsies can have significant effect on the mortality and morbidity of patients.

References

1. Buursma, A.R., et al., *[18F]FHPG positron emission tomography for detection of herpes simplex virus (HSV) in experimental HSV encephalitis.* J Virol, 2005. **79**(12): p. 7721-7.
2. Weinstein, E.A., et al., *Imaging Enterobacteriaceae infection in vivo with 18F-fluorodeoxysorbitol positron emission tomography.* Sci Transl Med, 2014. **6**(259): p. 259ra146.
3. Li, Z.B., et al., *The synthesis of 18F-FDS and its potential application in molecular imaging.* Mol Imaging Biol, 2008. **10**(2): p. 92-8.
4. Cook, S.H. and D.E. Griffin, *Luciferase imaging of a neurotropic viral infection in intact animals.* J Virol, 2003. **77**(9): p. 5333-8.
5. Hwang, S., et al., *Persistent gammaherpesvirus replication and dynamic interaction with the host in vivo.* J Virol, 2008. **82**(24): p. 12498-509.
6. Luker, G.D., et al., *Noninvasive bioluminescence imaging of herpes simplex virus type 1 infection and therapy in living mice.* J Virol, 2002. **76**(23): p. 12149-61.

7. Luker, G.D., et al., *In vitro and in vivo characterization of a dual-function green fluorescent protein--HSV1-thymidine kinase reporter gene driven by the human elongation factor 1 alpha promoter.* Mol Imaging, 2002. **1**(2): p. 65-73.
8. Zaitseva, M., et al., *Application of bioluminescence imaging to the prediction of lethality in vaccinia virus-infected mice.* J Virol, 2009. **83**(20): p. 10437-47.
9. Luker, K.E., et al., *Bioluminescence imaging of vaccinia virus: effects of interferon on viral replication and spread.* Virology, 2005. **341**(2): p. 284-300.
10. Raaben, M., et al., *Non-invasive imaging of mouse hepatitis coronavirus infection reveals determinants of viral replication and spread in vivo.* Cell Microbiol, 2009. **11**(5): p. 825-41.
11. Kang, H.R., et al., *Persistent infection of a gammaherpesvirus in the central nervous system.* Virology, 2012. **423**(1): p. 23-9.
12. Li, X.F., et al., *Noninvasive bioluminescence imaging of dengue virus infection in the brain of A129 mice.* Appl Microbiol Biotechnol, 2013. **97**(10): p. 4589-96.
13. Phillips, A.T., et al., *Bioluminescent imaging and histopathologic characterization of WEEV neuroinvasion in outbred CD-1 mice.* PLoS One, 2013. **8**(1): p. e53462.
14. D'Archivio, S., et al., *Non-invasive in vivo study of the Trypanosoma vivax infectious process consolidates the brain commitment in late infections.* PLoS Negl Trop Dis, 2013. **7**(1): p. e1976.
15. Dellacasa-Lindberg, I., N. Hitziger, and A. Barragan, *Localized recrudescence of Toxoplasma infections in the central nervous system of immunocompromised mice assessed by in vivo bioluminescence imaging.* Microbes Infect, 2007. **9**(11): p. 1291-8.
16. Mook-Kanamori, B.B., et al., *Daptomycin in experimental murine pneumococcal meningitis.* BMC Infect Dis, 2009. **9**: p. 50.
17. Myburgh, E., et al., *In vivo imaging of trypanosome-brain interactions and development of a rapid screening test for drugs against CNS stage trypanosomiasis.* PLoS Negl Trop Dis, 2013. **7**(8): p. e2384.
18. Pichler, A., et al., *Generation of a highly inducible Gal4-->Fluc universal reporter mouse for in vivo bioluminescence imaging.* Proc Natl Acad Sci U S A, 2008. **105**(41): p. 15932-7.
19. Yull, F.E., et al., *Bioluminescent detection of endotoxin effects on HIV-1 LTR-driven transcription in vivo.* J Histochem Cytochem, 2003. **51**(6): p. 741-9.
20. Kadurugamuwa, J.L., et al., *Reduction of astrogliosis by early treatment of pneumococcal meningitis measured by simultaneous imaging, in vivo, of the pathogen and host response.* Infect Immun, 2005. **73**(12): p. 7836-43.
21. Venneti, S., et al., *Longitudinal in vivo positron emission tomography imaging of infected and activated brain macrophages in a macaque model of human immunodeficiency virus encephalitis correlates with central and peripheral markers of encephalitis and areas of synaptic degeneration.* Am J Pathol, 2008. **172**(6): p. 1603-16.
22. Doorduin, J., et al., *[11C]-DPA-713 and [18F]-DPA-714 as new PET tracers for TSPO: a comparison with [11C]-(R)-PK11195 in a rat model of herpes encephalitis.* Mol Imaging Biol, 2009. **11**(6): p. 386-98.
23. Fujita, M., et al., *PET reveals inflammation around calcified Taenia solium granulomas with perilesional edema.* PLoS One, 2013. **8**(9): p. e74052.
24. Lee, D.E., et al., *Lack of neuroinflammation in the HIV-1 transgenic rat: an [(18)F]-DPA714 PET imaging study.* J Neuroinflammation, 2015. **12**(1): p. 171.
25. Owen, D.R., et al., *An 18-kDa translocator protein (TSPO) polymorphism explains differences in binding affinity of the PET radioligand PBR28.* J Cereb Blood Flow Metab, 2012. **32**(1): p. 1-5.
26. Zanotti-Fregonara, P., et al., *Synthesis and evaluation of translocator 18 kDa protein (TSPO) positron emission tomography (PET) radioligands with low binding sensitivity to human single nucleotide polymorphism rs6971.* ACS Chem Neurosci, 2014. **5**(10): p. 963-71.
27. Haugh, O., et al., *The emerging role of the cannabinoid receptor family in peripheral and neuro-immune interactions.* Curr Drug Targets, 2016. **17**: p. 1-8.

28. Ahmad, R., et al., *Whole-body biodistribution and radiation dosimetry of the cannabinoid type 2 receptor ligand [11C]-NE40 in healthy subjects.* Mol Imaging Biol, 2013. **15**(4): p. 384-90.
29. Savonenko, A.V., et al., *Cannabinoid CB2 Receptors in a Mouse Model of Abeta Amyloidosis: Immunohistochemical Analysis and Suitability as a PET Biomarker of Neuroinflammation.* PLoS One, 2015. **10**(6): p. e0129618.
30. Slavik, R., et al., *Discovery of a high affinity and selective pyridine analog as a potential positron emission tomography imaging agent for cannabinoid type 2 receptor.* J Med Chem, 2015. **58**(10): p. 4266-77.
31. von Zur Muhlen, C., et al., *A contrast agent recognizing activated platelets reveals murine cerebral malaria pathology undetectable by conventional MRI.* J Clin Invest, 2008. **118**(3): p. 1198-207.
32. Schwarz, M., et al., *Conformation-specific blockade of the integrin GPIIb/IIIa: a novel antiplatelet strategy that selectively targets activated platelets.* Circ Res, 2006. **99**(1): p. 25-33.
33. Schaeffer, M., et al., *Dynamic imaging of T cell-parasite interactions in the brains of mice chronically infected with Toxoplasma gondii.* J Immunol, 2009. **182**(10): p. 6379-93.
34. Shaw, T.N., et al., *Perivascular Arrest of CD8+ T Cells Is a Signature of Experimental Cerebral Malaria.* PLoS Pathog, 2015. **11**(11): p. e1005210.

Chapter 9
Pharmacokinetic and Pharmacodynamics Relationships

Zhuo Zhang, Kayla R. Gogarty, Fereidoon Daryaee, and Peter J. Tonge

9.1 Introduction

Drugs work by binding to their therapeutic targets in the human body. However, before a drug can work, it has to reach the site of action and this process, described by the pharmacokinetics (PK) of the drug (viz. what the body does to the drug), involves absorption, distribution, metabolism, and excretion (ADME) of the drug [1, 2]. Drugs can be administered by several routes, the most common being oral administration in which the drug is ingested through the mouth and absorbed from the digestive system into the blood [3]. Once the drug is absorbed into the blood stream, it distributes throughout the body and rapidly equilibrates throughout the central compartment which is normally defined as the total blood volume or plasma [1]. Subsequently, the drug then equilibrates into the tissue, including highly perfused tissues such as the heart, lungs, liver, brain, and kidneys and poorly perfused tissues such as muscles, lean tissue, fat, and bone [1, 2, 4]. Many drugs are large molecules that are lipophilic and/or only partially ionized, which hinders their excretion through the kidneys. Thus, in order for drugs to be eliminated, they must be metabolized into polar, water-soluble compounds that are fully ionized at physiological pH [3–5]. Consequently, metabolism is the first phase of drug clearance and involves modifications to the drug such as the introduction of polar groups usually by enzymes in the liver [3]. Drug metabolites are often less active than the parent compound and can also be responsible for unwanted (toxic) side effects [5], although in some cases

Z. Zhang • K.R. Gogarty • F. Daryaee • P.J. Tonge (✉)
Institute for Chemical Biology and Drug Discovery, Department of Chemistry,
Stony Brook University, Stony Brook, NY, USA

Department of Radiology, Stony Brook University School of Medicine,
Stony Brook, NY, USA
e-mail: peter.tonge@stonybrook.edu

S.K. Jain (ed.), *Imaging Infections*, DOI 10.1007/978-3-319-54592-9_9

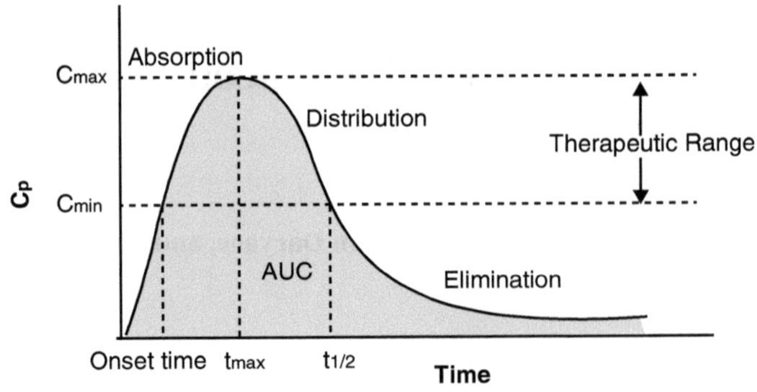

Figure 9.1 A hypothetical concentration-time curve [1]

metabolism can generate the active therapeutic compound, for example, if drugs are administered as prodrugs [3]. The second phase of drug clearance involves elimination of the metabolites as well as parent drug typically by the kidneys but also through the intestines and occasionally the lungs [3].

Since the concentration of drug at the target site will directly influence the therapeutic outcome, it is critical to quantify drug concentration in the human body as a function of time and to relate drug PK to the drug pharmacodynamics (PD) (viz. what the drug does to the body). In this chapter we first introduce the basic aspects of drug PK and then describe models to correlate drug PK and PD. Most existing approaches estimate drug concentration at the site of action using experimental measurements of plasma drug concentration. However, it is clear that direct knowledge of tissue drug concentration would have a major impact on the predictive power of PK/PD models, and we describe how positron emission tomography (PET) can fulfill this goal.

9.2 Drug Pharmacokinetics

The change in drug concentration as a function of time following administration is normally described by a drug concentration-time curve (Figure 9.1). Analysis of this curve yields several PK parameters including the minimum ($C_{\min}$) and maximum ($C_{\max}$) drug concentration in the plasma; the time at which the drug concentration in the plasma (C_p) reaches a maximum ($t_{\max}$); the area under the concentration-time curve (AUC) [1]; the volume of distribution (V_d), which is the ratio of total drug in the body and the plasma drug concentration at the same time point [1]; and the half-life of the drug ($t_{1/2}$), which is the time taken for half of the drug concentration to be eliminated from the body [3].

9.2.1 Pharmacokinetic and Pharmacodynamics Relationships

The main purpose of analyzing drug PK is to determine the drug concentration as a function of time and then correlate drug PK with drug PD [1]. The PK/PD relationship determines the relationship between drug dose, response, and toxicity and is used to predict drug efficacy, to design drug dosing regimens, and even to predict the outcome of treatment. PK/PD relationships are established by first determining drug concentration as a function of time following administration. Most commonly these studies focus on the plasma drug concentration and primarily involve techniques based on mass spectrometry (MS). Historically, gas chromatography/MS (GC/MS) was used, and only volatile molecules could be analyzed with low selectivity and sensitivity [6]. The coupling of liquid chromatography (LC) with soft ionization techniques, such as electrospray ionization (ESI) or atmospheric pressure chemical ionization (APCI) together with triple quadruple mass analysis (MS/MS), has dramatically broadened the types of compounds that can be quantified [6]. LC-MS/MS, which is commonly referred to as tandem-mass spectrometry, can simultaneously generate weight and structural and quantitative information with high sensitivity, is fairly rapid, and can selectively detect less than 1 ng/mL of drug in samples such as plasma, urine, and CSF [6].

Once the drug plasma concentration has been determined, the variation in drug concentration as a function of time is analyzed using mathematical models that calculate the PK parameters (Figure 9.1). These PK parameters are then correlated with drug PD, usually after taking into account plasma protein binding, so that the relationship to PD is with the free drug concentration rather than the total drug concentration. In addition, PK/PD relationships for antibiotics usually utilize the minimum inhibitory concentration (MIC) as a metric for antibiotic activity, which is the lowest drug concentration that completely inhibits the growth of a microorganism in vitro.

Antibiotics are normally classified depending on which PK parameter best describes antibacterial activity [7, 8]. Antibiotics such as β-lactams [9], and erythromycin [10], demonstrate time-dependent killing in which the maximum effect depends on how long the drug concentration remains above the MIC. For these antibiotics, time above MIC ($t >$ MIC) is the most applicable driver of in vivo antibacterial activity [11], and dosing regimens are designed to maximize the duration of exposure (i.e., the time that the blood/plasma drug concentration remains above MIC). In contrast, antibiotics such as aminoglycosides [12] and fluoroquinolones [10] show concentration-dependent killing in which the rate and extent of bacterial kill depends on the concentration of drug. For this group of antibiotics, C_{max} or AUC governs in vivo drug efficacy, and dosing regimens are designed to maximize C_{max}/MIC or AUC/MIC [13]. A third class of antibiotics, which includes vancomycin [10], streptogramins, and macrolides such as azithromycin, show time-dependent killing but also have persistent effects (post-antibiotic effect). In this case AUC/MIC is the driver of in vivo antibacterial activity and dosing regimens maximize the total amount of drug given to maximize the duration of the PAE.

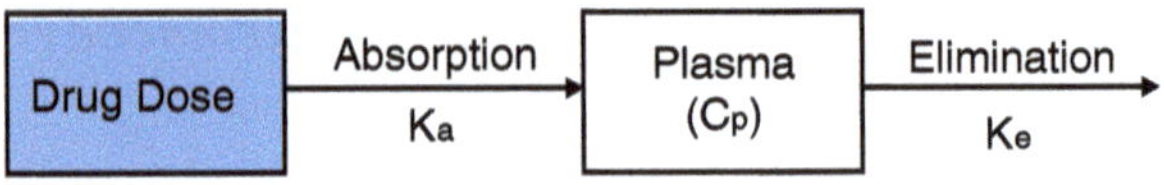

Figure 9.2 A single-compartment PK model [1]

9.2.2 *Single and Multi-Compartment PK Models*

A critical step in establishing a PK/PD relationship depends on the PK model used to estimate drug concentration in the human body. The simplest analysis uses a single compartment to describe the time course of drug concentration (Figure 9.2). This model assumes that the human body is one homogenous kinetic unit in which the drug rapidly equilibrates between the blood and tissues [1]. This model also assumes that drug elimination follows first-order kinetics [14]. One of the limitations of the single-compartment model is the assumption that the drug rapidly equilibrates throughout the body [1, 15]. Often there is a delay in the distribution of drug between plasma and tissue, and consequently drug concentration in the target tissue can be lower (or potentially higher) than estimates based on plasma concentration [16]. This is critical for antibacterial agents since most infections occur in tissues, and therefore a more accurate correlation between PK and PD requires direct knowledge of drug concentration at the site of infection.

In general there are several challenges to directly determining drug tissue concentration, not least of which is the difficulty of acquiring tissue samples from humans as well as the possibility that drug concentrations may be below the detection limit of standard analytical methods. Consequently, the current strategy is to estimate drug concentration in the target tissue using a multi-compartment PK model which is populated with measurements of plasma drug concentration as a function of time [17] (Figure 9.3). The multi-compartment PK model estimates the difference between plasma and tissue drug concentration by adding one or more peripheral tissue compartments: homogenous units representative of the site of action [1, 2]. Drug distribution between the different compartments is then described by a series of rate constants: in Figure 9.3, k_{12} and k_{21} are used to describe drug exchange between plasma and a tissue compartment. Although multi-compartment models are more realistic representations of drug distribution, it is sometimes difficult to decide which model to use, while in most cases there is no direct experimental proof to validate predictions made by the models.

Thus, the challenge remains to determine tissue drug concentration directly and then to use the tissue drug concentration for PK/PD correlations or to fit the tissue drug concentration to a multi-compartment model and couple it to a PD model. As we describe below, this challenge can be met by positron emission tomography (PET).

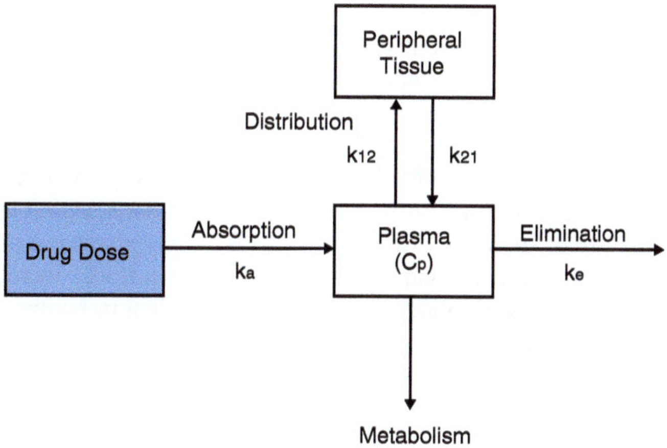

Figure 9.3 A multi-compartment PK model [1]

9.3 Positron Emission Tomography

PET is a powerful method for rapidly determining drug bio-distribution and quantifying the concentration of molecules of interest in different tissues and organs. The method is noninvasive and very sensitive, providing key advantages over methods such as LC-MS/MS which require tissue samples and are less sensitive. Typically, the detection limit for LC-MS/MS is around 0.1 ng/ml [6], whereas PET can detect 0.1 nCi/mL which is 10^{-5} ng/mL assuming a specific activity of 1 Ci/μmol and a molecular weight of 400 g/mol [18]. Although the spatial resolution of PET is generally only 1–2 mm, the ability of this method to locate specific tissues and organs, and thus generate the necessary data for multi-compartment PK analysis, is significantly improved by combining PET with other imaging techniques such as computed tomography (CT) or magnetic resonance imaging (MRI) that have higher anatomical accuracy. In addition, PET imaging can also be used to assess drug-target occupancy, and thus this method is an excellent tool for informing mechanism-based PK/PD modeling and assisting in predictions of drug efficacy, designing drug regimens, and predicting drug candidate outcome.

There are also hurdles that have to be overcome in the application of PET to determining drug PK, the principal being the necessity to develop synthetic methods in which the PET radionuclide is introduced very rapidly in high yield and as late as possible in the synthesis. This is because ^{11}C and ^{18}F, the two PET isotopes that are often used for radiotracer synthesis, have half-lives of only 20.4 and 110 min, respectively. The fraction of drug that contains a radiolabel is often very small due to the specific activity of the tracer: for example, ^{18}F-fluoride is usually only $\leq 1\%$ ^{18}F, the remainder of the material being ^{19}F-fluoride. In general the specific activity that can be achieved from a daily radiosynthesis run ranges from less than 0.01 Ci/μmol to higher than 100 Ci/μmol. For a typical rodent preclinical PET imaging study, usually about 500 μCi of tracer is injected. This means that only 0.5 nmol of the investigational compound will be injected, and for a compound with a MW of 400 g/mol, this translates to a dose of 0.2 μg (1 μg/kg for a 200 g rat), which is much lower than a normal therapeutic dose of 1–100 mg/kg. Thus, one key question is whether drug PK obtained with a microdose of PET radiotracer scales linearly with concentration since one or more events involved in drug ADME can have saturable processes. Conversely, the use of such low drug doses in a PET study also has a major advantage: since the amount of compound used is so much lower than a therapeutic dose, PET imaging can be used to obtain first-in-human PK data in humans—so called Phase 0 clinical trials [19–21].

9.3.1 Carbon-11

The application of PET to PK analysis was recognized not long after the PET method was developed, and PET has been heavily used to generate PK data for investigational compounds. However, there are relatively few examples of attempts to monitor the concentration of antibacterial agents in infected tissues. An early study involved an analysis of ^{11}C-labeled erythromycin in patients with lobular pneumonia [22]. In this study, [^{11}C]-erythromycin was diluted with nonradioactive erythromycin, and 270 mg of total erythromycin was administered to patients via intravenous injection. The concentration of the drug in both blood and the lungs was determined by PET, and it was found that the average drug concentration in the entire lungs was above the MIC. In addition, no significant difference was observed between the density-normalized drug concentrations in pneumonic and healthy lungs. However, due to the limitations of PET scanners used in the early 1980s, including low anatomical resolution, it was not possible to determine the drug concentration at different locations in the lungs and in particular in the infected areas of the lungs.

9.3.2 Fluorine-18

If the objective is to capture the entire distribution and elimination time course for a complete PK analysis, then it is likely that the imaging time window provided by ^{11}C is insufficient for most antibiotics. Instead, ^{18}F, which has a half-life of 110 min, is a better choice for many drugs. However, given that not all drugs contain fluorine and that the addition of a fluorine atom might significantly alter drug ADME, the use of ^{18}F is usually limited to the drugs that already contain fluorine or those whose PK profile may not be significantly altered by the addition of a fluorine atom. ^{18}F is a very popular PET tracer and several approaches are available for ^{18}F labeling including $^{18}F/^{19}F$ exchange [23], as well as more recent methods such as nickel-/platinum-catalyzed fluorination [24, 25].

Increasing numbers of studies have shown that the disease state can influence the distribution of drugs [26–32]. This is particularly true for infectious diseases, where the inflammatory response to infection can alter the expression and activity of metabolic enzymes such as cytochrome P450s [31, 32] as well as proteins involved in drug uptake and efflux [30], thus changing drug transport and metabolism [27, 30]. For instance, in rabbits it was observed that tuberculosis (TB) infection alters the concentration of drug in infected, diseased areas of the lung compared to uninfected sites [33]. However, the distribution of drugs in infected animals or humans is not widely studied due to the challenge of acquiring infected tissue samples and lack of proper tools to analyze the samples even if the tissue samples are accessible. As a result, for some infectious diseases, it is not even known whether the prescribed drug can actually reach the site of infection, and treatment is thus based on trial and error. This is a significant problem in life-threatening infections, such as osteomyelitis, where information concerning drug distribution is urgently needed. Clearly in these cases PET imaging can play a major role in informing therapeutic options.

9.3.3 2-^{18}F-Fluoroisonicotinic Acid Hydrazide

The use of PET to determine the PK of drugs in infected tissue was demonstrated by imaging a fluoro analog of isoniazid (INH), a front-line drug for the treatment of tuberculosis infection [34]. INH was radiolabeled at the 2′ position with ^{18}F to give 2-[^{18}F]-fluoroisonicotinic acid hydrazide (2-^{18}F-INH), and this radiotracer was imaged for 2 h in mice infected with *Mycobacterium tuberculosis*. Analysis of the PET/CT data demonstrated that 2-^{18}F-INH accumulated in the liver of both infected and uninfected mice (Figure 9.4). However, compared with uninfected mice (Figure 9.4a), 2-^{18}F-INH significantly accumulated in the lungs of infected mice (Figure 9.4b). In particular, foci of activity were observed in necrotic pulmonary tuberculosis lesions indicating that the drug accumulated specifically at the site of infection (Figure 9.4b). While previous ex vivo studies using LC-MS/MS or MALDI technology have already shown that INH accumulates in the lungs [35, 36], the accumulation of the drug into TB lesions has not been observed. The PET/CT imaging of 2-^{18}F-INH provides quantitative INH concentrations in TB-infected lung tissues including TB lesions. In addition, unlike the ex vivo methods which only provide drug concentration at a single time point from each tissue biopsy, continuous dynamic monitoring of 2-^{18}F-INH concentration in infected lung tissues was achieved with a single PET scan. The 2-^{18}F-INH study strongly supports the ability of PET/CT to noninvasively determine antibiotic levels at the site of infection. The 2-^{18}F-INH imaging study indicates that drug distribution can be affected by infection: in this case significantly higher levels of drug were observed at the site of infection (Figure 9.5). It is already generally accepted that infection can affect drug PK, and in a standard drug discovery program, PK studies are

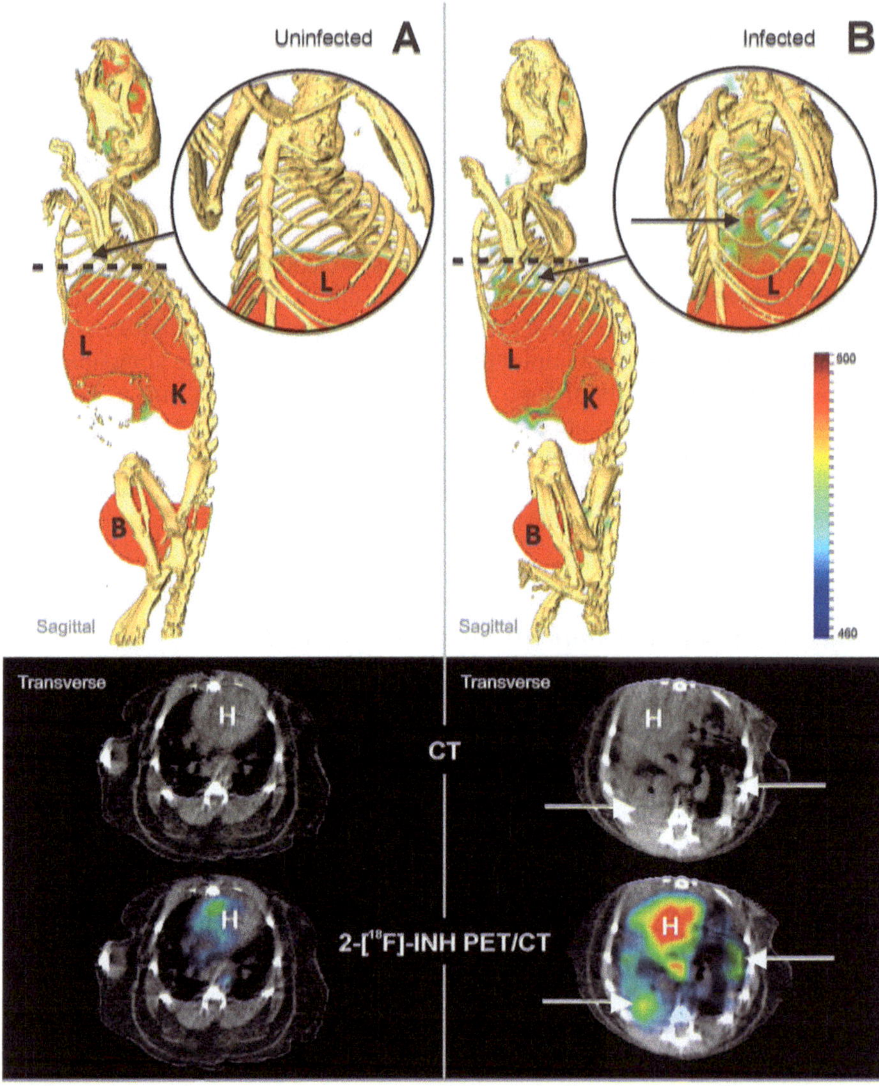

Figure 9.4 Distribution of 2-^{18}F-INH in uninfected (**a**) and *Mycobacterium tuberculosis*-infected mice (**b**). The foci of 2-^{18}F-INH accumulation are indicated by *arrows*. Adapted from Weinstein and Liu et al. [34]

performed in infected animals [37, 38]. However, these studies often only focus on the PK determined from levels of drug in plasma, and our PET/CT study underlines the importance of not only performing PK studies in infected animals and subjects but actually determining the levels of drugs at their site of action. In the 2-^{18}F-INH study, we observe an increase in drug levels in the TB-infected lungs; however, in principal infection could also reduce the ability of drug to reach the

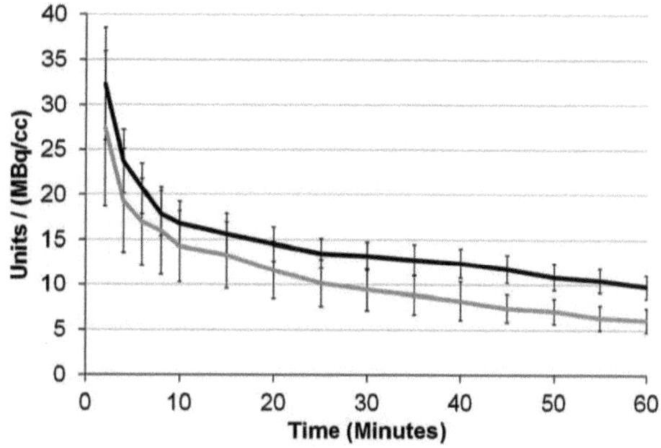

Figure 9.5 Accumulation of 2-^{18}F-INH in healthy (*gray*) and *Mycobacterium tuberculosis*-infected lungs (*black*). Adapted from Weinstein and Liu et al. [34]

infectious agent, resulting in lower drug levels in infected tissue than expected [39], leading to reduced efficacy and triggering the emergence of drug resistance [40]. Interestingly, due to its accumulation in *M. tuberculosis* bacteria, 2-^{18}F-INH may have potential as a biomarker for clinical TB imaging in addition to its effectiveness as a PET tracer for pharmacokinetic studies.

9.3.4 ^{11}C-Isonicotinic Acid Hydrazide (^{11}C-INH)

Having established that PET imaging can be used to determine drug concentration at the site of infection, the next step is to demonstrate how this information can inform multi-compartment PK analysis. However, currently there is only a limited amount of PET imaging data that can be used. In attempt to use PET data to model drug concentration, we used a multi-compartment PK model to analyze drug bio-distribution data for ^{11}C-labeled isoniazid (^{11}C-INH) in nonhuman primates [18]. In this study, the concentration of ^{11}C-INH in plasma was obtained as a function of time from blood samples, while dynamic tracer accumulation in the lungs and other tissues was determined by PET/CT imaging. The PK of INH was then analyzed in two ways: based solely on the plasma drug concentration and based on the tissue concentration (Figure 9.6). Initially a traditional two-compartment PK model was used to fit the plasma drug concentration data. Using previously reported values of k_e (0.005 min^{-1}) and V_d (12.5 L) in nonhuman primates [41], Eq. 1 gave values for k_{12} and k_{21} of 0.032 and 0.0175 min^{-1}, respectively. The values of k_{12} and k_{21} were then used to predict the tissue concentration of the drug (Eq. 2) (Figure 9.6b). However, this approach gave relatively poor agreement between predicted and experimental tissue concentrations including the lungs, which is one of the primary sites of action of INH. We used INH concentration in the lungs determined by PET imaging as

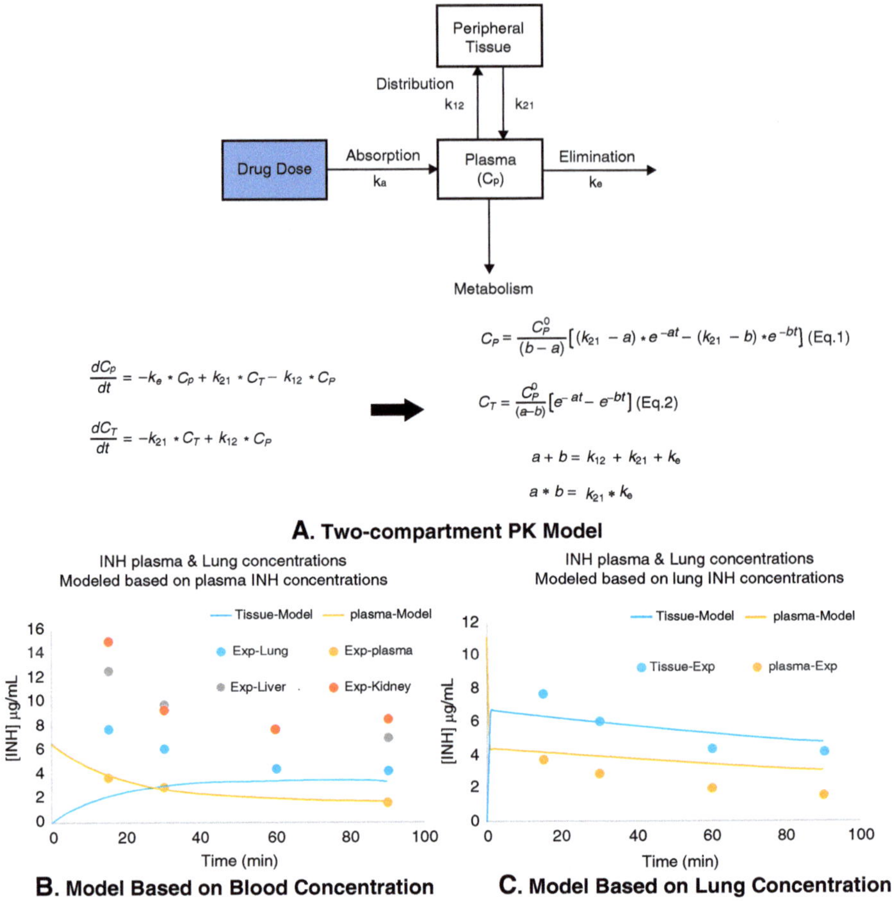

$$\frac{dC_P}{dt} = -k_e * C_P + k_{21} * C_T - k_{12} * C_P$$

$$\frac{dC_T}{dt} = -k_{21} * C_T + k_{12} * C_P$$

$$C_P = \frac{C_P^0}{(b-a)}[(k_{21}-a) * e^{-at} - (k_{21}-b) * e^{-bt}] \text{ (Eq.1)}$$

$$C_T = \frac{C_P^0}{(a-b)}[e^{-at} - e^{-bt}] \text{ (Eq.2)}$$

$$a + b = k_{12} + k_{21} + k_e$$

$$a * b = k_{21} * k_e$$

Figure 9.6 Multi-compartment PK models of INH drug concentration in blood and tissues. (**a**) The two-compartment PK model. (**b**) Predicted drug concentration based on plasma drug concentration. (**c**) Predicted drug concentration based on the experimentally observed concentration of drug in the lungs. Adapted from Liu et al. [44]

input to Eq. 2 (Figure 9.6) to calculate k_{12} and k_{21}. However, the model is not able to reliably fit the tissue data nor predict the plasma drug concentration (Figure 9.6c). In this case the short data collection window provided by the ^{11}C tracer is likely not long enough to capture the complete drug elimination process, reinforcing the importance of using tracers with longer half-lives such as ^{18}F. In this regard, we note that ^{18}F-ciprofloxacin enabled distribution and elimination of this drug to be monitored over 5 h, from which an elimination rate (k_e) of drug from infected tissues could be calculated ($k_e = 0.693/t_{1/2}$, and $t_{1/2}$ was reported to be 87 ± 24 min) [42].

9.3.5 *^{18}F-C-SNAT*

Although only a limited number of ^{18}F radiotracers have been analyzed by PET imaging in infection, there are many examples where ^{18}F PET has been used in other diseases. For example, PET was used to determine the bio-distribution uptake and accumulation of the apoptosis tracer ^{18}F-C-SNAT in tumor tissues [43]. The PK of the tracer in tumor tissues was modeled using a three-compartment PK model, in which the two tissue compartments represented free tracer in the tissue and the tracer "retained" in the tissue. In this case, the model was able to accurately fit the experimental tissue data. The investigators also compared tracer PK with and without drug treatment and showed that both the rate of tracer delivery to the tumor tissue (k_1) and the rate of accumulation of tracer in the tissue (k_3) increased significantly after treatment. This example illustrates how ^{18}F PET imaging can inform multi-compartment PK analysis to understand the relationship between dose, plasma drug concentration, and tissue drug concentration.

9.4 Summary

PET imaging is likely to be a valuable tool for informing multi-compartment PK analysis by directly providing tissue drug concentration as a function of time, enabling a better understanding of the quantitative relationship between drug doses, time, and drug concentrations at the site of infection. Improved PK models coupled with real-time noninvasive PET imaging will support the design of drug regimens and allow the effect of drug dose on tissue drug concentrations to be directly monitored.

References

1. Rowe, P., *Pharmacokinetics*. 1 ed. 2012: Bookboon.
2. Ruiz-Garcia, A., et al., *Pharmacokinetics in drug discovery*. J Pharm Sci, 2008. **97**(2): p. 654-90.
3. Kerns, E. and L. Di, *Drug-like properties: concepts, structure design and methods: from ADME to toxicity optimization*. 2008: Academic Press.
4. Reddy, M.B., et al., *Physiologically Based Pharmacokinetic Modeling: A Tool for Understanding ADMET Properties and Extrapolating to Human*. New Insights into Toxicity and Drug Testing. 2013.
5. Singh, S.S., *Preclinical pharmacokinetics: an approach towards safer and efficacious drugs*. Curr Drug Metab, 2006. **7**(2): p. 165-82.
6. Marzo, A. and L.D. Bo, *Tandem mass spectrometry (LC-MS-MS): a predominant role in bioassays for pharmacokinetic studies*. Arzneimittelforschung, 2007. **57**(2): p. 122-8.
7. Craig, W.A., *Choosing an antibiotic on the basis of pharmacodynamics*. Ear Nose Throat J, 1998. **77**(6 Suppl): p. 7-11; discussion 11-2.
8. Drusano, G.L., *Antimicrobial pharmacodynamics: critical interactions of 'bug and drug'*. Nat Rev Microbiol, 2004. **2**(4): p. 289-300.

9. MacVane, S.H., J.L. Kuti, and D.P. Nicolau, *Prolonging beta-lactam infusion: a review of the rationale and evidence, and guidance for implementation.* Int J Antimicrob Agents, 2014. **43**(2): p. 105-13.
10. Mehrotra, R., R. De Gaudio, and M. Palazzo, *Antibiotic pharmacokinetic and pharmacodynamic considerations in critical illness.* Intensive Care Med, 2004. **30**(12): p. 2145-56.
11. Vogelman, B., et al., *Correlation of antimicrobial pharmacokinetic parameters with therapeutic efficacy in an animal model.* J Infect Dis, 1988. **158**(4): p. 831-47.
12. Craig, W.A., J. Redington, and S.C. Ebert, *Pharmacodynamics of amikacin in vitro and in mouse thigh and lung infections.* J Antimicrob Chemother, 1991. **27 Suppl C**: p. 29-40.
13. Moise, P.A. and J.J. Schentag, *Pharmacokinetic and pharmacodynamic modelling of antibiotic therapy.* Curr Opin Infect Dis, 1998. **11**(6): p. 673-80.
14. Jones, A.W., A. Eklund, and R. Kronstrand, *Concentration-time profiles of gamma-hydroxybutyrate in blood after recreational doses are best described by zero-order rather than first-order kinetics.* J Anal Toxicol, 2009. **33**(6): p. 332-5.
15. Zhao, L., N. Li, and H. Yang, *A new stochastic approach to multi-compartment pharmacokinetic models: probability of traveling route and distribution of residence time in linear and nonlinear systems.* J Pharmacokinet Pharmacodyn, 2011. **38**(1): p. 83-104.
16. Mouton, J.W., et al., *Tissue concentrations: do we ever learn?* J Antimicrob Chemother, 2008. **61**(2): p. 235-7.
17. de Araujo, B.V., et al., *PK-PD modeling of beta-lactam antibiotics: in vitro or in vivo models?* J Antibiot (Tokyo), 2011. **64**(6): p. 439-46.
18. Liu, L., et al., *Radiosynthesis and Bioimaging of the Tuberculosis Chemotherapeutics Isoniazid, Rifampicin and Pyrazinamide in Baboons.* Journal of Medicinal Chemistry, 2010. **53**(7): p. 2882-2891.
19. Bauer, M., et al., *A positron emission tomography microdosing study with a potential antiamyloid drug in healthy volunteers and patients with Alzheimer's disease.* Clin Pharmacol Ther, 2006. **80**(3): p. 216-27.
20. Saleem, A., et al., *Plasma pharmacokinetic evaluation of cytotoxic agents radiolabelled with positron emitting radioisotopes.* Cancer Chemother Pharmacol, 2008. **61**(5): p. 865-73.
21. Wagner, C.C., et al., *A combined accelerator mass spectrometry-positron emission tomography human microdose study with 14C- and 11C-labelled verapamil.* Clin Pharmacokinet, 2011. **50**(2): p. 111-20.
22. Wollmer, P., et al., *Measurement of pulmonary erythromycin concentration in patients with lobar pneumonia by means of positron tomography.* Lancet, 1982. **2**(8312): p. 1361-4.
23. Blom, E., F. Karimi, and B. Långström, *[18F]/19F exchange in fluorine containing compounds for potential use in 18F-labelling strategies.* Journal of Labelled Compounds and Radiopharmaceuticals, 2009. **52**(12): p. 504-511.
24. Lee, E., et al., *A fluoride-derived electrophilic late-stage fluorination reagent for PET imaging.* Science, 2011. **334**(6056): p. 639-42.
25. Lee, E., J.M. Hooker, and T. Ritter, *Nickel-mediated oxidative fluorination for PET with aqueous [18F] fluoride.* J Am Chem Soc, 2012. **134**(42): p. 17456-8.
26. Gandhi, A., B. Moorthy, and R. Ghose, *Drug disposition in pathophysiological conditions.* Curr Drug Metab, 2012. **13**(9): p. 1327-44.
27. Aitken, A.E., T.A. Richardson, and E.T. Morgan, *Regulation of drug-metabolizing enzymes and transporters in inflammation.* Annu Rev Pharmacol Toxicol, 2006. **46**: p. 123-49.
28. Danhof, M., *Kinetics of drug action in disease states: towards physiology-based pharmacodynamic (PBPD) models.* J Pharmacokinet Pharmacodyn, 2015.
29. Kato, R., *Drug metabolism under pathological and abnormal physiological states in animals and man.* Xenobiotica, 1977. **7**(1-2): p. 25-92.
30. Morgan, E.T., et al., *Regulation of drug-metabolizing enzymes and transporters in infection, inflammation, and cancer.* Drug Metab Dispos, 2008. **36**(2): p. 205-16.
31. Renton, K.W., *Alteration of drug biotransformation and elimination during infection and inflammation.* Pharmacol Ther, 2001. **92**(2-3): p. 147-63.

32. Renton, K.W., *Cytochrome P450 regulation and drug biotransformation during inflammation and infection.* Curr Drug Metab, 2004. **5**(3): p. 235-43.
33. Prideaux, B., et al., *High-sensitivity MALDI-MRM-MS imaging of moxifloxacin distribution in tuberculosis-infected rabbit lungs and granulomatous lesions.* Anal Chem, 2011. **83**(6): p. 2112-8.
34. Weinstein, E.A., et al., *Noninvasive determination of 2-[18F]-fluoroisonicotinic acid hydrazide pharmacokinetics by positron emission tomography in Mycobacterium tuberculosis-infected mice.* Antimicrob Agents Chemother, 2012. **56**(12): p. 6284-90.
35. Manier, M.L., et al., *Reagent precoated targets for rapid in-tissue derivatization of the anti-tuberculosis drug isoniazid followed by MALDI imaging mass spectrometry.* J Am Soc Mass Spectrom, 2011. **22**(8): p. 1409-19.
36. Kjellsson, M.C., et al., *Pharmacokinetic evaluation of the penetration of antituberculosis agents in rabbit pulmonary lesions.* Antimicrob Agents Chemother, 2012. **56**(1): p. 446-57.
37. Berkhout, J., et al., *Pharmacokinetics and penetration of ceftazidime and avibactam into epithelial lining fluid in thigh- and lung-infected mice.* Antimicrob Agents Chemother, 2015. **59**(4): p. 2299-304.
38. He, J., et al., *Pharmacokinetics and efficacy of liposomal polymyxin B in a murine pneumonia model.* Int J Antimicrob Agents, 2013. **42**(6): p. 559-64.
39. DeMarco, V.P., et al., *Determination of [11C]Rifampin Pharmacokinetics within Mycobacterium tuberculosis-Infected Mice by Using Dynamic Positron Emission Tomography Bioimaging.* Antimicrob Agents Chemother, 2015. **59**(9): p. 5768-74.
40. Buerger, C., et al., *Pharmacokinetics of unbound linezolid in plasma and tissue interstitium of critically ill patients after multiple dosing using microdialysis.* Antimicrob Agents Chemother, 2006. **50**(7): p. 2455-63.
41. Kumar Verma, R., et al., *Partial biodistribution and pharmacokinetics of isoniazid and rifabutin following pulmonary delivery of inhalable microparticles to rhesus macaques.* Mol Pharm, 2012. **9**(4): p. 1011-6.
42. Langer, O., et al., *In vitro and in vivo evaluation of [18F]ciprofloxacin for the imaging of bacterial infections with PET.* Eur J Nucl Med Mol Imaging, 2005. **32**(2): p. 143-50.
43. Palner, M., et al., *Preclinical Kinetic Analysis of the Caspase-3/7 PET Tracer 18F-C-SNAT: Quantifying the Changes in Blood Flow and Tumor Retention After Chemotherapy.* J Nucl Med, 2015. **56**(9): p. 1415-21.
44. Liu, L., et al., *Radiosynthesis and bioimaging of the tuberculosis chemotherapeutics isoniazid, rifampicin and pyrazinamide in baboons.* J Med Chem, 2010. **53**(7): p. 2882-91.

Chapter 10
Biodistribution and Pharmacokinetics of Antimicrobials

Alvaro A. Ordonez, Lauren E. Bambarger, Sanjay K. Jain, and Edward A. Weinstein

10.1 Introduction

Traditional techniques to study the pharmacokinetics and biodistribution of antimicrobial drugs are performed by measuring drug concentrations in the blood. These data are often complemented by drug measurement from direct tissue sampling, but given the difficulties in obtaining such tissues in humans, the studies are mostly limited to animal models. However, drug concentrations at the target tissues, i.e., the site of infection can often differ markedly from those measured in blood. Since the success of a drug is highly dependent on the bioavailability and pharmacokinetic properties, information about drug distribution in the target tissues, early in the drug development pathway, is essential. Low-energy isotope (^{14}C, ^{3}H)-labeled antimicrobials have been utilized extensively for pharmacokinetic studies in animal models for more than 50 years [1]. However, these isotopes can only be measured by invasive sampling and/or radioactivity quantification of the tissues harvested from

A.A. Ordonez • L.E. Bambarger
Department of Pediatrics, Johns Hopkins University School of Medicine, Baltimore, MD, USA

Center for Infection and Inflammation Imaging Research, Johns Hopkins University School of Medicine, Baltimore, MD, USA

S.K. Jain
Department of Pediatrics, Johns Hopkins University School of Medicine, Baltimore, MD, USA

Center for Infection and Inflammation Imaging Research, Johns Hopkins University School of Medicine, Baltimore, MD, USA

Department of International Health, Johns Hopkins Bloomberg School of Public Health, Baltimore, MD, USA

E.A. Weinstein (✉)
Department of Medicine, Johns Hopkins University School of Medicine, Baltimore, MD, USA

Center for Infection and Inflammation Imaging Research, Johns Hopkins University School of Medicine, Baltimore, MD, USA
e-mail: edward.a.weinstein@gmail.com

S.K. Jain (ed.), *Imaging Infections*, DOI 10.1007/978-3-319-54592-9_10

the animal models. Autoradiography provides useful two-dimensional information of the drug concentration in a specific section of the tissue, but its results are limited, requiring different animals for multiple time points.

The development of nuclear imaging techniques allowed the noninvasive assessment of deep tissue from multiple different compartments simultaneously. Many drugs can be radiolabeled without alteration (or minimal effects) of the chemical properties of the original compound and evaluated using two-dimensional planar gamma scintigraphy, single-photon emission computed tomography (SPECT), or positron emission tomography (PET). Due to the improvements in resolution and sensitivity of these imaging techniques, ^{11}C- or ^{18}F-radiolabeled molecules can be detected with PET in the nanomolar to picomolar concentration range. Nuclear imaging can also use targeted agents or activatable probes to evaluate the distribution and function of the target of a specific drug. This has been a very valuable tool for the discovery and development of central nervous system drugs [2]. The translational potential is a major driving force promoting nuclear imaging in pharmaceutical research. PET is the most widely available quantitative noninvasive technique that can be used to study distribution of drug in tissue in humans at multiple time points. Therefore, its use in preclinical and clinical phases could facilitate the development process for new antimicrobials.

10.1.1 Microdosing

Most PET pharmacokinetic studies use microdosing, where only microgram amounts of the radiolabeled and unlabeled drug are administered to the testing subject [3]. In contrast to regular antibiotic therapy, concentration of these radiolabeled drugs in tissues is typically in the nanomolar range. Using these very small amounts of drug, valuable pharmacokinetic and distribution information can be obtained without inducing pharmacological effects, thereby reducing or even preventing unwanted side effects [4]. Although they provide useful data in the drug distribution and pharmacokinetic parameters, these early studies are not meant to replace traditional phase 1 studies, where safety and tolerability are determined.

10.2 Antibacterials

A large number of antimicrobial drugs have been radiolabeled in the last several decades (Table 10.1). Nuclear imaging has been used in a handful of publications where biodistribution was studied in animal models; however, most of these investigations were designed to evaluate the potential of the radiolabeled antibiotic as a bacteria-specific imaging agent. Therefore, pharmacokinetic parameters have been analyzed only for a small number of these compounds.

Table 10.1 Radiolabeled antimicrobials

Antibiotic	Radioisotope	Imaging modality	Stage	Reference
Antibacterials				
Fluoroquinolones				
Ciprofloxacin	^{99m}Tc, ^{18}F	Scintigraphy, SPECT, PET	Clinical	[9, 40]
Clinafloxacin	^{99m}Tc	[a]	Preclinical	[41]
Difloxacin	^{99m}Tc	[a]	Preclinical	[42]
Enrofloxacin	^{99m}Tc	SPECT	Preclinical	[43]
Fleroxacin	^{18}F, ^{19}F	PET, MRS	Clinical	[14]
Garenoxacin	^{99m}Tc	[a]	Preclinical	[44]
Gatifloxacin	^{99m}Tc	[a]	Preclinical	[45]
Gemifloxacin	^{99m}Tc	[a]	Preclinical	[46]
Levofloxacin	^{99m}Tc	Scintigraphy	Preclinical	[47, 48]
Lomefloxacin	^{99m}Tc, ^{18}F	Scintigraphy, rectilinear scanning	Clinical	[18, 48, 49]
Moxifloxacin	^{99m}Tc	Scintigraphy	Preclinical	[50]
Norfloxacin	^{99m}Tc	Scintigraphy, SPECT	Preclinical	[48, 51, 52]
Ofloxacin	^{99m}Tc-tricarbonyl	Scintigraphy	Preclinical	[48, 53]
Pefloxacin	^{99m}Tc	[a]	Preclinical	[42]
Rufloxacin	^{99m}Tc	[a]	Preclinical	[54]
Sarafloxacin	^{99m}Tc	[a]	Preclinical	[55]
Sitafloxacin	^{99m}Tc	Scintigraphy	Preclinical	[56, 57]
Sparfloxacin	^{99m}Tc	SPECT	Preclinical	[58]
Trovafloxacin	^{18}F	PET	Clinical	[16, 17]
β-Lactams				
Cefazolin	^{99m}Tc	[a]	Preclinical	[59]
Cefepime	^{99m}Tc	[a]	Preclinical	[45]
Cefoperazone	^{99m}Tc	[a]	Preclinical	[60]
Cefotaxime	^{99m}Tc	Scintigraphy	Preclinical	[61]
Ceftazidime	^{99m}Tc	Scintigraphy	Preclinical	[62]
Ceftizoxime	^{99m}Tc	Scintigraphy	Preclinical[b]	[63]
Ceftriaxone	^{99m}Tc	SPECT	Clinical	[64]
Cefuroxime	^{99m}Tc	Scintigraphy	Preclinical	[65, 66]
Meropenem	^{99m}Tc	SPECT	Preclinical	[67]
Inhibitors of protein synthesis				
Azithromycin	^{99m}Tc	[a]	Preclinical	[68]
Clarithromycin	^{99m}Tc	[a]	Preclinical	[69]
Clindamycin	^{99m}Tc	Scintigraphy	Preclinical	[70]
Doxycycline	^{99m}Tc	Scintigraphy	Preclinical	[71]
Erythromycin	^{11}C	PET	Clinical	[5]
Kanamycin	^{99m}Tc	Scintigraphy	Preclinical	[72]
Tetracycline	^{131}I	Scintigraphy	Preclinical	[73]

(continued)

Table 10.1 (continued)

Antibiotic	Radioisotope	Imaging modality	Stage	Reference
Vibramycin	^{99m}Tc	[a]	Preclinical	[74]
Antimycobacterials				
Ethambutol	^{99m}Tc	Scintigraphy	Clinical	[75]
Isoniazid	^{99m}Tc, ^{11}C, ^{18}F	Scintigraphy, PET	Preclinical	[22, 76–78]
Pyrazinamide	^{11}C	PET	Preclinical	[78]
Rifampin	^{99m}Tc, ^{11}C	Scintigraphy, PET	Preclinical	[25, 78, 79]
Other				
Alafosfalin	^{99m}Tc	Scintigraphy	Preclinical	[80]
Amoxicillin	^{99m}Tc	Scintigraphy	Preclinical	[81]
Linezolid	^{131}I	[a]	Preclinical	[82]
Nitrofurantoin	^{99m}Tc	Scintigraphy	Preclinical	[83]
Novobiocin	^{99m}Tc	[a]	Preclinical	[83]
Sulfanilamide	^{99m}Tc	[a]	Preclinical	[84]
Vancomycin	^{99m}Tc, ^{201}Tl, IRDye800CW	SPECT, optical imaging	Preclinical	[85–87]
Antifungals				
Fluconazole	^{18}F	PET	Clinical	[27, 28]
Antivirals				
Ganciclovir	^{18}F	PET	Preclinical	[33, 34]
Oseltamivir	^{11}C	PET	Preclinical	[36–38]
Stavudine	^{11}C	PET	Preclinical	[31]
Tenofovir	^{18}F	PET	Preclinical	[30]
Zanamivir	^{11}C	PET	Clinical	[35]
Zidovudine	^{11}C	PET	Preclinical	[32]

[a]In vivo imaging of the compound has not been reported
[b]Case report of a patient evaluated with 99mTc-ceftizoxime scintigraphy [88]

10.2.1 Macrolides

Erythromycin was the first antibiotic used for PET pharmacokinetic analysis. *N*-demethyl erythromycin was radiolabeled using a single-step reaction with ^{11}C, and the final product was injected into healthy volunteers and infected patients with lobar pneumonia [5]. An effective concentration of erythromycin was reached in the infected lung tissue within 10 min postinjection. This short equilibration time allowed the acquisition of enough data to determine the pharmacokinetic parameters during the 60 min PET scan.

10.2.2 Fluoroquinolones

10.2.2.1 Ciprofloxacin

Ciprofloxacin was initially developed as a bacteria-specific imaging agent. Due to its broad spectrum with gram-negative bacteria, easy radiolabeling method, and low cost, ^{99m}Tc-ciprofloxacin (commercialized as Infecton) was extensively studied in clinical and preclinical models [6, 7]. Although initial investigations were promising, subsequent research reported lack of specificity [8]. PET studies in humans with ^{18}F-ciprofloxacin provided information on tissue distribution and pharmacokinetics [9] but showed nonspecific accumulation in the infection site [10]. More recently, Langer et al. used a PET/microdialysis combination to measure the intracellular pharmacokinetics of ^{18}F-ciprofloxacin with unlabeled drug in the skeletal muscle of healthy human volunteers [11]. This is a promising approach that could be used to evaluate other antibiotics with intracellular sites of action.

10.2.2.2 Fleroxacin

^{18}F-labeled fleroxacin was used in PET imaging to evaluate the pharmacokinetic parameters of this fluoroquinolone in *E. coli*-infected mice, rats, and rabbits [12]. Subsequently, the pharmacokinetics of ^{18}F-fleroxacin were evaluated in healthy human volunteers [13] and patients with chronic bronchitis and complicated urinary tract infection [14]. Using ^{19}F magnetic resonance spectroscopy (MRS), Jynge et al. described the concentration of fleroxacin in the liver and muscle over time, providing support for the use of ^{19}F MRS as a way to noninvasively monitor fluorine-containing antibiotics [15].

10.2.2.3 Other Fluoroquinolones

Similar studies describing the biodistribution and pharmacokinetics of ^{18}F-trovafloxacin in humans and animal models were published by Fischman et al. [16, 17]. ^{18}F-Lomefloxacin has also been synthesized and the time-activity curves for major organs were obtained from rectilinear scans in healthy patients [18]. Other fluoroquinolones have also been radiolabeled but in vivo imaging data and/or pharmacokinetic analyses are not available (Table 10.1). A comprehensive review on the potential of fluoroquinolones as bacterial imaging agents was recently published by Auletta et al. [19].

10.2.3 *β-Lactams*

Multiple cephalosporins have been radiolabeled to determine their ability to detect infection and differentiate it from inflammation (Table 10.1). For example, ^{99m}Tc-ceftriaxone scintigraphy was used to evaluate *S. aureus* infection in rabbits and detect bacterial infection in orthopedic patients [20]. These radiolabels can also be used for study antimicrobial pharmacokinetics.

10.2.4 *Antimycobacterials*

Previously, in preclinical animal studies, direct measurement of drug concentration in necrotic lung lesions associated with pulmonary tuberculosis (TB) could only be accomplished via necropsy, which limits the number of time points assessable per animal and is only accomplishable in humans in extreme circumstances of lung resection. However, there is an urgent need to understand the pharmacokinetics of TB drugs at the site of disease, where the mycobacteria reside. PET imaging of radiolabeledantimycobacterials could provide valuable information for optimizing drug use for different forms of TB and for shortening TB treatments.

10.2.4.1 Isoniazid

Isoniazid, also known as isonicotinic acid hydrazide, is a first-line antibiotic agent for the prevention and treatment of latent and active TB. In initial preclinical studies, isoniazid was radiolabeled with ^{11}C and examined using PET imaging in healthy baboons [21]. These studies revealed that isoniazid, and/or the radiolabeled metabolites are rapidly cleared from circulation and most tissues, concentrating in the bladder over time. Subsequently, a radiofluorinated analog of isoniazid was developed, 2-^{18}F-fluoroisonicotinic acid hydrazide (2-^{18}F-INH), to examine the pharmacokinetic properties of the drug in TB-infected mice compared to healthy, uninfected mice [22]. When compared with uninfected mice, dynamic PET revealed that 2-^{18}F-INH significantly accumulates at the site of necrotic pulmonary TB lesions in infected mice [22].

10.2.4.2 Rifampin

Rifampin (also known as rifampicin) plays a key role in the treatment of a variety of bacterial infections including *M. tuberculosis*. Recent studies have suggested that increased rifampin dose could lead to a more rapid culture conversion rates in cases of pulmonary TB [23] and survival in patients with tuberculous meningitis [24]. ^{11}C-Rifampin was initially developed and used for PET-imaging pharmacokinetic

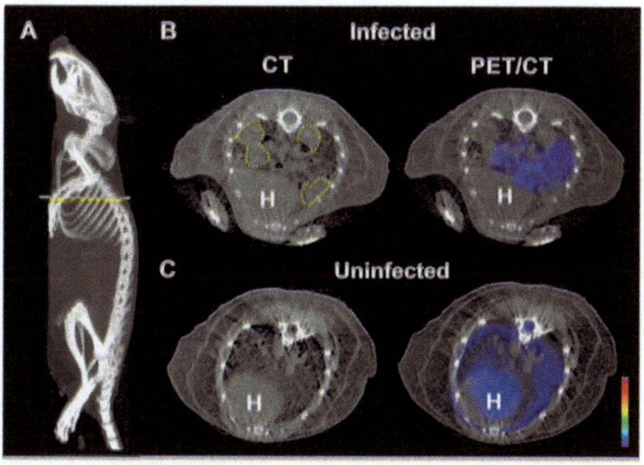

Figure 10.1 Pulmonary ^{11}C-rifampin PET/CT imaging of *Mycobacterium tuberculosis*-infected mice. (**a**) Three-dimensional CT reconstruction of a representative mouse is shown. The *yellow line* marks the location of transverse PET/CT images in (**b**, **c**). (**b**) Transverse images from a representative mouse 10 weeks after infection with *M. tuberculosis* demonstrate a much lower ^{11}C-rifampin PET signal (*purple*) in the areas of consolidation seen on CT (*gray areas, outlined*) than in uninfected areas. (**c**) More-uniform ^{11}C-rifampin PET signal is noted in the lung of an uninfected mouse. PET signal is also noted in the heart (H). Adapted from DeMarco and Ordonez et al. [25]

studies in healthy baboons [21]. Rifampin and/or the radiolabeled metabolites were determined to rapidly clear from tissue while concentrating in the liver and gallbladder. These findings supported previously identified drug excretion routes. Recently, ^{11}C-rifampin PET imaging was employed as a noninvasive and real-time alternative to study pharmacokinetics in live *Mycobacterium tuberculosis*-infected mice that develops necrotic and hypoxic granulomas [25]. In this study, lower concentrations of ^{11}C-rifampin were noted in lesions of infected mice that suggested lack of penetration into the necrotic tissue (Figure 10.1). AUC-time curves were similar between infected and uninfected mice in the liver and blood and were uniformly low in brain (10–20% of blood values) compartments. However, lower concentrations were noted in necrotic lung tissues of infected mice than in healthy lungs (Figure 10.2). Rifampin concentrations, derived from PET imaging, were analyzed using a noncompartmental intravenous bolus model (WinNonlin Standard) and shown in Table 10.2.

10.2.4.3 Pyrazinamide

Pyrazinamide is a prodrug used in the treatment of TB. ^{11}C-Pyrazinamide was generated by Liu et al. for in vivo real-time PET imaging of pyrazinamide pharmacokinetics and biodistribution in healthy baboons [21]. Preclinical studies with a radiolabeled analog, 5-^{18}F-pyrazinamide, were also recently reported in *M. tuberculosis*-infected mice [26].

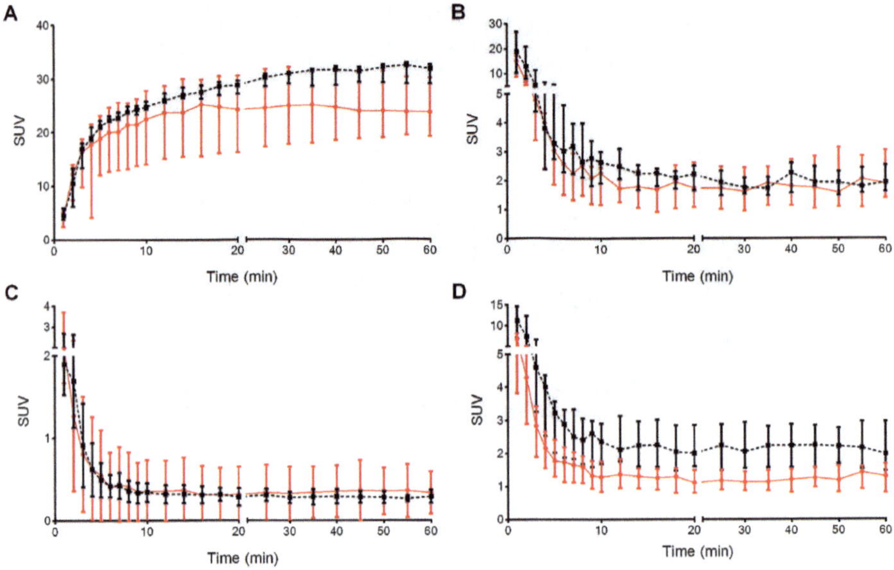

Figure 10.2 Dynamic ^{11}C-rifampin PET imaging. Dynamic ^{11}C-rifampin PET imaging in live animals over 60 min. Standardized uptake values (SUV) for liver (**a**), blood (**b**), brain (**c**), and lung (**d**) compartments in *Mycobacterium tuberculosis*-infected (*red*) and uninfected (*black*) mice are shown. Adapted from DeMarco and Ordonez et al. [25]

Table 10.2 Noncompartmental pharmacokinetic analyses for ^{11}C-rifampin

Parameter	Mean ± SD for animal type		*P* value
	Mycobacterium tuberculosis infected	Uninfected	
Weight (g)	30.54 ± 1.90	34.18 ± 2.50	0.07
Injected dose (ng)	0.07 ± 0.02	0.07 ± 0.02	0.80
Injected dose (MBq)	8.61 ± 2.09	8.26 ± 2.51	0.80
Blood			
C_{max} (ng/ml)	0.0622 ± 0.0289	0.0591 ± 0.0447	0.90
AUC_{0-60} (ng h/ml)	0.0056 ± 0.0015	0.0061 ± 0.0021	0.68
Brain			
C_{max} (ng/ml)	0.0086 ± 0.0085	0.0050 ± 0.0022	0.39
AUC_{0-60} (ng h/ml)	0.0012 ± 0.0013	0.0008 ± 0.0025	0.53
Liver			
C_{max} (ng/ml)	0.0608 ± 0.0167	0.0656 ± 0.0156	0.65
AUC_{0-60} (ng h/ml)	0.0583 ± 0.01406	0.0538 ± 0.0168	0.65
Lung			
C_{max} (ng/ml)	0.0221 ± 0.0095	0.0326 ± 0.0205	0.33
AUC_{0-60} (ng h/ml)	0.0034 ± 0.0008	0.0054 ± 0.0015	0.03

Peak concentrations (C_{max}) and areas under the concentration-time curve for the first 60 min (AUC_{0-60}) for different compartments are shown as means ± standard deviations. Adapted from DeMarco and Ordonez et al. [25]

10.3 Antifungals

The biodistribution of fluconazole was determined in rabbits with candida infections and healthy human volunteers by Fischman et al. using PET scans of ^{18}F-fluconazole [27, 28]. These studies provided useful information in the drug pharmacokinetics in multiple tissues, which can be used to determine the dose of drug needed to treat infection at different sites. Despite the significant need to understand the pharmacokinetic properties of other systemic antifungal agents, there is a lack of publications with radiolabeled antifungals. Preliminary chemistry validation has been published for ^{99m}Tc-voriconazole and ^{125}I-caspofungin [29].

10.4 Antivirals

The pharmacokinetics of a radiolabeled analog of the antiretroviral drug tenofovir, ^{18}F-PMPA, was studied using PET imaging in rats. The increased concentration in the renal cortex appeared to correspond to the drug's nephrotoxicity occasionally reported in humans [30]. Tissue distribution of ^{11}C-labeled antiretroviral drugsstavudine and zidovudine has also been evaluated using PET in animal models [31, 32].

Due to the increased interest in the herpes simplex virus thymidine kinase (HSV-tk), radiolabeled versions of multiple antiviral drugs and their analogs have been developed and their biodistribution evaluated using PET imaging. Two ^{18}F-labeled analogs of ganciclovir, 8-^{18}F-fluoroganciclovir and ^{18}F-FHPG, have been reported [33, 34].

PET imaging has also been used to evaluate the biodistribution of ^{11}C-zanamivir in nasal passages and lungs of human patients after inhalation. The high-quantitative accuracy and good-spatial resolution provided by nuclear imaging allowed the observation that less than 2% of the inhaled drug was detected in the lower respiratory tract [35]. Similarly, the anti-influenza drugoseltamivir was radiolabeled with ^{11}C, injected into mice and rats, and PET scanned in an effort to understand the neurologic side effects associated with this drug [36, 37]. ^{11}C-Oseltamivir PET was also performed in juvenile macaques to evaluate the effect of innate immune activation on the CNS uptake of oseltamivir [38].

10.5 Limitations

Unlike plasma and tissue sampling, PET in vivo measurements do not allow the possibility to discern if the radionuclide is attached to the native drug or possible metabolites. However, if there is information on the metabolites, kinetic models can be used to adjust the imaging findings. Moreover, depending on the radiochemistry resources, imaging equipment, and chemical structure of the drug, multiple different radionuclides can be used for radiolabeling. Labeling with ^{11}C has the advantage of not changing the molecular structures. However, a drawback of ^{11}C use for pharmacokinetic studies is its short radioactive half-life (20 min). This allows for a maximum observation time in most studies of 60 min, which limits its use for drugs with long elimination half-life. Molecules with fluorine atoms can be radiolabeled with ^{18}F, which is widely available and affordable, and provides excellent spatial resolution. Other radionuclides with longer half-life could also be used for PET imaging (^{68}Ga, ^{64}Cu, ^{76}Br, ^{89}Zr, ^{124}I) or SPECT (^{99m}Tc, ^{123}I, ^{111}In, ^{67}Ga).

10.6 Summary

Inadequate drug concentrations in target tissues can lead to treatment failure and/or selection of drug-resistant organisms. Additionally, altered pharmacokinetics in diseased patients may elevate tissue drug levels leading to organ toxicity or failure. A major advantage of PET-based bioimaging is its ability to measure in situ biodistribution of antimicrobials in real time and simultaneously in multiple organ system/compartments in live animals, with relatively unaltered physiology. This technology overcomes some fundamental limitations of current methodologies and could provide detailed preclinical data for appropriate dosing of new and existing antimicrobials. Such tracers could also enable the first-in-human clinical (phase 0) studies that are recognized by the US Food and Drug Administration to support Investigational New Drug Applications [39]. Human subject safety may be improved by using a PET tracer microdosing approach in early drug development which could eliminate the development of drugs with an unfavorable pharmacokinetic profiles and potential toxicities at higher doses. The approach can be extended to drug-drug interaction studies and to vulnerable populations, such as hepatically or renally impaired patients. Finally, PET tracers could also be adapted to study pharmacogenetics or personalized medicine approaches in the practice of medicine.

References

1. Keberle, H., H. Meyer-Brunot, and K. Schmid, *Pharmacokinetic and metabolic studies with labeled rifamycin antibiotics.* Antimicrob Agents Chemother (Bethesda), 1966. **6**: p. 365-70.
2. Rudin, M. and R. Weissleder, *Molecular imaging in drug discovery and development.* Nat Rev Drug Discov, 2003. **2**(2): p. 123-31.
3. Bauer, M., C.C. Wagner, and O. Langer, *Microdosing studies in humans: the role of positron emission tomography.* Drugs R D, 2008. **9**(2): p. 73-81.
4. Bergstrom, M., A. Grahnen, and B. Langstrom, *Positron emission tomography microdosing: a new concept with application in tracer and early clinical drug development.* Eur J Clin Pharmacol, 2003. **59**(5-6): p. 357-66.
5. Wollmer, P., et al., *Measurement of pulmonary erythromycin concentration in patients with lobar pneumonia by means of positron tomography.* Lancet, 1982. **2**(8312): p. 1361-4.

6. Britton, K.E., et al., *Imaging bacterial infection with (99m)Tc-ciprofloxacin (Infecton).* J Clin Pathol, 2002. **55**(11): p. 817-23.
7. Sonmezoglu, K., et al., *Usefulness of 99mTc-ciprofloxacin (infecton) scan in diagnosis of chronic orthopedic infections: comparative study with 99mTc-HMPAO leukocyte scintigraphy.* J Nucl Med, 2001. **42**(4): p. 567-74.
8. Siaens, R.H., et al., *Synthesis and comparison of 99mTc-enrofloxacin and 99mTc-ciprofloxacin.* J Nucl Med, 2004. **45**(12): p. 2088-94.
9. Brunner, M., et al., *[18F]Ciprofloxacin, a new positron emission tomography tracer for noninvasive assessment of the tissue distribution and pharmacokinetics of ciprofloxacin in humans.* Antimicrob Agents Chemother, 2004. **48**(10): p. 3850-7.
10. Langer, O., et al., *In vitro and in vivo evaluation of [18F]ciprofloxacin for the imaging of bacterial infections with PET.* Eur J Nucl Med Mol Imaging, 2005. **32**(2): p. 143-50.
11. Langer, O., et al., *Combined PET and microdialysis for in vivo assessment of intracellular drug pharmacokinetics in humans.* J Nucl Med, 2005. **46**(11): p. 1835-41.
12. Fischman, A.J., et al., *Pharmacokinetics of 18F-labeled fleroxacin in rabbits with Escherichia coli infections, studied with positron emission tomography.* Antimicrob Agents Chemother, 1992. **36**(10): p. 2286-92.
13. Fischman, A.J., et al., *Pharmacokinetics of [18F]fleroxacin in healthy human subjects studied by using positron emission tomography.* Antimicrob Agents Chemother, 1993. **37**(10): p. 2144-52.
14. Fischman, A.J., et al., *Pharmacokinetics of [18F]fleroxacin in patients with acute exacerbations of chronic bronchitis and complicated urinary tract infection studied by positron emission tomography.* Antimicrob Agents Chemother, 1996. **40**(3): p. 659-64.
15. Jynge, P., et al., *In vivo tissue pharmacokinetics by fluorine magnetic resonance spectroscopy: a study of liver and muscle disposition of fleroxacin in humans.* Clin Pharmacol Ther, 1990. **48**(5): p. 481-9.
16. Fischman, A.J., et al., *Pharmacokinetics of [18F]trovafloxacin in healthy human subjects studied with positron emission tomography.* Antimicrob Agents Chemother, 1998. **42**(8): p. 2048-54.
17. Fischman, A.J., et al., *Pharmacokinetics of 18F-labeled trovafloxacin in normal and Escherichia coli-infected rats and rabbits studied with positron emission tomography.* Clin Microbiol Infect, 1997. **3**(1): p. 63-72.
18. Tewson, T.J., et al., *The synthesis of fluorine-18 lomefloxacin and its preliminary use in human studies.* Nucl Med Biol, 1996. **23**(6): p. 767-72.
19. Auletta, S., et al., *Imaging bacteria with radiolabelled quinolones, cephalosporins and siderophores for imaging infection: a systematic review.* Clin Transl Imaging, 2016. **4**: p. 229-252.
20. Kaul, A., et al., *Preliminary evaluation of technetium-99m-labeled ceftriaxone: infection imaging agent for the clinical diagnosis of orthopedic infection.* Int J Infect Dis, 2013. **17**(4): p. e263-70.
21. Liu, L., et al., *Radiosynthesis and bioimaging of the tuberculosis chemotherapeutics isoniazid, rifampicin and pyrazinamide in baboons.* J Med Chem, 2010. **53**(7): p. 2882-91.
22. Weinstein, E.A., et al., *Noninvasive determination of 2-[18F]-fluoroisonicotinic acid hydrazide pharmacokinetics by positron emission tomography in Mycobacterium tuberculosis-infected mice.* Antimicrob Agents Chemother, 2012. **56**(12): p. 6284-90.
23. Steingart, K.R., et al., *Higher-dose rifampin for the treatment of pulmonary tuberculosis: a systematic review.* Int J Tuberc Lung Dis, 2011. **15**(3): p. 305-16.
24. Heemskerk, A.D., et al., *Intensified Antituberculosis Therapy in Adults with Tuberculous Meningitis.* N Engl J Med, 2016. **374**(2): p. 124-34.
25. DeMarco, V.P., et al., *Determination of [11C]rifampin pharmacokinetics within Mycobacterium tuberculosis-infected mice by using dynamic positron emission tomography bioimaging.* Antimicrob Agents Chemother, 2015. **59**(9): p. 5768-74.

26. Zhang, Z., et al., *The Biodistribution of 5-[18F]fluoropyrazinamide in Mycobacterium tuberculosis-infected Mice determined by Positron Emission Tomography.* PLoS One 2017. **(in press)**.
27. Fischman, A.J., et al., *Pharmacokinetics of 18F-labeled fluconazole in rabbits with candidal infections studied with positron emission tomography.* J Pharmacol Exp Ther, 1991. **259**(3): p. 1351-9.
28. Fischman, A.J., et al., *Pharmacokinetics of 18F-labeled fluconazole in healthy human subjects by positron emission tomography.* Antimicrob Agents Chemother, 1993. **37**(6): p. 1270-7.
29. Wareham, D., J. Michael, and S. Das, *Advances in bacterial specific imaging.* Brazilian Archives of Biology and Technology, 2005. **48**: p. 145-152.
30. Di Mascio, M., et al., *Antiretroviral tissue kinetics: in vivo imaging using positron emission tomography.* Antimicrob Agents Chemother, 2009. **53**(10): p. 4086-95.
31. Livni, E., et al., *Preparation and pharmacokinetics of 11C labeled stavudine (d4T).* Nucl Med Biol, 2004. **31**(5): p. 613-21.
32. Tahara, T., et al., *A novel (11)C-labeled thymidine analog, [(11)C]AZT, for tumor imaging by positron emission tomography.* EJNMMI Res, 2015. **5**(1): p. 124.
33. Gambhir, S.S., et al., *Imaging adenoviral-directed reporter gene expression in living animals with positron emission tomography.* Proc Natl Acad Sci U S A, 1999. **96**(5): p. 2333-8.
34. Buursma, A.R., et al., *[18F]FHPG positron emission tomography for detection of herpes simplex virus (HSV) in experimental HSV encephalitis.* J Virol, 2005. **79**(12): p. 7721-7.
35. Bergstrom, M., et al., *Deposition and disposition of [11C] Zanamivir following administration as an intranasal spray.* Clinical pharmacokinetics, 1999. **36**(1): p. 33-39.
36. Hatori, A., et al., *Biodistribution and metabolism of the anti-influenza drug [11C]oseltamivir and its active metabolite [11C]Ro 64-0802 in mice.* Nucl Med Biol, 2009. **36**(1): p. 47-55.
37. Hatori, A., et al., *Determination of radioactivity in infant, juvenile and adult rat brains after injection of anti-influenza drug [(1)(1)C]oseltamivir using PET and autoradiography.* Neurosci Lett, 2011. **495**(3): p. 187-91.
38. Seki, C., et al., *Evaluation of [(11)C]oseltamivir uptake into the brain during immune activation by systemic polyinosine-polycytidylic acid injection: a quantitative PET study using juvenile monkey models of viral infection.* EJNMMI Res, 2014. **4**: p. 24.
39. FDA. *Guidance for Industry, Investigators, and Reviewers: Exploratory IND Studies.* 2006 [cited November 10, 2012; Available from: http://www.fda.gov/downloads/Drugs/GuidanceComplianceRegulatoryInformation/Guidances/ucm078933.pdf.
40. Vinjamuri, S., et al., *Comparison of 99mTc infecton imaging with radiolabelled white-cell imaging in the evaluation of bacterial infection.* Lancet, 1996. **347**(8996): p. 233-5.
41. Shah, S.Q., M.R. Khan, and S.M. Ali, *Radiosynthesis of 99mTc (CO) 3-Clinafloxacin Dithiocarbamate and Its Biological Evaluation as a Potential Staphylococcus aureus Infection Radiotracer.* Nuclear Medicine and Molecular Imaging, 2011. **45**(4): p. 248-254.
42. Motaleb, M., *Radiochemical and biological characteristics of 99mTc-difloxacin and 99mTc-pefloxacin for detecting sites of infection.* Journal of Labelled Compounds and Radiopharmaceuticals, 2010. **53**(3): p. 104-109.
43. Siaens, R.H., et al., *Synthesis and comparison of 99mTc-enrofloxacin and 99mTc-ciprofloxacin.* Journal of Nuclear Medicine, 2004. **45**(12): p. 2088-2094.
44. Shah, S.Q., A.U. Khan, and M.R. Khan, *Radiosynthesis and biodistribution of 99m TcN–garenoxacin dithiocarbamate complex a potential infection imaging agent.* Journal of Radioanalytical and Nuclear Chemistry, 2011. **288**(1): p. 59-64.
45. Motaleb, M., et al., *Study on the preparation and biological evaluation of 99mTc–gatifloxacin and 99mTc–cefepime complexes.* Journal of Radioanalytical and Nuclear Chemistry, 2011. **289**(1): p. 57-65.
46. Shah, S.Q. and M.R. Khan, *Radiolabeling of gemifloxacin with technetium-99m and biological evaluation in artificially Streptococcus pneumoniae infected rats.* Journal of Radioanalytical and Nuclear Chemistry, 2011. **288**(1): p. 307-312.

47. El-ghany, E., et al., *Technetium-99m labeling and freeze-dried kit formulation of levofloxacin (L-Flox): a novel agent for detecting sites of infection.* Journal of Labelled Compounds and Radiopharmaceuticals, 2007. **50**(1): p. 25-31.
48. Nayak, D.K., et al., *Evaluation of 99mTc(i)-tricarbonyl complexes of fluoroquinolones for targeting bacterial infection.* Metallomics, 2012. **4**(11): p. 1197-1208.
49. Motaleb, M.A., *Preparation and biodistribution of 99mTc-lomefloxacin and 99mTc-ofloxacin complexes.* Journal of Radioanalytical & Nuclear Chemistry, 2007. **272**(1): p. 95-99.
50. Chattopadhyay, S., et al., *Synthesis and evaluation of 99mTc-moxifloxacin, a potential infection specific imaging agent.* Applied Radiation and Isotopes, 2010. **68**(2): p. 314-316.
51. Ibrahim, I., M. Motaleb, and K. Attalah, *Synthesis and biological distribution of 99m Tc–norfloxacin complex, a novel agent for detecting sites of infection.* Journal of radioanalytical and nuclear chemistry, 2010. **285**(3): p. 431-436.
52. Zhang, S., et al., *Synthesis and biodistribution of a novel ((9)(9)m)TcN complex of norfloxacin dithiocarbamate as a potential agent for bacterial infection imaging.* Bioconjug Chem, 2011. **22**(3): p. 369-75.
53. Erfani, M., et al., *99mTc-tricabonyl labeling of ofloxacin and its biological evaluation in Staphylococcus aureus as an infection imaging agent.* Journal of Labelled Compounds and Radiopharmaceuticals, 2013. **56**(12): p. 627-631.
54. Motaleb, M.A. and S.M. Ayoub, *Preparation, quality control, and biodistribution of 99mTc-rufloxacin complex as a model for detecting sites of infection.* Radiochemistry, 2013. **55**(6): p. 610-614.
55. Moustapha, M.E., et al., *Synthesis and biological evaluation of technetium-sarafloxacin complex for infection imaging.* Journal of Radioanalytical and Nuclear Chemistry, 2016. **307**(1): p. 699-705.
56. Shah, S.Q., A.U. Khan, and M.R. Khan, *Radiosynthesis and biological evaluation of 99mTcN-sitafloxacin dithiocarbamate as a potential radiotracer for Staphylococcus aureus infection.* Journal of Radioanalytical and Nuclear Chemistry, 2011. **287**(3): p. 827-832.
57. Qaiser, S.S., A.U. Khan, and M.R. Khan, *Synthesis, biodistribution and evaluation of 99mTc-sitafloxacin kit: a novel infection imaging agent.* Journal of Radioanalytical and Nuclear Chemistry, 2010. **284**(1): p. 189-193.
58. Singh, A., et al., *99m labeled sparfloxacin: a specific infection imaging agent.* WJ Nucl Med, 2003. **2**(2): p. 103-109.
59. El-Tawoosy, M., *Preparation and biological distribution of 99mTc-cefazolin complex, a novel agent for detecting sites of infection.* Journal of Radioanalytical and Nuclear Chemistry, 2013. **298**(2): p. 1215-1220.
60. Motaleb, M., *Preparation of 99m Tc-cefoperazone complex, a novel agent for detecting sites of infection.* Journal of Radioanalytical and Nuclear Chemistry, 2007. **272**(1): p. 167-171.
61. Mirshojaei, S., et al., *Radio labeling, quality control and biodistribution of 99mTc-cefotaxime as an infection imaging agent.* Journal of Radioanalytical and Nuclear Chemistry, 2011. **287**(1): p. 21-25.
62. Mirshojaei, S.F., M. Erfani, and M. Shafiei, *Evaluation of 99mTc-ceftazidime as bacterial infection imaging agent.* Journal of Radioanalytical and Nuclear Chemistry, 2013. **298**(1): p. 19-24.
63. Gomes Barreto, V., et al., *[99mTc-ceftizoxime scintigraphy in normal rats and abscess induced rats].* Rev Esp Med Nucl, 2005. **24**(5): p. 312-8.
64. Kaul, A., et al., *Preliminary evaluation of technetium-99m-labeled ceftriaxone: infection imaging agent for the clinical diagnosis of orthopedic infection.* International Journal of Infectious Diseases, 2013. **17**(4): p. e263-e270.
65. Yurt Lambrecht, F., et al., *Evaluation of 99m Tc-Cefuroxime axetil for imaging of inflammation.* Journal of Radioanalytical and Nuclear Chemistry, 2008. **277**(2): p. 491-494.
66. Chattopadhyay, S., et al., *Preparation and evaluation of 99mTc-cefuroxime, a potential infection specific imaging agent: A reliable thin layer chromatographic system to delineate impurities from the 99mTc-antibiotic.* Applied Radiation and Isotopes, 2012. **70**(10): p. 2384-2387.

67. Sakr, T., M. Motaleb, and I. Ibrahim, *99mTc–meropenem as a potential SPECT imaging probe for tumor hypoxia.* Journal of Radioanalytical and Nuclear Chemistry, 2012. **292**(2): p. 705-710.
68. Sanad, M.H., *Labeling and biological evaluation of 99m Tc-azithromycin for infective inflammation diagnosis.* Radiochemistry, 2013. **55**(5): p. 539-544.
69. Borai, E.H., M.H. Sanad, and A.S.M. Fouzy, *Optimized chromatographic separation and biological evaluation of 99m Tc-clarithromycin for infective inflammation diagnosis.* Radiochemistry, 2016. **58**(1): p. 84-91.
70. Hina, S., et al., *Preparation, biodistribution, and scintigraphic evaluation of (99m) Tc-clindamycin: an infection imaging agent.* Appl Biochem Biotechnol, 2014. **174**(4): p. 1420-33.
71. İlem-Özdemir, D., et al., *99mTc-Doxycycline hyclate: a new radiolabeled antibiotic for bacterial infection imaging.* Journal of Labelled Compounds and Radiopharmaceuticals, 2013: p. n/a-n/a.
72. Roohi, S., et al., *Synthesis, quality control and biodistribution of 99m Tc-Kanamycin.* Journal of radioanalytical and nuclear chemistry, 2006. **267**(3): p. 561-566.
73. Hagan, P., et al., *Comparison of 131I-tetracycline and 67Ga-citrate as abscess localizing agents.* Nuklearmedizin Archive, 1977. **16**(2): p. 76-78.
74. Hina, S., et al., *Labeling, quality control and biological evaluation of 99m Tc-vibramycin for infection sites imaging.* Bulg Chem Comm, 2015. **47**: p. 747-754.
75. Singh, N. and A. Bhatnagar, *Clinical Evaluation of Efficacy of 99mTC -Ethambutol in Tubercular Lesion Imaging.* Tuberculosis Research and Treatment, 2010. **2010**.
76. Roohi, S., et al., *Direct labeling of isoniazid with technetium-99m for diagnosis of tuberculosis*, in *Radiochimica Acta.* 2006. p. 147.
77. Amartey, J.K., et al., *2-[(18)F]-fluoroisonicotinic acid hydrazide: biological evaluation in an acute infection model.* Appl Radiat Isot, 2004. **60**(6): p. 839-43.
78. Liu, L., et al., *Radiosynthesis and Bioimaging of the Tuberculosis Chemotherapeutics Isoniazid, Rifampicin and Pyrazinamide in Baboons.* Journal of Medicinal Chemistry, 2010. **53**(7): p. 2882-2891.
79. Shah, S.Q., A.U. Khan, and M.R. Khan, *Radiosynthesis and biodistribution of 99mTc-rifampicin: A novel radiotracer for in-vivo infection imaging.* Applied Radiation and Isotopes, 2010. **68**(12): p. 2255-2260.
80. Tsopelas, C., et al., *99mTc-alafosfalin: an antibiotic peptide infection imaging agent.* Nucl Med Biol, 2003. **30**(2): p. 169-75.
81. Shahzadi, S.K., et al., *99mTc-amoxicillin: A novel radiopharmaceutical for infection imaging.* Arabian Journal of Chemistry.
82. Yurt Lambrecht, F., et al., *Preparation and biodistribution of [131 I] linezolid in animal model infection and inflammation.* Journal of radioanalytical and nuclear chemistry, 2009. **281**(3): p. 415-419.
83. Shah, S., A. Khan, and M. Khan, *Radiosynthesis of 99mTc-nitrofurantoin a novel radiotracer for in vivo imaging of Escherichia coli infection.* Journal of Radioanalytical and Nuclear Chemistry, 2011. **287**(2): p. 417-422.
84. Essouissi, I., et al., *Synthesis and evaluation of 99mTc-N-sulfanilamide ferrocene carboxamide as bacterial infections detector.* Nucl Med Biol, 2010. **37**(7): p. 821-9.
85. van Oosten, M., et al., *Real-time in vivo imaging of invasive- and biomaterial-associated bacterial infections using fluorescently labelled vancomycin.* Nat Commun, 2013. **4**: p. 2584.
86. Sadeghi, M., *Preparation and biodistribution of [201Tl](III) vancomycin complex in normal rats.* Nukleonika, 2006. **51**(4): p. 203-208.
87. Roohi, S., A. Mushtaq, and S.A. Malik, *Synthesis and biodistribution of 99mTc-Vancomycin in a model of bacterial infection.* Radiochimica Acta, 2005. **93**(7): p. 415-418.
88. Martin-Comin, J., et al., *[Diagnosis of bone infection with 99mTc-ceftizoxime].* Rev Esp Med Nucl, 2004. **23**(5): p. 357.

Chapter 11
Image Analyses

Ziyue Xu, Georgios Z. Papadakis, Daniel J. Mollura, and Ulas Bagci

11.1 Introduction

Radiological imaging of infectious lung diseases poses a diagnostic challenge due to the multitude of pathological events and the high degree of heterogeneity of infections processes. Anatomic/morphologic imaging modalities such as conventional radiography, ultrasound (US), computed tomography (CT), and magnetic resonance (MR) imaging, which have been employed in the diagnostic work-up of infectious diseases, are based on the identification of infection-induced anatomical/structural changes. Complementary to structural imaging modalities, nuclear medicine imaging techniques such as positron emission tomography (PET), single photon emission tomography (SPECT), etc., have also been used for imaging infectious lung diseases for decades [1]. Current practice in diagnostic and treatment guidance of infectious lung diseases relies on radiologic image evaluation combined with clinical information (Figure 11.1). These tasks are challenging because radiologic manifestations of infections are associated with a large spectrum of nonspecific abnormal imaging patterns. The qualitative judgments of radiologists can be improved by quantitative image analysis techniques by providing reliable markers such as volumetric, density, shape, and pattern-based metrics [2–5]. Therefore, automated and computer-aided image analysis tools can make valuable contributions to early recognition of parenchymal lesions by increasing sensitivity and specificity, as well as by providing quantitative measures of disease severity,

Z. Xu • G.Z. Papadakis • D.J. Mollura
Center for Infectious Disease Imaging, U.S. National Institutes of Health, Bethesda, MD, USA

Department of Radiology and Imaging Sciences, Clinical Center, U.S. National Institutes of Health, Bethesda, MD, USA

U. Bagci (✉)
Center for Research in Computer Vision, University of Central Florida, Orlando, FL, USA
e-mail: bagci@crcv.ucf.edu

S.K. Jain (ed.), *Imaging Infections*, DOI 10.1007/978-3-319-54592-9_11

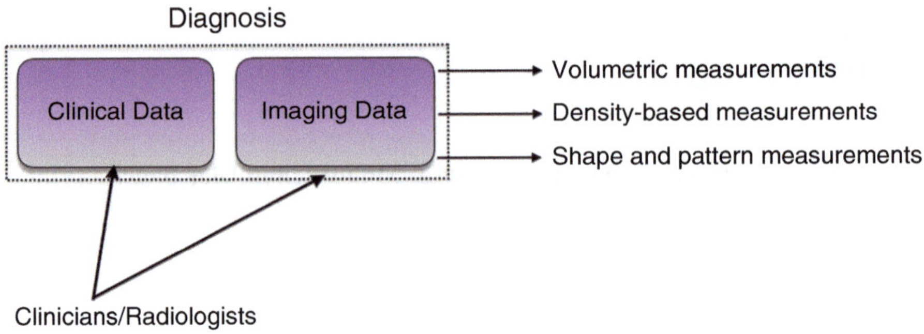

Figure 11.1 Contemporary diagnosis strategies combine clinical and imaging information as a routine task

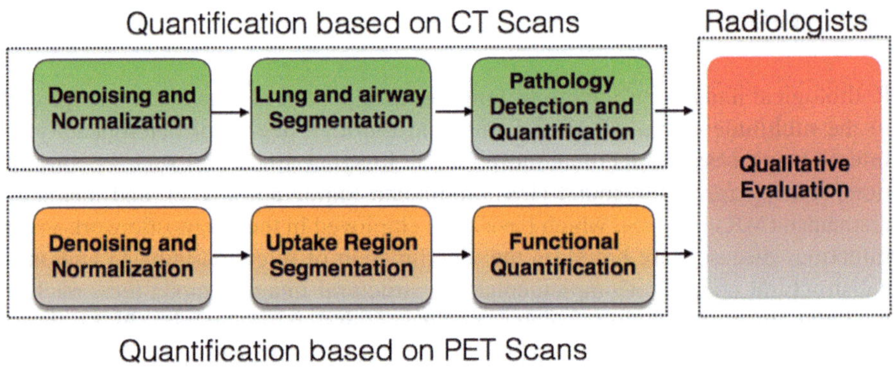

Figure 11.2 Steps for quantifying infectious lung diseases from CT and PET scans are shown

and assessing treatment response [6]. We will provide various analysis techniques from pulmonary imaging as an example of what may be possible for infectious diseases.

11.2 Anatomic Imaging

CT imaging is a common anatomic imaging modality used to assess the pulmonary system. Details of the infectious pathologies, such as location, size, and shape of the infiltrate, can be qualitatively and quantitatively assessed via CT imaging system. Some approaches of image analysis are described: (1) image denoising and enhancement for improved perception and diagnostic workout, (2) segmentation for lung and airway capacity measurements, and (3) pathology detection for quantification of abnormalities based on their location, type, number of lesions, etc. Figure 11.2 (upper panel) shows these three approaches and their semantic relationships to radiologists' final diagnostic decision(s).

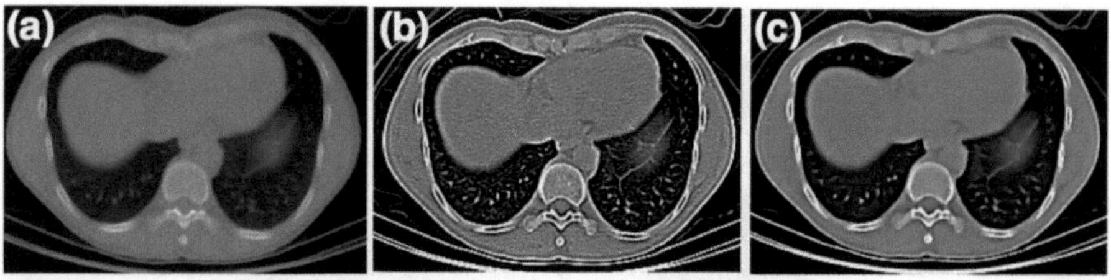

Figure 11.3 Image enhancements. For a given non-contrast CT image (**a**), an example contrast enhancement procedure is illustrated in (**b**). Note that noise is amplified with this process. An edge-preserving smoothing method is then applied and used to reduce noise (**c**)

11.2.1 Denoising and Enhancement

Although more definitive diagnosis of pulmonary diseases can be obtained by thin-section high-resolution CT (HRCT) scans, routine clinical assessment is generally based on a standard CT scanning procedure where low dose is often used, and separation of the regions with pathology from nearby structures can be demanding when using non-contrast protocols. In non-contrast CT scans, a priori use of contrast enhancement filtering can enhance visual information. However, contrast enhancement amplifies the level of noise; hence, denoising process should be performed after contrast enhancement operation. Last, but not least, the criteria for accurately denoising CT images is to minimize noise while preserving image structures such as edges (i.e., to avoid cross-boundary blurring between different tissues). Figure 11.3 illustrates a contrast enhancement procedure for a non-contrast CT scan followed by an edge-preserving denoising method. Resulting image can be used for qualitative and quantitative evaluation of pulmonary infections.

11.2.2 Segmentation

Identification of lung boundaries from CT scans (called delineation/segmentation) is a vital first step in pulmonary image analysis [7]. Any errors in this step could generate unreliable information such as incorrect lung volume and inaccurate identification of diseased areas. Hence, precise segmentation is critical for reliable quantification. Literature related to lung segmentation and subsequent pathology detection algorithms is rich [6]. However, most lung image segmentation algorithms apply well only when the lungs exhibit minimal or no pathologic conditions. Moderate to high disease burden often causes these segmentation algorithms to fail to depict pathological regions, thus leading to inaccurate image-based quantification results. Infected lungs often display moderate to large volumes of abnormal imaging patterns but also a wide range of abnormal imaging patterns such as ground-glass opacity (GGO), consolidation, tree-in-bud, nodule, pleural effusion, etc. (Figure 11.4). Therefore, it is necessary to develop automated computerized

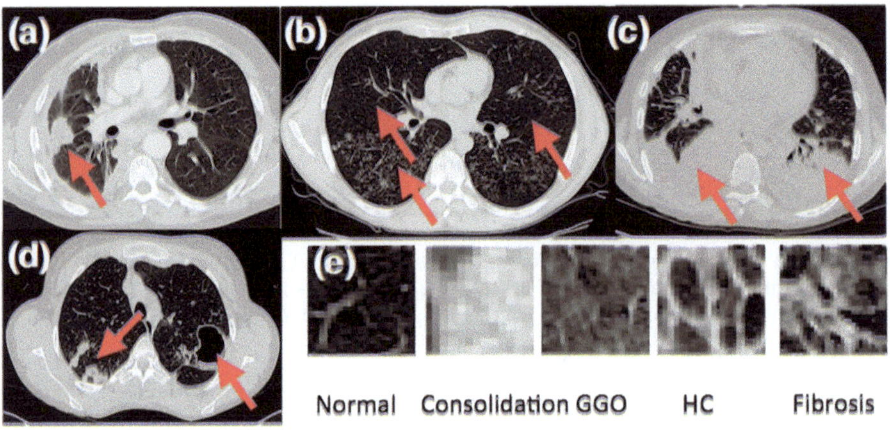

Figure 11.4 Pattern detection. A wide spectrum of abnormal imaging patterns can be observed in CT images pertaining to subjects with infectious lung diseases: (**a**) consolidation, (**b**) tree-in-bud, (**c**) pleural effusion, (**d**) mass and cavity, (**e**) normal lung parenchyma and other common pathologies including fibrosis, ground-glass opacity (GGO), and honeycombing (HC)

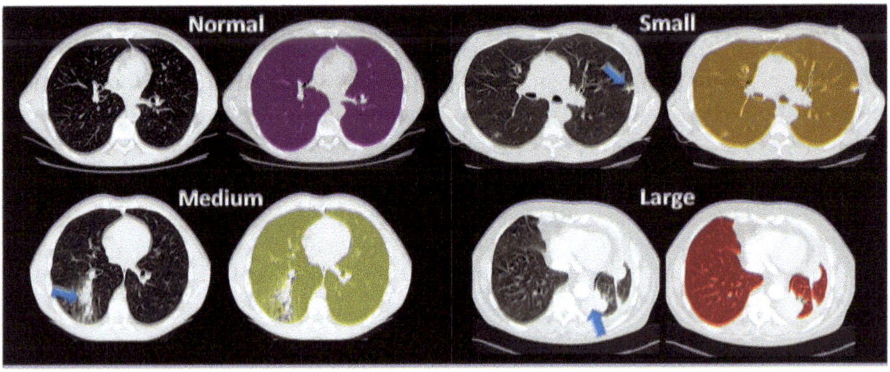

Figure 11.5 Lung segmentation algorithm. CT images with commonly used lung segmentation algorithm (i.e., region growing) are shown with different type and varying amounts of pathologies (normal-no disease, small, medium, and large)

mathematical methods for identification, classification, and quantification of all abnormal imaging patterns along with lung region delineation. There is almost no general method for handling detection of all pulmonary abnormalities. In [8], our group has proposed a generic lung segmentation algorithm to address this problem, called pathological lung segmentation (PLS), considering wide-range abnormalities to be detected in parallel to the lung segmentation process (Figure 11.5).

Airways (trachea, bronchi, bronchioles, and alveolar ducts and sacs) are pathologically involved in several respiratory infections. Typically, infections cause thickening and irregular (or uniform) narrowing in airways. Measurements of bronchial wall thickening and identification of its position are important markers to be extracted for quantitative evaluation of airway diseases. Conventionally, qualitative and quantitative assessment of airway structures is manually performed at limited locations on the CT images. However, as a treelike structure with complex bifurcation patterns, such characterization, is often labor-intensive and time-consuming for practical clinical investigation. Therefore, semi- and fully automatic airway segmentation methods could facilitate understanding of the mechanism of airway-related pathologies. Several airway segmentation algorithms have been investigated. Among them, region growing (RG) is widely used because of its high efficiency and accuracy. Other general methods are the following: rule based [9], morphology based [10], and classification based [11]. All these methods are not entirely useful for extracting airway structures when a significant amount of pathologies exist on or nearby airway structures. It is because irregularities in the appearance of airway structure in CT such as broken airway wall boundaries can lead delineation algorithms to leak into non-airway territories. Hence, in the presence of pathologies, an intensity-based RG strategy can easily leak into the neighboring lung parenchyma through the broken boundaries. To address the difficulty of airway-tree extraction when infection presents in the respiratory tract, a method based on fuzzy connectedness (FC) was designed in our group's previous publication [12]. This method incorporates both shape and appearance information of airways in order to enhance the capability of conventional RG method in segmentation. Specifically, the tubular shape of airway branches can be enhanced by vesselness computation based on Hessian analysis. Meanwhile, the appearance of airways can be regarded as local intensity minima within CT image, which can be recognized by gray-scale morphological reconstruction. Complementary strengths of the three measurements, i.e., intensity, vesselness, and morphological reconstruction, can then be combined within the proposed FC framework to delineate airways. Figure 11.6 (left panel)

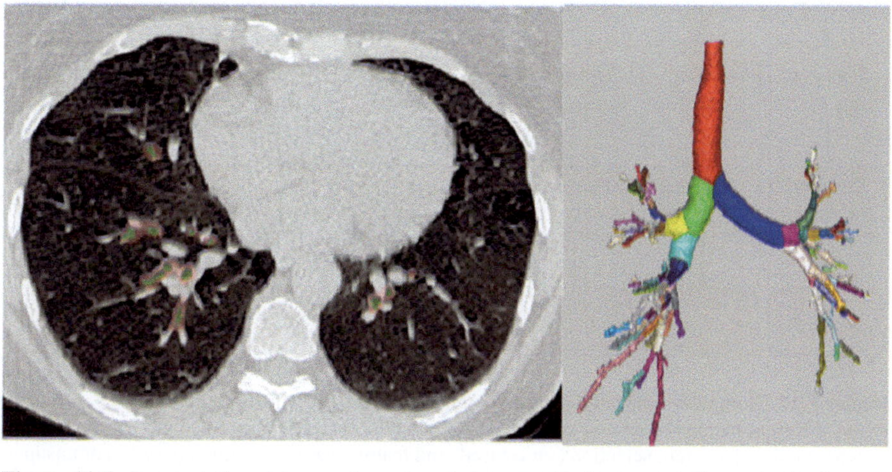

Figure 11.6 Segmentation. Airways (*green*) and airway walls (*red*) are delineated with the proposed algorithm (*left*). Reconstructed lumen is illustrated with multiple branches; each branch has a different color

shows an axial slice of a CT image in which both large and small airways and their walls are delineated using the proposed approach. Delineation results are shown on the right with different colors, indicating different branches of the airway tree. The proposed algorithm successfully handles delineation process without leaking into non-airway regions.

11.2.3 Detection and Quantification of Imaging Patterns

The development of image analysis systems using CT imaging requires *detection* and *identification* of a wide spectrum of abnormal imaging patterns pertaining to the infectious lung diseases such as GGO, consolidation, tree-in-bud, cavities, etc. (Figure 11.4), and a specific algorithm has been published for almost each abnormal imaging pattern in the literature. Moreover, it is has been shown that it is quite difficult to have a universal algorithm for detection and classification of abnormal imaging patterns. In general, a typical analysis system includes a machine-learning algorithm where imaging features are used to train the classifier, and when a new image is tested, similar imaging features are extracted and tested over this classifier. Based on similarities of the extracted imaging features, an automatic detection process is conducted. Figure 11.7 shows an overview of available analysis systems and their characteristics on feature training, selection, and type of learning classifiers.

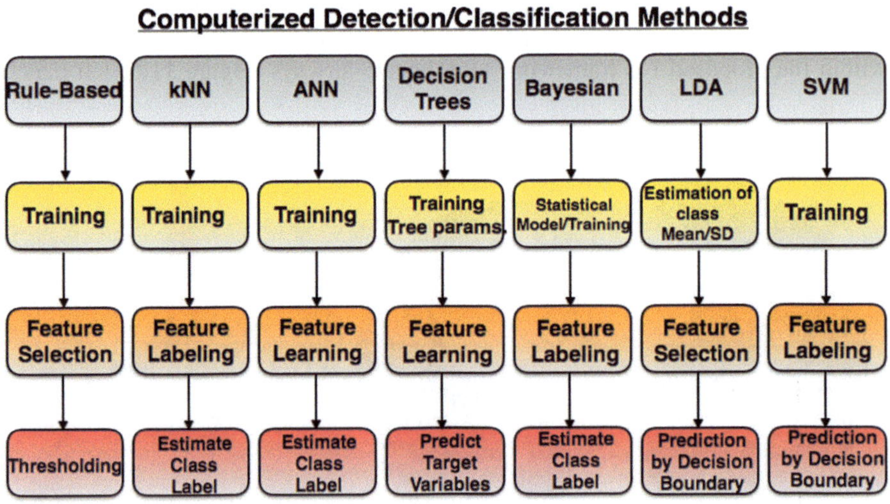

Figure 11.7 Computer-assisted detection/diagnosis (CAD) systems for lung diseases. *First row* shows different machine-learning classifiers. *Second row* indicates how machine-learning classifiers are modeled. Feature selection (supervised) and feature learning (semi-supervised or unsupervised) are two main components of CAD design as shown in *third row*. Final decision boundary for pathology detection may depend on different criteria including thresholding, statistical estimations, and predictions

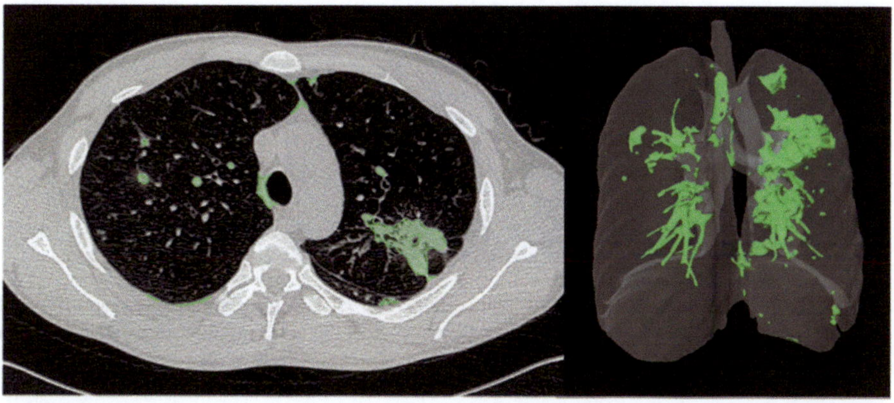

Figure 11.8 Detection and quantification of imaging patterns. An example of CAD system is shown where pathology regions are detected automatically (*left*, *green* boundaries). The resulting pathology distribution within the lung volume is visualized for qualitative evaluation (*right*)

Figure 11.8 shows a sample output for a CAD system that our group previously developed [8], which is trained to detect wide range of abnormal imaging patterns pertaining to pulmonary infections. In terms of imaging features, statistical, textural, and shape-based features extracted from local windows are used in random forest (RF) decision tree-based machine-learning classifier.

11.3 Functional Imaging

PET is a common functional imaging modality used in the clinic and often combined with CT imaging for anatomic reference. PET/CT using ^{18}F-2-fluoro-deoxy-D-glucose (^{18}F-FDG) (glucose analog) is a common nuclear medicine technique used for the management of infections. The list of ^{18}F-FDG PET/CT imaging applications in the assessment of both acute and chronic disease entities is growing, while its main weakness lies on the limited specificity which does not allow confident differentiation between infection, aseptic inflammation, and malignant processes. The development of novel infection-specific PET tracers can however overcome this limitation and holds promise for even better diagnostic accuracy.

11.3.1 Denoising and Partial Volume Correction

Normalization of PET images prior to quantitative image analysis mainly includes two tasks, denoising and partial volume correction (PVC) [13, 14]. Unlike CT images, the noise in PET images follows non-Gaussian distribution that degrades

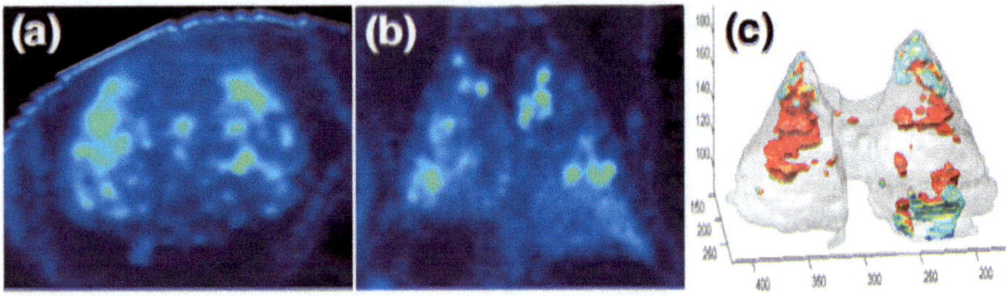

Figure 11.9 Quantification. Sagittal (**a**) and coronal (**b**) PET slices pertaining to a rabbit infected with *Mycobacterium tuberculosis* are shown. Delineation of the uptake regions due to the infection within the lung is visualized in (**c**)

the sensitivity of image-based quantitative metrics due to distorting structural integrity of tissue appearances. Despite this fact, most approaches in the literature still assume the presence of Gaussian noise. In [13], it was shown by our group both in phantom and real clinical images that the nature of the noise in PET images follows a mixed Poisson-Gaussian distribution. It should be noted that inaccurately denoising PET images could lead to misdiagnosis or misinterpretation of the lesions or erroneous severity assessment. The straightforward approach for enhancing PET images is to gaussianize the images followed by an edge-preserving denoising, filtering, and transforming the image back into its original image domain. Further technical details and mathematics behind this approach can be found in [13, 15]. Partial volume effect is the apparent loss of activity in small objects or regions because of the limited resolution of the imaging systems. Specifically, if the object or region to be imaged is less than twice the full width at half maximum (FWHM) resolution in any dimension, the resultant activity in the object or region is underestimated. Measurements of activity, i.e., standardized uptake value (SUV)-based metrics (SUVmax, SUVmean, etc.), are vital for quantitative analysis of lesions and directly affected by partial volume effects. Common techniques for partial volume correction are based on deconvolution strategies from a signal-processing field where point spread function of the imaging device is assumed to be known a priori. This information is used to estimate original signal from its degraded counterpart in an iterative fashion such that degraded signal is enhanced in each iteration. As long as edge-preserving denoising and precise partial volume correction methods are used, resulting enhanced PET images can be used for quantification in (near) optimal settings. Since PET images pertaining to infectious lung diseases may include highly multifocal and varying sizes of lesions spread over the lungs (Figure 11.9), it is necessary to conduct partial volume correction prior to lesion quantification because small lesions are affected most from partial volume effects. This procedure should be followed by a denoising algorithm as partial volume correction amplifies the noise artificially.

11.3.2 Quantification

Once PET images are denoised and partial volume correction has been applied, quantification and visual evaluation can be performed. Lesions (significant uptake regions) in PET images can be quantified in the following manner: (1) metabolic lesion volume, (2) texture analysis of the lesions, (3) signal strengths of the lesion (i.e., SUVmax, SUVmean, etc.), and (4) number and spreadness of lesions. Larger metabolic lesion volumes and higher SUVs are considered to be associated with higher (disease) severity [16]. Similarly, heterogeneous textures are considered to be highly likely more severe than the homogeneous regions [17]. Lastly, it has been recently shown that number and spreadness of the multifocal lesions are predictive of severity better than volume or any other quantitative metrics [18, 19]. All the markers defined in (1)–(4) require precise delineation of lesions in PET images. Although numerous methods have been proposed for PET image segmentation [20], most of them are designed for (focal) solid tumor analysis. However, in pulmonary infections, it is common to see *multifocal* and widely spread lesions in lung regions (Figure 11.9a, b). Therefore, conventional methods do not optimally segment these lesions. Specific to PET image analysis in pulmonary infections, a clustering-based image segmentation algorithm has been developed by our group handling multifocal and wide spreadness nature of infectious lesions [1]. A sample result for the proposed algorithm is illustrated in Figure 11.9c. Our proposed delineation method utilized an unsupervised clustering algorithm in order to determine high- and low-uptake regions precisely using a novel similarity metric between clustered objects. The proposed method is superior to other PET image segmentation methods such as thresholding, fuzzy locally Bayesian, region growing, and others. It is worth noting that integrated information from high-uptake regions and nearby regions with less activities can give further insights on the severity and morphological evolution of lesions over time.

11.3.3 Co-Registration for Longitudinal Evaluation

Image registration is the process of transforming two different images into the same image space by considering the spatial image correspondences and is needed in many medical image processing tasks [21]. Two types of registration are often required for quantitative analysis. First, an alignment is necessary to bring the two different modalities into the same image domain in order to correlate anatomical information from CT and functional information from PET. Second, longitudinal registration is needed to correlate image findings at same anatomical locations from different time points in order to track the progression of infection over time (Figure 11.10). Different challenges posed by both imaging characteristics and infection pathologies need to be addressed in designing proper registration strategies. Two major components are critical for registration algorithms: similarity measurement and transformation model. Similarity measurement determines the degree

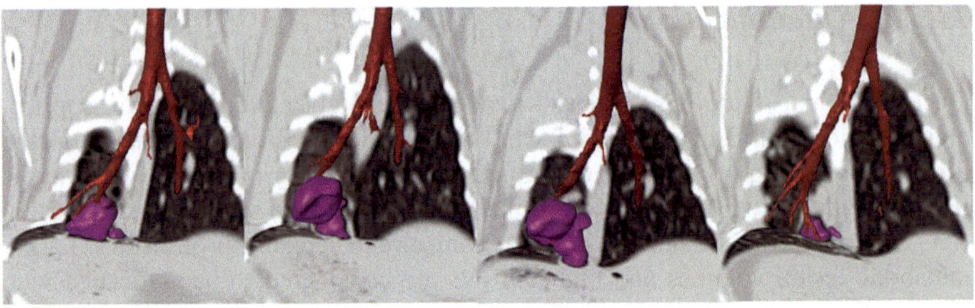

Figure 11.10 Co-registration for longitudinal evaluation. The temporal evolution of cavitary disease in an animal model is illustrated (from *left* to *right*). Cavity, airways, and CT images should be in alignment for precise longitudinal evaluation. Similar steps are necessary when PET images are involved in the longitudinal evaluations

of agreement between the two images to be registered, which further drives the convergence of registration. Similarity measurement is the essential driving force of registration algorithms; hence, it is crucial for the performance. Several measurements have been proposed to tackle challenges under various scenarios. The most basic measurement is the sum of squared difference between intensity values. The assumption behind the use of this metric is that two images have approximately the same intensities at the corresponding locations. Therefore, it is often suitable for registrations between two CT images. If intensities are different but can be related by a linear transformation, normalized correlation could be used. For two binary images, Kappa statistic is often utilized for its effectiveness in the same exact value. If two sets of landmarks can be identified, the Euclidean distance can be included in the evaluation. For multimodal image registration, since the intensities are different at the corresponding locations, mutual information is often the metric of choice [22]. For imaging applications in infectious lung diseases, mutual information is used to align PET into CT image, and squared difference can be used for longitudinal studies for registering CT images at different time points. The transformation model, as the other critical component of image registration, determines how one image space is related to the other space. It controls the degree of freedom for the space warping. For different applications, commonly used models include two types: *linear* and *deformable* transformations. Linear deformation covers rotation, translation, scaling, shearing, and other affine transformations. Since it is global, i.e., all voxels are transformed in the same manner, it is not capable of modeling the local geometric deformations. On the other hand, deformable transformations allow each individual voxel to move on its own and thus can model the local changes. Both models are needed in infectious disease-imaging applications. Since PET and CT images are acquired either simultaneously or sequentially, the local discrepancy is negligible; linear transformation is a common choice for this purpose.

For a longitudinal study, it is often necessary to register CT images at different time points. In this case, we could have significant local deformations between the two, especially for pulmonary images. Thus, a deformable transformation model should be employed [23]. Not only does a lung have significant local deformation during scanning, but also the presence of abnormal imaging patterns pertaining to the infectious lung diseases increases the level of variation. At different time points, the breathing motion and different breathing functionalities lead to two changes in the image: a local shape difference and intensity difference within lung regions. Therefore, to properly model the change within the lung region longitudinally, a deformable image registration method should preferably be used to find the correspondence between images. A relevant preclinical study shows plausible results on longitudinal evaluation of infectious lung disease progression [24].

11.4 Other Developments in Image Analyses

Several different groups have utilized methods for longitudinal assessments. A novel diffeomorphic image registration method was used to monitor the spatial evolution of individual pulmonary lesions in a cohort of infected mice that were serially imaged through pretreatment, TB treatment, and subsequent development of relapse [25]. To accurately follow the evolution of lesions across time points, all imaging sets were co-registered, such that voxels from each image set matched the imaging sets from all other time points using the Large Deformation Diffeomorphic Metric Matching (LDDMM) algorithm [26, 27]. This allowed for accurate monitoring of the temporal evolution of each lesion by accounting for any morphometric differences, e.g., due to positioning or other anatomical changes, such as aging [28]. In another study to monitor TB treatments in adults with multidrug-resistant TB, a quantitative software algorithm was developed to computationally extract the volume of a diseased lung from CT images. Lung regions were segmented by sequential removal of external contiguous structures (bone, soft tissues, etc.). Quantitative changes in lesion volumes on CT imaging were predictive of treatment responses [29]. More recently, a similar approach was used to quantify changes in low-radiation exposure pulmonary CT imaging and to guide an individualized drug regimen in a 2-year-old child with extensively drug-resistant TB [30].

Since multi-detector row CT imaging remains the gold standard for diagnosis and interpretation of the general lung diseases, the most of the current automated image analysis efforts focus on developing new, fast, and accurate computerized algorithms for characterizing the imaging patterns pertaining to pathological formations observed in CT scans [31]. Such efforts can be categorized under two groups: radiomics and deep-learning-based approaches. In radiomics approaches [32], first, second, and higher-order image-derived statistics are used to extract high-throughput low-level quantitative features (edge, texture, shape, density, etc.) from CT scans, and these features are combined with other patient data to improve diagnostic, prognostic, and predictive accuracy. Radiomics features often include handcrafted, carefully designed markers to conduct aforementioned tasks; therefore, it has a natural limitation that there may be a high-level relationship, which is not easily captured by radiomics approaches. Noticeable studies include radiomics-based differentiations of tuberculosis, cystic fibrosis, and lung carcinomas [33] and radiomics-based outcome prediction of multidrug-resistant tuberculosis using PET/CT images [29]. Alternative to the radiomics approaches, there has been a tremendous increase in the use of deep-learning-based approaches almost in every subfield of quantitative radiology, including infectious lung disease analysis [34]. In deep-learning strategies [35], the main premise comes from several layers of the neural network classifiers that provide both low and high level of feature representation (i.e., hierarchical representation), which was not possible to learn with the conventional approaches before. With deep representation of CT images, dramatic improvements have been obtained compared to the state-of-the-art image analysis techniques [36]. Although deep-learning strategies are shown to be promising, the lack of big data in radiology and nuclear medicine leads to logistic difficulties such as data collection, annotation of those big data by multiple users, and their ground-truth correlations. Some studies in this group include automated classification and quantification of CT imaging patterns pertaining to tuberculosis and interstitial lung diseases [37].

Molecular-imaging methodologies, particularly PET and SPECT, have been proven "useful" for diagnostic imaging modality for infection and inflammation. In 2013, a guideline on the use of ^{18}F-FDG in infection and inflammation was announced jointly by the Society of Nuclear Medicine and Molecular Imaging and the European Association of Nuclear Medicine [38]. However, there is still not enough evidence-based data available to draw a conclusion whether ^{18}F-FDG PET/CT provides a significant advantage over other imaging modalities [39]. One reason is that imaging patterns of infection (and inflammation) are not substantially different than imaging biomarkers of cancer [40]. Therefore, several groups in imaging infection field aim at exploring molecular-imaging biomarkers that can differentiate patterns of infectious diseases from other diseases. Noteworthy studies include the development of novel imaging systems or imaging tracers (for PET/SPECT) for rapid assessment of bacterial infections [41–45] and development of post-processing methods utilizing texture, shape, density, intensity, and location-based unique signatures both for bacterial and viral infections in the lungs [16, 46–48].

11.5 Summary

Technological advancements in imaging have revolutionized noninvasive imaging, enabling improvements in diagnosis and prognosis of lung diseases in general and infectious lung diseases in particular. In parallel to these imaging developments, there have been important improvements in radiological image analysis techniques that provide accurate quantifiable information to help clinicians in their diagnostic decisions. Current quantitative image analysis approaches have some limitations, and novel image analysis techniques could provide automated and quantitative information that could be even more beneficial for the clinicians.

References

1. Foster, B., et al., *Segmentation of PET images for computer-aided functional quantification of tuberculosis in small animal models.* IEEE Trans Biomed Eng, 2014. **61**(3): p. 711-24.
2. Martinez, C.H., et al., *Relationship between quantitative CT metrics and health status and BODE in chronic obstructive pulmonary disease.* 2012. **67**(5): p. 399-406.
3. Brightling, C.E., et al., *Lung damage and airway remodelling in severe asthma.* 2011. **42**(5): p. 638-649.
4. Bayouth, J.E., et al., *Image-based biomarkers in clinical practice.* Semin Radiat Oncol, 2011. **21**(2): p. 157-66.
5. Galban, C.J., et al., *The parametric response map is an imaging biomarker for early cancer treatment outcome.* 2009. **15**(5): p. 572-576.
6. Bagci, U., et al., *Computer-assisted detection of infectious lung diseases: a review.* Comput Med Imaging Graph, 2012. **36**(1): p. 72-84.
7. Mansoor, A., et al., *Segmentation and Image Analysis of Abnormal Lungs at CT: Current Approaches, Challenges, and Future Trends.* Radiographics, 2015. **35**(4): p. 1056-76.
8. Mansoor, A., et al., *A generic approach to pathological lung segmentation.* IEEE Trans Med Imaging, 2014. **33**(12): p. 2293-310.
9. Sonka, M., W. Park, and E.A. Hoffman, *Rule-based detection of intrathoracic airway trees.* IEEE Trans Med Imaging, 1996. **15**(3): p. 314-26.
10. Aykac, D., et al., *Segmentation and analysis of the human airway tree from three-dimensional X-ray CT images.* IEEE Trans Med Imaging, 2003. **22**(8): p. 940-50.
11. Lo, P., et al., *Vessel-guided airway tree segmentation: A voxel classification approach.* Med Image Anal, 2010. **14**(4): p. 527-38.
12. Xu, Z., et al., *A hybrid method for airway segmentation and automated measurement of bronchial wall thickness on CT.* Med Image Anal, 2015. **24**(1): 1-17.
13. Mansoor, A., U. Bagci, and D.J. Mollura, *Optimally stabilized PET image denoising using trilateral filtering.* Med Image Comput Comput Assist Interv, 2014. **17**(Pt 1): p. 130-7.
14. Xu, Z., et al., *Segmentation based denoising of PET images: an iterative approach via regional means and affinity propagation.* Med Image Comput Comput Assist Interv, 2014. **17**(Pt 1): p. 698-705.
15. Bagci, U. and D.J. Mollura, *Denoising PET images using singular value thresholding and Stein's unbiased risk estimate.* Med Image Comput Comput Assist Interv, 2013. **16**(Pt 3): p. 115-22.
16. Bagci, U., et al., *Predicting future morphological changes of lesions from radiotracer uptake in 18F-FDG-PET images.* PLoS One, 2013. **8**(2): p. e57105.
17. Camp, J.V., et al., *Lower Respiratory Tract Infection of the Ferret by 2009 H1N1 Pandemic Influenza A Virus Triggers Biphasic, Systemic, and Local Recruitment of Neutrophils.* J Virol, 2015. **89**(17): p. 8733-48.
18. Kubler, A., et al., *Mycobacterium tuberculosis dysregulates MMP/TIMP balance to drive rapid cavitation and unrestrained bacterial proliferation.* J Pathol, 2015. **235**(3): p. 431-44.
19. Luna, B., et al., *In vivo prediction of tuberculosis-associated cavity formation in rabbits.* J Infect Dis, 2015. **211**(3): p. 481-5.
20. Foster, B., et al., *A review on segmentation of positron emission tomography images.* Comput Biol Med, 2014. **50**: p. 76-96.
21. Bagci, U. and L. Bai, *Automatic best reference slice selection for smooth volume reconstruction of a mouse brain from histological images.* IEEE Trans Med Imaging, 2010. **29**(9): p. 1688-96.
22. Zhang, Z., et al., *Multi-modality medical image registration using support vector machines.* Conf Proc IEEE Eng Med Biol Soc, 2005. **6**: p. 6293-6.
23. Cunliffe, A.R., et al., *Effect of deformable registration on the dose calculated in radiation therapy planning CT scans of lung cancer patients.* Med Phys, 2015. **42**(1): p. 391-9.

24. Bagci, U., et al., *A computational pipeline for quantification of pulmonary infections in small animal models using serial PET-CT imaging.* EJNMMI Res, 2013. **3**(1): p. 55.
25. Murawski, A.M., et al., *Imaging the evolution of reactivation pulmonary tuberculosis in mice using 18F-FDG PET.* J Nucl Med, 2014. **55**(10): p. 1726-9.
26. Vidal, C., et al., *Template Registration with Missing Parts: Application to the Segmentation of M. Tuberculosis Infected Lungs.* 2009 Ieee International Symposium on Biomedical Imaging: From Nano to Macro, Vols 1 and 2, 2009: p. 718-721.
27. Vidal, C., et al. *Incorporating user input in template-based segmentation.* in *Biomedical Imaging: From Nano to Macro, 2011 IEEE International Symposium on.* 2011.
28. Beg, M.F., et al., *Computing large deformation metric mappings via geodesic flows of diffeomorphisms.* International Journal of Computer Vision, 2005. **61**(2): p. 139-157.
29. Chen, R.Y., et al., *PET/CT imaging correlates with treatment outcome in patients with multidrug-resistant tuberculosis.* Sci Transl Med, 2014. **6**(265): p. 265ra166.
30. Salazar-Austin, N., et al., *Extensively drug-resistant tuberculosis in a young child after travel to India.* Lancet Infect Dis, 2015. **15**(12): p. 1485-91.
31. Hoffman, E.A., et al., *Characterization of the interstitial lung diseases via density-based and texture-based analysis of computed tomography images of lung structure and function.* Acad Radiol, 2003. **10**(10): p. 1104-18.
32. Gillies, R.J., P.E. Kinahan, and H. Hricak, *Radiomics: Images Are More than Pictures, They Are Data.* Radiology, 2016. **278**(2): p. 563-77.
33. Szigeti, K., et al., *Radiomics-based differentiation of lung disease models generated by polluted air based on X-ray computed tomography data.* BMC Med Imaging, 2016. **16**: p. 14.
34. Cheng, J.Z., et al., *Computer-Aided Diagnosis with Deep Learning Architecture: Applications to Breast Lesions in US Images and Pulmonary Nodules in CT Scans.* Sci Rep, 2016. **6**: p. 24454.
35. LeCun, Y., Y. Bengio, and G. Hinton, *Deep learning.* Nature, 2015. **521**(7553): p. 436-44.
36. Buty, M., et al. *Characterization of Lung Nodule Malignancy Using Hybrid Shape and Appearance Features.* in *International Conference on Medical Image Computing and Computer-Assisted Intervention.* 2016. Springer International Publishing.
37. Gao, M., et al., *Holistic classification of CT attenuation patterns for interstitial lung diseases via deep convolutional neural networks.* Computer Methods in Biomechanics and Biomedical Engineering: Imaging & Visualization, 2016: p. 1-6.
38. Jamar, F., et al., *EANM/SNMMI guideline for 18F-FDG use in inflammation and infection.* J Nucl Med, 2013. **54**(4): p. 647-58.
39. Glaudemans, A.W., et al., *Molecular imaging of infectious and inflammatory diseases: a terra incognita.* J Nucl Med, 2015. **56**(5): p. 659-61.
40. Wang, L., et al., *Evaluation of candidate vaccine approaches for MERS-CoV.* Nat Commun, 2015. **6**: p. 7712.
41. Andreu, N., A. Zelmer, and S. Wiles, *Noninvasive biophotonic imaging for studies of infectious disease.* FEMS Microbiol Rev, 2011. **35**(2): p. 360-94.
42. Crepin, V.F., et al., *Citrobacter rodentium mouse model of bacterial infection.* Nat Protoc, 2016. **11**(10): p. 1851-76.
43. Jorgensen, N.P., et al., *Cholinergic PET imaging in infections and inflammation using 11C-donepezil and 18F-FEOBV.* Eur J Nucl Med Mol Imaging, 2016.
44. Heuker, M., et al., *Preclinical studies and prospective clinical applications for bacteria-targeted imaging: the future is bright.* Clin Transl Imaging, 2016. **4**: p. 253-264.
45. Vilche, M., et al., *(6)(8)Ga-NOTA-UBI-29-41 as a PET Tracer for Detection of Bacterial Infection.* J Nucl Med, 2016. **57**(4): p. 622-7.
46. Carles, M., et al., *Evaluation of PET texture features with heterogeneous phantoms: complementarity and effect of motion and segmentation method.* Phys Med Biol, 2016. **62**(2): p. 652-668.

47. Desseroit, M.C., et al., *Reliability of PET/CT shape and heterogeneity features in functional and morphological components of Non-Small Cell Lung Cancer tumors: a repeatability analysis in a prospective multi-center cohort.* J Nucl Med, 2016.
48. Chan, S.C., et al., *Tumor heterogeneity measured on F-18 fluorodeoxyglucose positron emission tomography/computed tomography combined with plasma Epstein-Barr Virus load predicts prognosis in patients with primary nasopharyngeal carcinoma.* Laryngoscope, 2017. **127**(1): p. E22-E28.

Chapter 12
Imaging in the Developing World

Thomas Ebenhan and Mike Sathekge

12.1 Introduction

In developing countries, infectious diseases continue to be the leading cause of death in children and adolescents and one of the leading causes in adults. Most of these deaths are attributable to preventable or treatable diseases such as diarrhea, pneumonia, malaria, human immunodeficiency virus (HIV/AIDS), and tuberculosis (TB) [1]. TB remains a leading cause of death among people, especially those coinfected with HIV, accounting for one in five AIDS-related deaths globally [2, 3]. While significant advances have been made to prevent and treat these diseases, these interventions are often unavailable to the populations most in need. Imaging is among these critical technologies, which could save lives and prevent new infections [4]. The potential benefits arising from the introduction of imaging in developing countries are numerous, and several have argued that advanced imaging is a viable solution to some of the ongoing problems and healthcare challenges experienced by these countries.

12.2 Imaging Services

Developing countries present nuclear physicians, radiologists, and clinicians with substantial challenges—massive disease burden, cost, accessing care, poor infrastructure, human resource shortages, political instability, and migration [5]. Developing countries also experience extremes of climate, which may affect the operation of equipment, and can cause malfunction [6]. The International Atomic

T. Ebenhan (✉) • M. Sathekge
Department of Nuclear Medicine, Steve Biko Academic Hospital, University of Pretoria, Pretoria, South Africa
e-mail: thomas.ebenhan@gmail.com

S.K. Jain (ed.), *Imaging Infections*, DOI 10.1007/978-3-319-54592-9_12

Energy Agency (IAEA) via the Nuclear Medicine Section provides advice on establishing and operating nuclear medicine facilities and encourages appropriate use and quality management approaches for obtaining the best results from the practice of nuclear medicine. Dondi et al. performed a survey in mid- and lower-income countries to identify challenges for the use of advanced technologies such as nuclear imaging [7]. While the shortage of equipment was an important challenge, equally important were the lack of education or training and insufficient human resources.

During the past decade, imaging practices have evolved through remarkable advances in radiopharmacy, instrumentation, and information technology. Advanced imaging is expanding rapidly in several developing countries, especially the BRICS nations (Brazil, Russia, India, China, South Africa), and widely available in large cities in these countries [8, 9]. Moreover, costs of advanced imaging are substantially lower than in the USA and sometimes (paradoxically) equivalent to the costs of standard testing (microbiology or molecular) at reputed private, for-profit laboratories [10–12]. Recent developments, such as the marketing of ^{68}Ge/^{68}Ga generators, negate the need of a cyclotron and could be adopted in remote areas [13–15].

12.3 Advanced Imaging Techniques

^{18}F-2-fluoro-deoxy-D-glucose (^{18}F-FDG) positron emission tomography (PET) is widely used globally and improving our understanding of diseases pathogenesis in humans. There is increasing body of evidence that ^{18}F-FDG PET is promising in monitoring of TB therapy and detection of active disease and extrapulmonary TB [16, 17]. PET imaging can also be utilized to assess long-term outcomes [18]. In addition, the potential of longitudinal assessments can aid in the discovery of new TB drug regimens [18]. Nuclear imaging has also emerged as an efficient preclinical tool to facilitate the development of new TB drugs and to assist in the fundamental understanding of the disease [19–23]. As TB lesions may present with complex pathophysiologic changes, valuable insight was gained by using imaging for understanding glucose-independent mechanisms in animal infection models such as lesion hypoxia, enzymatic expression, lesion calcification, and drug treatment [22, 24–26].

12.3.1 Extrapulmonary Tuberculosis

The AIDS epidemic has led to a higher incidence of TB, with varied disease patterns and increased extrapulmonary dissemination. Extrapulmonary TB may affect any organ and is an AIDS-defining condition indicative of stage 4 disease in adults [27–29]. The most frequently affected sites include lymph nodes (Figure 12.1), pleura, musculoskeletal, gastrointestinal, and genitourinary tract [30, 31]. Despite recent advances, the diagnosis of extrapulmonary TB remains problematic, as obtaining

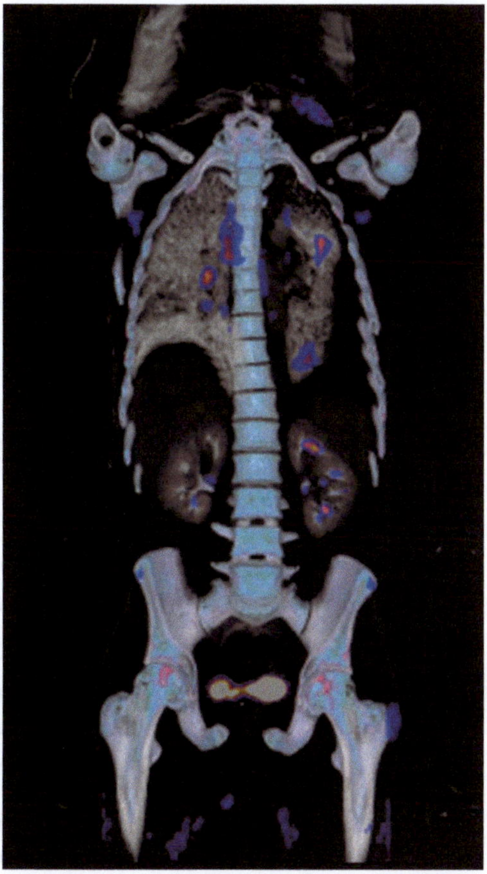

Figure 12.1 ^{18}F-FDG PET/CT image from a patient presenting with lymph node tuberculosis

tissue or fluid for analysis from these sites is often challenging. The correct assessment of the disease extent is important when deciding on the correct treatment regimen. ^{18}F-FDG PET studies performed on TB patients have demonstrated that PET detects more TB lesions, especially extrapulmonary, than CT [32].

12.3.2 Evaluation of Treatment Response

Treatment response is potentially the most important clinical application of ^{18}F-FDG PET/CT in TB. Morphological changes often take significantly longer than molecular changes to manifest, and it is in this context that PET may have a role, emphasizing the need for further evaluation. In developing countries, multidrug-resistant (MDR) and extensively drug-resistant (XDR) TB has serious consequences, and monitoring of therapy is thus essential. A major advantage of PET/CT is the ability to detect morphological changes and quantify the ^{18}F-FDG uptake simultaneously, allowing assessment of response to therapy and making treatment interventions in nonresponders [33]. TB treatment regimens can be complex in the settings of coinfection with HIV, where a high possibility of development of immune reconstitution inflammatory syndrome exists. Treatment duration may need to be between 3 and 9 months, and PET might provide an objective measure of treatment response and the optimal duration of treatment [17, 33]. For example, incomplete eradication of mycobacteria post-therapy was noted recently using nuclear imaging techniques [34]. In addition, a clinical study reported ^{18}FDG-PET to be superior to conventional microbiology in monitoring treatments in MDR-TB patients [18]. Similarly, low radiation dose CT imaging was utilized to monitor treatment in a 2-year-old child with XDR-TB [35].

12.3.3 Novel Technologies as a Solution to Better Infection Imaging

In recent years, molecular imaging efforts are now actively illuminating new biology in a broad range of conditions, including discriminating infection from sterile inflammation, spreading of infection, and therapy monitoring [36]. Although microorganisms have a distinctive metabolism which is highly diverse from eukaryotic cells, only few approaches were successful to achieve infection-selective imaging [37]. Biomarker and radiopharmaceuticals that interact with the microorganism are considered for selective infection imaging and not sterile inflammatory processes [38, 39]. Recently, several radiolabeled sugars—^{18}F-labeled maltohexaose, ^{18}F-fluoromaltose, and 2-^{18}F-fluorodeoxysorbitol (^{18}F-FDS)—were shown to be promising for the specific detection of bacterial infections [40–42]. Similarly, advances in imaging using immuno-PET and antimicrobial peptides have also shown promise in the specific detection of infections [43, 44]. The key problem persists with the clinical translation of the most desirable tracer candidates. A study in healthy volunteers showed that ^{18}F-FDS is safe, well tolerated, and rapidly cleared, following a single, intravenous dose [11], suggesting significant potential for use in humans. PET imaging can be introduced to detect infection using ^{68}Ga-bioconjugates such as novel peptide derivatives and other macromolecules or even by adapting existing radiodiagnostic agents (^{68}Ga-citrate) [13]. Ubiquicidin (UBI29-41), a cationic, synthetic antimicrobial peptide fragment that binds preferentially with the anionic microbial cell membrane at the site of infection, was labeled with ^{99m}Tc (Figure 12.2a). Recently, a ^{68}Ga-labeled UBI(29-41)-conjugate was shown to be specific for the detection of bacterial infections in vivo [43] (Figure 12.2b). ^{99m}Tc-UBI(29-41)-SPECT has shown promising results for detecting infections in patients [45], and the development of the freeze-dried instant kit formulations has shown a high labeling yield with proven stability [46–48]. Similarly, a novel depsipeptide derivative was developed and successfully radiolabeled with ^{68}Ga [49]. This bioconjugate (Figure 12.3a) comprises of a peptide structure, inherited from a class of antimicrobial-active depsipeptides, which was

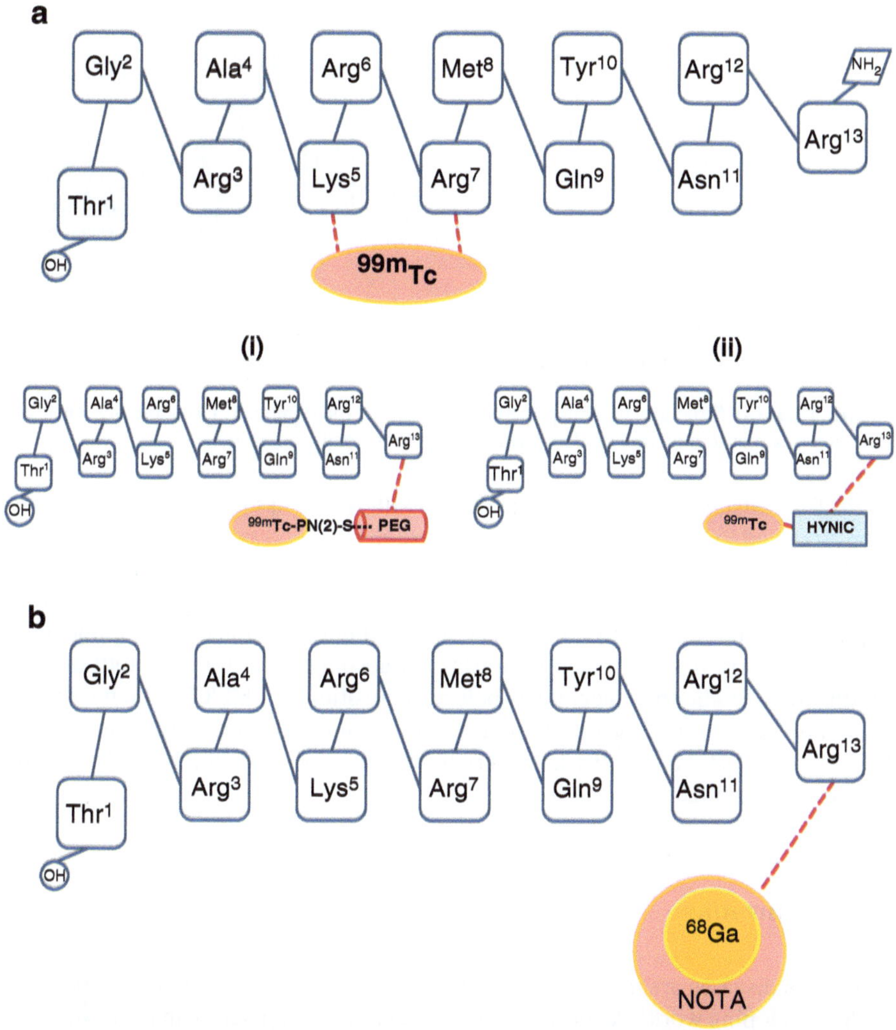

Figure 12.2 Schematic display of (**a**) a ^{99m}Tc-labeled ubiquicidin fragment (^{99m}Tc-UBI-29-41) and its alternatives using (*i*) derivatized polyethylene glycol (PEG) or (*ii*) hydrazinonicotinic acid (HYNIC) as linking structures. (**b**) A ^{68}Ga-labeled ubiquicidin (^{68}Ga-NOTA-UBI29-41) using the bifunctional chelator molecule 1,4,7-triazacyclononane-1,4,7-triacetic acid (NOTA) to complex ^{68}Ga

extended by a ^{68}Ga complexing moiety (-Gly-Gly-DOTA (1,4,7,10-tetraazacyclodo decane-1,4,7,10-tetraacetic acid)). Despite the structural extension, the depsipeptide vector was able to locate the infection site using PET imaging (Figure 12.3b) in a mouse myositis model.

The development of ^{68}Ga-PET radiopharmaceuticals may be considered a true landmark in molecular imaging which will allow diverse molecules and receptor analogs to be used in clinical practice [50]. Moreover, PET imaging is superior to

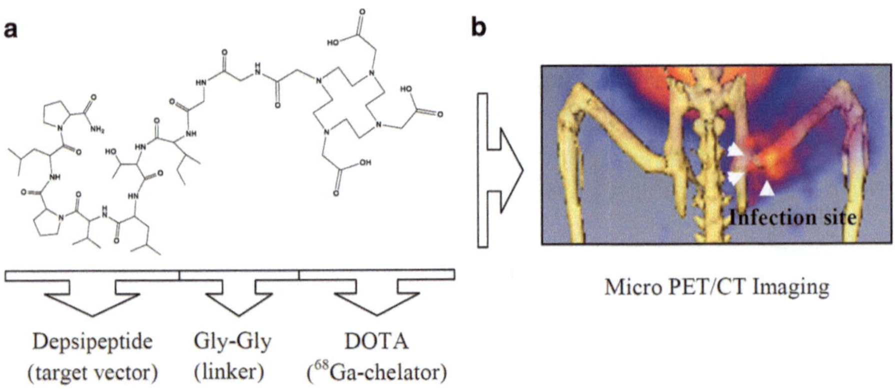

Figure 12.3 (**a**) Structure of a depsipeptide-based ^{68}Ga-bioconjugate (**b**) targeting muscular infection in a mouse infection model. Adapted from Mokaleng et al. [49]

SPECT in sensitivity and resolution. Since South Africa has gained access to generator-produced ^{68}Ga, novel strategies for freeze-dried, good manufacturing practice-produced, kit-formulated PET radiopharmaceuticals have emerged [13, 51–53]. Collaborative research to develop new ^{68}Ga-based radiopharmaceuticals for PET application will be a reality in the near future in developed and developing countries. This effort may also help to bypass the absolute need for a cyclotron-based production of radiopharmaceuticals before acquisition of PET/CT which seems to be an impediment in some developing countries. Similarly, due to the much longer half-life of ^{124}I (4.2 days), ^{124}I-labeled radiopharmaceuticals could be easily distributed from centralized pharmacies.

12.4 Summary

Infectious diseases are major causes of global morbidity and mortality, particularly in the developing world. A considerable segment of the population in the developing countries has a disease spectrum similar to those of the industrialized countries. Given the considerable size of people living in big cities in the developing world, advanced imaging could become a powerful clinical tool for the early diagnosis and monitoring of infectious diseases in developing countries.

References

1. WHO, *World health statistics 2016: monitoring health for the SDGs, sustainable development goals*. 2016, World Health Organization: WHO Library Cataloguing-in-Publication Data. p. 1-136.
2. UNAIDS, *Global AIDS Response Progress Reporting*. WHO Library Cataloguing-in-Publication Data, 2014: p. 1-264.

3. WHO, *Global tuberculosis report 2016*. 2016, World Health Organization: WHO Library Cataloguing-in-Publication Data. p. 1-214.
4. Sathekge, M., *The potential role of 68Ga-labeled peptides in PET imaging of infection.* Nucl Med Commun, 2008. **29**(8): p. 663-5.
5. Andronikou, S., et al., *Paediatric radiology seen from Africa. Part I: providing diagnostic imaging to a young population.* Pediatr Radiol, 2011. **41**(7): p. 811-25.
6. Creeden, A. *Advice on Donating Equipment Overseas*. 2002.; Available from: http://idcsig.org/page6.html.
7. Dondi, M., et al., *Trends in nuclear medicine in developing countries.* J Nucl Med, 2011. **52 Suppl 2**: p. 16S-23S.
8. Jankharia, G.R., *Commentary - radiology in India: the next decade.* The Indian journal of radiology & imaging, 2008. **18**(3): p. 189-91.
9. Jha, S. *(2015) Radiology in India: Trends in medical imaging technology*. 2015 December 28, 2016]; Available from: http://www.auntminnie.com/index.aspx?sec=ser&sub=def&pag=dis&ItemID=110035.
10. Mosessian, S., et al., *INDs for PET molecular imaging probes-approach by an academic institution.* Mol Imaging Biol, 2014. **16**(4): p. 441-8.
11. Zhu, W., et al., *Biodistribution and radiation dosimetry of the Enterobacteriaceae-specific imaging probe [18F]fluorodeoxysorbitol determined by PET/CT in healthy human volunteers.* Mol Imaging Biol, 2016.
12. Wakabayashi, H., et al., *Initial preclinical evaluation of 18F-fluorodeoxysorbitol PET as a novel functional renal imaging agent.* J Nucl Med, 2016.
13. Vorster, M., et al., *A modified technique for efficient radiolabeling of 68Ga-citrate from a SnO2-based 68Ge/68Ga generator for better infection imaging.* Hell J Nucl Med, 2013. **16**(3): p. 193-8.
14. Ebenhan, T., et al., *Antimicrobial Peptides: Their Role as Infection-Selective Tracers for Molecular Imaging.* European Cells and Materials, 2014. **2014**.
15. Fani, M., J.P. Andre, and H.R. Maecke, *68Ga-PET: a powerful generator-based alternative to cyclotron-based PET radiopharmaceuticals.* Contrast Media Mol Imaging, 2008. **3**(2): p. 67-77.
16. Sathekge, M., A. Maes, and C. Van de Wiele, *FDG-PET imaging in HIV infection and tuberculosis.* Semin Nucl Med, 2013. **43**(5): p. 349-66.
17. Sathekge, M. and J.R. Buscombe, *Can positron emission tomography work in the African tuberculosis epidemic?* Nucl Med Commun, 2011. **32**(4): p. 241-4.
18. Chen, R.Y., et al., *PET/CT imaging correlates with treatment outcome in patients with multidrug-resistant tuberculosis.* Sci Transl Med, 2014. **6**(265): p. 265ra166.
19. Lin, P.L., et al., *Sterilization of granulomas is common in active and latent tuberculosis despite within-host variability in bacterial killing.* Nat Med, 2014. **20**(1): p. 75-9.
20. Murawski, A.M., et al., *Imaging the evolution of reactivation pulmonary tuberculosis in mice using 18F-FDG PET.* J Nucl Med, 2014. **55**(10): p. 1726-9.
21. Ordonez, A.A., et al., *Radioiodinated DPA-713 imaging correlates with bactericidal activity of tuberculosis treatments in mice.* Antimicrob Agents Chemother, 2015. **59**(1): p. 642-9.
22. Davis, S.L., et al., *Noninvasive pulmonary [18F]-2-fluoro-deoxy-D-glucose positron emission tomography correlates with bactericidal activity of tuberculosis drug treatment.* Antimicrob Agents Chemother, 2009. **53**(11): p. 4879-84.
23. Johnson, D.H., et al., *Nuclear imaging: A powerful novel approach for tuberculosis.* Nuclear Medicine and Biology, 2014. **41**: p. 777-784.
24. Weinstein, E.A., et al., *Noninvasive determination of 2-[18F]-fluoroisonicotinic acid hydrazide pharmacokinetics by positron emission tomography in Mycobacterium tuberculosis-infected mice.* Antimicrob Agents Chemother, 2012. **56**(12): p. 6284-90.
25. Harper, J., et al., *Mouse Model of Necrotic Tuberculosis Granulomas Develops Hypoxic Lesions.* Journal of Infectious Diseases, 2012. **205**: p. 595-602.
26. Ordonez, A.A., et al., *Imaging Chronic Tuberculous Lesions Using Sodium [(18)F]Fluoride Positron Emission Tomography in Mice.* Mol Imaging Biol, 2015. **17**(5): p. 609-14.

27. Peto, H.M., et al., *Epidemiology of extrapulmonary tuberculosis in the United States, 1993-2006.* Clin Infect Dis, 2009. **49**(9): p. 1350-7.
28. Chaisson, R.E. and N.A. Martinson, *Tuberculosis in Africa--combating an HIV-driven crisis.* N Engl J Med, 2008. **358**(11): p. 1089-92.
29. WHO, *Global Tuberculosis Control: surveillance, planning, financing*, in *WHO Report*. 2008, WHO Press. p. 304.
30. Golden, M.P. and H.R. Vikram, *Extrapulmonary tuberculosis: an overview.* Am Fam Physician, 2005. **72**(9): p. 1761-8.
31. Arciniegas, W. and D.L. Orjuela, *[Extrapulmonary tuberculosis: a review of 102 cases in Pereira, Colombia].* Biomedica, 2006. **26**(1): p. 71-80; discussion 81.
32. Vorster, M., M.M. Sathekge, and J. Bomanji, *Advances in imaging of tuberculosis: the role of (1)(8)F-FDG PET and PET/CT.* Curr Opin Pulm Med, 2014. **20**(3): p. 287-93.
33. Sathekge, M., et al., *Use of 18F-FDG PET to predict response to first-line tuberculostatics in HIV-associated tuberculosis.* J Nucl Med, 2011. **52**(6): p. 880-5.
34. Malherbe, S.T., et al., *Persisting positron emission tomography lesion activity and Mycobacterium tuberculosis mRNA after tuberculosis cure.* Nat Med, 2016. **22**(10): p. 1094-1100.
35. Salazar-Austin, N., et al., *Extensively drug-resistant tuberculosis in a young child after travel to India.* Lancet Infect Dis, 2015. **15**(12): p. 1485-91.
36. Palestro, C.J., *Radionuclide imaging of osteomyelitis.* Semin Nucl Med, 2015. **45**(1): p. 32-46.
37. Hooker, J.M., *Modular strategies for PET imaging agents.* Curr Opin Chem Biol, 2010. **14**(1): p. 105-11.
38. Bunschoten, A., et al., *Development and prospects of dedicated tracers for the molecular imaging of bacterial infections.* Bioconjug Chem, 2013. **24**(12): p. 1971-89.
39. Ordonez, A.A., et al., *A Systematic Approach for Developing Bacteria-Specific Imaging Tracers.* J Nucl Med, 2017. **58**(1): p. 144-150.
40. Gowrishankar, G., et al., *Investigation of 6-[18F]-fluoromaltose as a novel PET tracer for imaging bacterial infection.* PLoS One, 2014. **9**(9): p. e107951.
41. Ning, X., et al., *PET imaging of bacterial infections with fluorine-18-labeled maltohexaose.* Angew Chem Int Ed Engl, 2014. **53**(51): p. 14096-101.
42. Weinstein, E.A., et al., *Imaging Enterobacteriaceae infection in vivo with 18F-fluorodeoxysorbitol positron emission tomography.* Sci Transl Med, 2014. **6**(259): p. 259ra146.
43. Ebenhan, T., et al., *Preclinical evaluation of 68Ga-labeled 1,4,7-triazacyclononane-1,4,7-triacetic acid-ubiquicidin as a radioligand for PET infection imaging.* J Nucl Med, 2014. **55**(2): p. 308-14.
44. Rolle, A.M., et al., *ImmunoPET/MR imaging allows specific detection of Aspergillus fumigatus lung infection in vivo.* Proc Natl Acad Sci U S A, 2016. **113**(8): p. E1026-33.
45. Arteaga de Murphy, C., F. Gemmel, and J. Balter, *Clinical trial of specific imaging of infections.* Nucl Med Commun, 2010. **31**(8): p. 726-33.
46. Martin, E., T. Ganz, and R.I. Lehrer, *Defensins and other endogenous peptide antibiotics of vertebrates.* J Leukoc Biol, 1995. **58**(2): p. 128-36.
47. Breeman, W.A., et al., *Effect of dose and specific activity on tissue distribution of indium-111-pentetreotide in rats.* J Nucl Med, 1995. **36**(4): p. 623-7.
48. Epand, R.M. and H.J. Vogel, *Diversity of antimicrobial peptides and their mechanisms of action.* Biochim Biophys Acta, 1999. **1462**(1-2): p. 11-28.
49. Mokaleng, B.B., et al., *Synthesis, 68Ga-radiolabeling, and preliminary in vivo assessment of a depsipeptide-derived compound as a potential PET/CT infection imaging agent.* Biomed Res Int, 2015. **2015**: p. 284354.
50. Al-Nahhas, A., et al., *What can gallium-68 PET add to receptor and molecular imaging?* Eur J Nucl Med Mol Imaging, 2007. **34**(12): p. 1897-901.
51. Ebenhan, T., et al., *Development of a Single Vial Kit Solution for Radiolabeling of 68Ga-DKFZ-PSMA-11 and Its Performance in Prostate Cancer Patients.* Molecules, 2015. **20**: p. 14860-14878.

52. Ebenhan, T., et al., *Evaluation of a Flexible NOTA-RGD Kit Solution Using Gallium-68 from Different 68Ge/68Ga-Generators: Pharmacokinetics and Biodistribution in Nonhuman Primates and Demonstration of Solitary Pulmonary Nodule Imaging in Humans.* Mol Imaging Biol, 2016.
53. Vorster, M., et al., *Fluorine-18-fluoroethylcholine PET/CT in the detection of prostate cancer: a South African experience.* Hell J Nucl Med, 2015. **18**(1): p. 53-9.

Index

S.K. Jain (ed.), *Imaging Infections*, DOI 10.1007/978-3-319-54592-9

G

J

MIX
Papier aus verantwortungsvollen Quellen
Paper from responsible sources
FSC® C105338

If you have any concerns about our products,
you can contact us on
ProductSafety@springernature.com

In case Publisher is established outside the EU,
the EU authorized representative is:
Springer Nature Customer Service Center GmbH
Europaplatz 3, 69115 Heidelberg, Germany

Printed by Libri Plureos GmbH
in Hamburg, Germany